Cannabis

A Clinician's Guide

Cannabis
A Clinician's Guide

Edited by
Betty Wedman-St. Louis

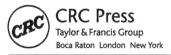

CRC Press
Taylor & Francis Group
Boca Raton London New York

CRC Press is an imprint of the
Taylor & Francis Group, an **informa** business

CRC Press
Taylor & Francis Group
6000 Broken Sound Parkway NW, Suite 300
Boca Raton, FL 33487-2742

International Standard Book Number-13: 978-1-138-30324-9 (Paperback)
978-1-138-30344-7 (Hardback)

Library of Congress Cataloging-in-Publication Data

Names: Wedman-St. Louis, Betty, author.
Title: Cannabis : a clinician's guide / Betty Wedman-St. Louis.
Description: Boca Raton : Taylor & Francis, 2018.
Identifiers: LCCN 2017061827| ISBN 9781138303249 (pbk. : alk. paper) | ISBN 9781138303447 (hardback : alk. paper)
Subjects: | MESH: Medical Marijuana--therapeutic use | Cannabis
Classification: LCC RM666.C266 | NLM WB 925 | DDC 615.3/23648--dc23
LC record available at https://lccn.loc.gov/2017061827

Visit the Taylor & Francis Web site at
http://www.taylorandfrancis.com

and the CRC Press Web site at
http://www.crcpress.com

*To the hospice patients who opened my eyes
to cannabis when they asked me to get them
some "weed" for their pain*

and

*many others denied to right to marijuana
as a remarkably safe medicine*

Contents

Section I: Cannabis Science

Section III: Regulations & Standards

Preface

Marijuana—A plant that spread throughout the world

Weed, pot, grass, Mary Jane—whatever name you call it, marijuana, or cannabis, originated thousands of years ago in Asia and has now been grown throughout the world. It was used as a medicine, in spiritual ventures, and has been legal in many regions of the world throughout its history [1].

An important distinction needs to be made between subspecies of the cannabis plant. Cannabis sativa, also called marijuana, has psychoactive properties from the active component tetrahydrocannabinol (THC). The other subspecies of Cannabis sativa is known as hemp, the nonpsychoactive form containing no more than 0.3% THC [2]. (Cannabis sativa L. is a subspecies with the "L" used to honor the botanist Carl Linnaeus). Hemp from the nonpsychoactive Cannabis sativa has been used in manufacturing oil, cloth, and fuel, along with hemp seed products sold in health food stores for over 20 years as a source of omega-3 fatty acids and vegetarian protein.

Cannabis indica is a second psychoactive species that was identified by Jean-Baptiste Lamarck, a French naturalist. The third species of cannabis is uncommon—Cannabis ruderalis. It was named in 1924 by the Russian botanist D.E. Janischevisky [3].

Hemp and psychoactive marijuana were used in China, with records of medical use dating back to 4000 BC where it was used as an anesthetic during surgery. From the Asian continent, marijuana traveled throughout the world for use in smoking and cooking.

From seed to consumer shelf

Louis Herbert, a French botanist in 1606, is credited with planting the first hemp crop in North America in Port Royal, Arcadia (present day Nova Scotia). By 1801, the lieutenant governor of the province of Upper Canada began distributing hemp seeds free to Canadian farmers for hemp fiber production [4], but by the early twentieth century, Canada and the United States confused Cannabis sativa with hemp, resulting in legal regulations on all production.

U.S. laws never recognized the difference between hemp and Cannabis sativa. Legal action against its use in the United States began in 1915 when it was outlawed in Utah. By 1930, with Harry Aslinger as the first commissioner of the Federal Bureau of Narcotics (FBN), action to make marijuana illegal in all states began. In 1937, the Marijuana Tax Act put cannabis under the regulation of the Drug Enforcement Agency (DEA) where possession of it became a crime.

Hemp has a long history of use. Mark Blumenthal, founder and executive director of the American Botanical Council (ABC) in Austin, Texas, has called CBD from Cannabis sativa "one of the most therapeutic compounds in cannabis" [5]. Chris Boucher, vice president of CannaVest Corporation in San Diego, California, described the difference between agricultural hemp and industrial hemp. The former is used primarily as a nutrition product and the latter as a source for wax, rope, paper, and fuel [5].

Hemp seed products have been sold in the natural foods industry for over two decades. Products such as hemp powder, hemp oil, and hemp snacks are marketed for their nutritional benefits—protein and omega-3 fatty acids. Examples of those products available in local health food stores follow.

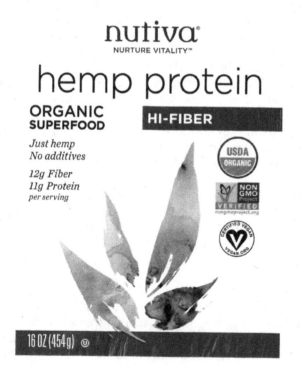

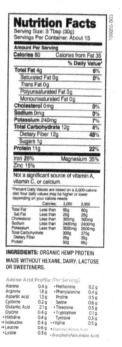

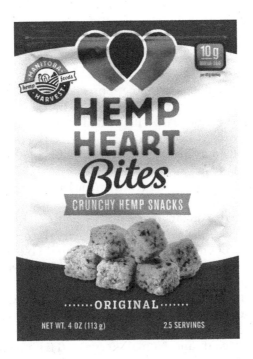

When is medicine not medicine?

In 1850, cannabis was listed in the U.S. Pharmacopoeia as a cure for many ailments, and by the early 1900's, Squibb Company, Eli Lilly, and Park-Davis were manufacturing drugs produced from marijuana for use as antispasmodics, sedatives, and analgesics.

The Controlled Substances Act of 1970 listed marijuana as a Schedule 1 drug that has no currently accepted medical use but excludes the seed and seed oil (CBD), according to American Herbal Products Association (AHPA) past president Michael McGuffin [5]. Hempseed and hemp oil products are available as capsules, chewables, emulsions, and softgels in addition to hulled hempseeds and hempseed burgers.

The same cannabis preparations once accepted as therapeutically useful drugs became illegal with marijuana, hashish, dagga, bhang, ganja, hash oil, sinsemilla, etc., comprising the world's most common and widely used group of illicit drugs. Worldwide about 300 million people are estimated to have used these drugs. In the United States, 36 million people have reported using some form of cannabis [6].

Marijuana politics

Cannabis grew popular for its medical properties and use in treating many ailments from insomnia, menstrual cramps, nausea, muscle spasms, and depression, but a 1936 film entitled *Reefer Madness* caused people to demonize it and believe its use could create drug zombies.

In the 1960's, Americans began smoking "weed" or cannabis as a political dissent over U.S. involvement in the Vietnam War. Thirty years later, California, Oregon, and Maine approved the medical use of cannabis as public opinion changed. Colorado became the first U.S. state to legalize cannabis in 2012, and the market flourished to over $100 million a month in revenue in just three years [7]. Since cannabis is illegal at the federal level, it forces marijuana operations to be an all-cash business because banks are federally regulated.

Cannabis sativa needs to be grown in the United States and reclassified from a narcotic to an agricultural crop. The federal law on hemp "has been a waste of taxpayer's dollars that ignores science, suppresses innovation, and subverts the will of states that have chosen to incorporate this versatile crop into their economies," Representative Jared Polis (D-Colorado) told the Huffington Post [8]. He is a co-sponsor of the Industrial Hemp Farming Act of 2015.

U.S. government policy is totally confused concerning cannabis. One agency, the Drug Enforcement Agency (DEA), says hemp and hemp extracts are a Schedule 1 drug with no medicinal use, while the U.S. Department of Health and Human Services (HHS) owns the patent on CBD use as an antioxidant, and the U.S. Food and Drug Administration (FDA) is reviewing cannabis as a prescription drug [9].

Research stymied

According to the *Handbook of Cannabis Therapeutics: From Bench to Bedside*, the discovery of the endocannabinoid system in the past 15 years has markedly stimulated research into the cannabis mechanisms of action, including CB receptors, antioxidant activity, and the role of natural lignands in medical use of cannabinoids [10].

Grotenherman explains that unlike opiates and other medicinal plant constituents, cannabinoids were not identified before the twentieth century so dosing oral cannabis extracts was a problem, but in 1964, Δ-9-tetrahydrocannabinol was defined and synthesized, which led to further research on cannabinoid receptors in mammals [11].

The federal government has not allowed farmers to grow hemp, and the only source of cannabis that can be legally produced in the United States is grown for research by the University of Mississippi [12]. Numerous studies reported throughout this book have used cannabis supplies that were confiscated by the DEA to further knowledge about cannabinoids. Individual states are currently passing legislation to legalize production and use of cannabis despite the threat of drug raids and prosecution.

Legalizing marijuana

According to the Pew Research Center in 2016, 57% of U.S. adults want to see the use of marijuana made legal, and 37% want it to remain illegal. Ten years ago, the statistics were the exact opposite—32% favored legalization, and 60% were opposed [13]. A 2012 National Survey on Drug Use and Health reported that 49% of Americans have tried marijuana with 12% indicating use in the past year. Four states—Colorado, Washington, Oregon, and Alaska—and the District of Columbia have passed legislation to legalize marijuana use.

Recent research by Bradford and Bradford [14] found that medical marijuana reduced prescription drug use. The University of Georgia study reviewed prescription drug use in 17 states with medical marijuana laws in place by 2013 and found prescriptions for painkillers and other drugs fell sharply compared to states without a medical cannabis law. In medical cannabis states, doctors wrote 265 fewer doses of antidepressants each year, 486 fewer doses of seizure medication, 541 fewer antinausea doses, and 562 fewer doses of antianxiety medications. Even more striking was that physicians in medical cannabis states prescribed 1826 fewer doses of painkillers in a given year.

According to the Bradford research, Medicare could save $468 million per year if marijuana was legalized in all U.S. states. The study calculated over $165 million had been saved in 2013 in the 18 states studied where medical cannabis is legal.

Denying patients their right to cannabis

Debate about the use of medical marijuana is challenging the accepted practice of medicine, as patients are demanding the right to any beneficial treatment available. Denying a patient knowledge of and access to a therapy to relieve pain, reduce seizures, modify nausea from toxic drugs, or to minimize suffering from a terminal illness violates the basic philosophy of healthcare [15].

Ethically, physicians have the right to prescribe a therapy that relieves pain and suffering for their patients without fear of retaliation from federal and state governments. Scientific research has shown that the benefits of medical cannabis greatly outweighs the risk from inadequate government legislation and lack of double-blind-controlled clinical studies.

Hemp versus marjuana

Cannabis sativa has been cultivated by humans throughout the world since antiquity, so it should come as no surprise that different species and subspecies of cannabis have different properties. Industrial hemp is produced from Cannabis sativa strains that have been cultivated to produce minimal levels of THC. These plants are taller and sturdier than the Cannabis sativa that is bred to maximize the concentration of cannabinoids—mainly THC, the psychoactive cannabinoid.

The major difference between industrial hemp and medical marijuana is that industrial hemp is exclusively bred to produce a low THC species. The tall, fibrous stalks have very few flowering buds compared to medical cannabis strains that are short, bushy, and contain many buds with high amounts of THC. Industrial hemp has a small amount of THC and a high amount of CBD, meaning that it is incapable of inducing an intoxicating effect or getting anyone "high" from ingesting it.

As Doug Fine discusses in *Hemp Bound*, many American farmers are waiting for the day when industrial cannabis farming is legalized. Fine writes that a fifth-generation Colorado rancher named Michael Bowman is willing to test his right to grow hemp in the U.S. legal system because "We can eat it, wear it, and slather it on out bodies, but we can't grow it?" [16].

His proclamation illustrates the ignorance that surrounds the marijuana debate.

References

1. Blaszczak-Boxe, A. Marijuana's history: How one plant spread through the world. www.livescience.com/48337.
2. Watts, G. Cannabis confusions. *BMJ*, 2006; 332(534): 175–176.
3. Warf, B. High points: an historical geography of cannabis. *Geographical Review*, 2014; 104(4): 414–438.
4. Canadian Hemp Trade Alliance. www.hemptrade.ca
5. Richman, A. Cannabis conundrum. *Nutraceuticals World*, March 2015.
6. Turner, C.E., ElSohly, M.A., and Boeren, E.G. Constituents of cannabis sativa L. XVII. A review of the natural constiuents. *J Nat Prod*, 1980; 43(2): 169–234.
7. Gupta, S. Weed. CNN. March 6, 2014.
8. Polis, J. Huffington Post, Jan 22, 2015.
9. Rules and Regulations—Department of Justice-Drug Enforcement Administration 21CFR Part 1308 (Docket No DEA-342) Federal Register, 2014; 81(240): 90194–90196.
10. Russo, E.B. and Grotenherman, F. (eds). *The Handbook of Cannabis Therapeutics: From Bench to Bedside*. Routledge, 2014.
11. Grotenherman, F. *Clinical Pharmacodynamics of Cannabinoids. Handbook of Cannabis Therapeutics*. The Haworth Press, 2006.
12. Fetterman, P.S., Keith, E.S., Waller, C.W. et al. Mississippi-grown Cannabis sativa L.: Preliminary observation on chemical definition of phenotype and veriations in tetrahydrocannabinol content versus age, sex, and plant part. *J Pharmaceutical Science*, 1971, 60(8): 1246–1249.
13. Support for marijuana legalization continues to rise. Pew Research Center. Oct 12, 2016. www.pewresearch.org.

14. Bradford, A.C. and Bradford, W.D. Medical marijuana laws reduce prescription medication use in Medicare Part D. *Health Affairs,* July 2016; 35(7): 1230–1236.
15. Clark, P.A., Capuzzi, K., and Fick, C. Medical marijuana: Medical necessity versus political agenda. *Med Sci Monit*, 2011; 17(12): RA249–RA261.
16. Fine, D. *Hemp Bound—Dispatches from the Front Lines of the Next Agricultural Revolution.* Chelsea Green Publishing, White River Junction, VT, 2014.

Acknowledgments

In addition to the 18 authors who contributed to this book, many others assisted in research and collaboration to bring *Cannabis: A Clinician's Guide* to completion.

My sincere gratitude goes to the hundreds of individuals who shared their cannabis stories. Many provided input but were fearful of retaliation should their story be told in print, but Casandra Stephen, Lilyann Baker's mother in Baltimore, Maryland, wanted everyone to know how grateful she was to share Lilyann's story so other mothers could have the courage to follow in her footsteps. Jennifer Rousch freely discussed her allopathic cancer treatments and why she moved to cannabis for help in cancer management. My interview with Rick Roos about his experience with his mother and sister was such an enlightening experience that I share their stories with patients regularly.

I am indebted to the hundreds of patients for whom I have served as adviser in using cannabis for their symptom management and the many healthcare professionals who contributed ideas and expertise in writing a book about a subject that has been condemned for over 50 years.

Creating a collaborative reference on therapeutic cannabis has been a labor of love and new learning. My sincere thanks goes to Randy Brehm for believing in this project and CRC Press/Taylor & Francis Group for providing healthcare professionals the opportunity to become advocators for every patient's right to cannabis as a medicine.

Introduction

Personal stories about cannabis use

In over 40 years of practice in clinical nutrition, I have had the privilege of hearing hundreds of thousands of patient stories and meeting some outstanding medical professionals who have come to realize that botanical products have health benefits. I respect the trust they place in me when they seek help to relieve their ailments and look to my guidance in helping their patients. Since beginning *Cannabis: A Clinicians Guide,* numerous individuals have shared their cannabis stories with me, and several have been chosen so healthcare providers can learn about their journey to use cannabis in disease management.

Since 1978, legislation has permitted patients with certain disorders to use cannabis/marijuana with a physician's approval through various "compassionate care" programs that were implemented but later abandoned due to bureaucratic issues. Even without those programs, patients have continued to learn about the health benefits cannabis provides and secure treatment by growing their own or purchasing prepared oils, creams, or extracts for

- Anticonvulsant benefits
- Muscle relaxation in spastic disorders
- Appetite stimulant in wasting syndrome of HIV (human immuno-deficiency virus)
- Relieving phantom limb pain
- Menstrual cramps
- Migraines

David Berger, MD, ventures in cannabis

Dr. Berger has been interested in cannabis and natural medicines since 1996 when he was a resident at Tampa General Hospital. Even as a freshman in college, he addressed the controversial topic of legalization of marijuana in an 11-page report. Today, he has a busy pediatric and family medical practice and medical cannabis clinic whereby he declares that "every patient with a chronic, debilitating disease should have the opportunity to use cannabis," and most will qualify under the Florida law.

He stays well informed about regulations and the certification process. An electronic medical charting system for patient assessment monitors patient care using the HER to streamline the process. Dr. Berger also evaluates for drug–cannabis interactions because patients referred by neurologists and psychiatrists may arrive with extensive medication lists.

Patient education is a key component of his patient assessment so they can determine which cannabis products would be the best choice for the individual. Dr. Berger emulates Sidney M. Baker, MD, a pediatrician and former faculty member of Yale Medical School whose philosophy is asking the most important question: "Have we done everything for this patient?" That philosophy of opening your mind to all treatment options and educating yourself comes across to those nurse practitioners who rotate through Dr. Berger's clinic as part of the University of South Florida curriculum.

Self-learning over the last 20 years has taught Dr. Berger how to help patients move toward "self-determination as healthcare consumers." His self-directed learning has enabled him to develop a comfort level doing things other physicians are waiting for the pharmaceutical industry to dictate. By expanding his learning, he can make life worth living for many people living with chronic disorders from seizures or constant pain needing to reduce their dependence on opioids.

David Berger, MD, FAAP
Owner and Medical Director, Family Medicine Cannabis Clinic
Owner and Director, Wholistic Pediatrics and Family Care
Assistant Professor, University of South Florida College of Nursing
Tampa, Florida

Lillyann Baker's story
Traumatic brain injury—seizures

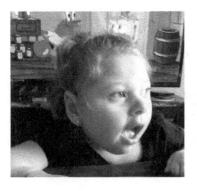

At 7 weeks old, Lillyann suffered a traumatic brain injury resulting in her being induced into a coma. Doctors then noticed she was having frequent seizures every day. Lilly was given two antiseizure medications that did not help or stop her seizures, and she continued to suffer multiple seizures every day. Lilly's neurologist suggested putting her on a third antiseizure medication, but I had already been doing research on medical marijuana oils and reading about how medical marijuana helped children with different conditions. When he suggested a third medication, I decided to try medical marijuana for Lilly.

As a mother, I wanted to see if a natural substance would stop her seizures so that I would not have to watch for side effects or worry about if I had given her too much or too little. Another concern was remembering different medications, proper doses, and being scared if she missed a dose or what side effects a third pharmaceutical could be having on her. With medical marijuana, I am in control of how much CBD oil she gets. I don't have to worry about watching for side effects.

I tried six different CBD oils from six different websites that did not work for her, but I refused to give up. That's when I found RSHO Hemp Oil through hempmeds.com. Almost immediately, her seizures started subsiding.

She has been seizure-free since February 10, 2016, and now that her seizures have stopped, she is able to make progress in her development. Following her coma, the doctor said Lilly would never walk, she would never talk or feed herself, and Lilly would always need a feeding tube along with needing assistance for the rest of her life. Since she has been on her RSHO oil, she is rolling, she is scooting herself, doing different baby babbling to start talking, eating off a spoon, and drinking out of a sippy cup. Lilly even reacts to hearing her name being called. Everything that doctors said she wouldn't ever do is now a part of her daily routine, and she is proving them wrong.

Lilly can interact with her big sister and little brother and is now in school and able to participate. Lilly's neurologist is very surprised that I took it upon myself to try a substance that he did not write a prescription for to help my daughter. One of Lilly's therapists did call child protective services on me for giving her the CBD oil, but that case was quickly closed after the social worker spoke to all her doctors. The doctors now support my decision to use CBD oil. Now that she is seizure-free and seizure activity in her brain has reduced, Lilly's neurologist is considering taking her off one of her medications.

Our family believes RSHO hempmeds is our medical miracle because we feel that doctors have the license to diagnose and prescribe medications, but mommy and daddy's decision to try CBD oil gave her a second chance to life. The progress Lilly has made and continues to make has changed our lives, and we would not have it any other way.

Casandra Stephan, Lillyann's mom

Jennifer's story

Breast cancer and brain cancer

At age 36, Jennifer was diagnosed with breast cancer and underwent a double mastectomy, chemotherapy, and radiation with a return to work in six months. A year later, lung cancer was diagnosed followed by more chemotherapy and a move to Colorado where medical cannabis (Charlotte's Web) was available. Two years later, a brain metastasis was discovered when she complained of head pressure and headaches. Surgery was successful in treating the tumor, but it reappeared nine months later.

Upon discovery of the tumor reappearance, she started on full plant cannabis, and the second brain surgery found no tumor and very few cancer cells. She was prescribed Avastin® (bevacizumab) but refused (cost can reach $100,000/year according to Mercola.com July 22,2008, and "The New York Times" July 6, 2008) because studies showed it only extends life a short time for breast and lung cancer.

Jennifer wanted to try hyperbariatric oxygen treatment, but three doctors, an oncologist, a brain surgeon, and a radiologist, refused to prescribe it. Her family physician ordered it, and she found another oncologist to monitor her disease every three months as she continued her cannabis treatment.

Her husband grows their own cannabis to insure it is 100% organic. Her dose of whole plant cannabis has been modified to meet her needs. Along the way, she has used capsules for high doses and suppositories for extended release but currently needs only the equivalent of two rice grains as maintenance for staying cancer-free. In addition to whole plant extract, they consume compounds from the whole cannabis plant as juice and edibles.

Judy's story

Traumatic brain injury: Aneurysm

Judy suffered a brain aneurysm while scraping snow off her car the week before Thanksgiving 2016. At 75 years old, she still worked full-time without any previous symptoms of blood vessel disruption in her brain— no eye pain, vision problems, neck or facial tingling, seizure, fatigue, or weakness, according to her son. When her husband saw her on the ground, paramedics transported her to the hospital where family members were told "she would not make it."

Eight days of an induced coma followed during which time her son fed her eye droppers of CBD cannabis daily. Medical staff kept advising the family that "she would not make it, and if she did, she would be transferred to the hospice floor." Realizing he had nothing to lose, her son began increasing the CBD concentrate administered by eye dropper. By the time the dose became a dropper two to three times daily, Judy started to become alert to her surroundings.

As Judy became more alert, she was moved to an extended care facility and even recognized her son when he came to visit, but the staff still did not give her any hope for regaining cognitive function and walking. One day her son took her to one of their favorite restaurants where he quizzed her about her mental and physical condition. Judy told him she "was faking being an invalid" so the staff would leave her alone. Doctors told her not to walk, and she wanted to regain her mobility, but the staff kept her confined to a wheelchair.

When doctors ask her about her miraculous recovery, she tells them about CBD, but they did not want her to continue using it since it "may interfere with other medications." Following their orders, she discontinued its use and suffered two seizures in one day.

Judy has now resumed her CBD regimen with a hidden bottle so no one knows her secret. It gives her a clear mind almost instantly after taking a dose and allows her to read everything she can get her hands on to stay sharp in her senior years.

Marcia's story

Multiple myeloma and neuropathy

Marcia developed multiple myeloma, a blood cancer that develops in the plasma cells of the bone marrow. The immune system is greatly compromised when white blood cells cannot produce antibodies to fight infections, and tumors can form in the bone marrow, which causes bone pain and fractures.

Her diagnosis came when she took an extensive physical exam with lab work following a divorce and symptoms of extreme fatigue. Marcia was given six months to live, her brother reported, so she underwent radiation and chemotherapy for six months and returned home with neuropathy. Her brother discovered research about cancer and CBD effectiveness that he passed on to her, but she declined to use it.

As her brother refined his techniques for producing CBD, he would send samples to Marcia, who has spent her life "being allergic to everything." The CBD oil he sent her stained her bedsheets, so he made it into a cream. Today she uses the oil and pain cream daily in her quest to regain her health.

Thomas's story

Traumatic brain injury and post-traumatic stress disorder

Thomas James Brennan wrote an op-ed in "The New York Times" on September 1, 2017, describing how an ambush in Afghanistan in

2010 left him with a traumatic brain injury and post-traumatic stress disorder. He was provided with prescriptions from the Department of Veterans Affairs—antidepressants, sedatives, amphetamines, and mood stabilizers—to control symptoms including a daily migraine.

A friend offered him a joint, which he smoked after some hesitation only to realize how much it helped control his symptoms. He tapered off his prescriptions to use cannabis only to realize it was illegal and the VA could not prescribe it for use.

Former Sergeant Thomas Brennan states, "If I hadn't begun self-medicating with it, I would have killed myself." He goes on to say, "Because of cannabis, I'm more hopeful, less woeful" and reports better relationships with his wife and daughter now that migraines and depression do not control his life, but like many cannabis users, he fears legal action because of using an illegal drug.

Editor

Betty Wedman-St. Louis, PhD, is a licensed nutritionist specializing in digestive diseases, diabetes, cancer, and environmental health issues who has been a practicing nutrition counselor for over 40 years. Her BS in foods and business from the University of Minnesota introduced her to how the food industry influences eating habits. Dr. Wedman-St. Louis completed her MS in nutrition at Northern Illinois University where she studied the relationship between prolonged bed rest and space flight weightlessness nutrient requirements. She had a private practice at the Hinsdale Medical Center before completing her PhD in nutrition and environmental health from The Union Institute in Cincinnati. Dr. Wedman-St. Louis completed her doctorate internship at WUSF-Tampa in multimedia production for distance learning and online course development.

Dr. Wedman-St. Louis is the author of numerous published articles on current nutrition topics including phosphates in food, folate, vitamin B12, seafood nutrition, alpha lipoic acid, and diabetes. She has authored columns for "The Hinsdale Doings," "Chicago Sun Times," and "Columbia Missourian" and has taught undergraduate and graduate courses on nutrition. She currently writes a personal health column for the "Tampa Bay Times" and maintains a private practice in Pinellas Park, Florida.

Origins and history of cannabis

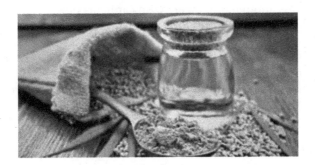

Chinese and Hindu pharmacology has indicated cannabis use for 12,000 years to:

- Relieve pain
- Reduce insomnia
- Treat wasting syndrome
- Reduce nausea
- Stop seizures

Early recorded history

3000 BC: Cannabis sativa burned seeds excavated in burial mound in Siberia.

2500 BC: Mummified marijuana found in tombs of aristocrats in Xinjiang, China.

1500 BC: Chinese Pharmacopeia references medical cannabis, called Rh-Ya.

1450 BC: Book of Exodus mentions "holy anointing oil" made of kaneh bosem (local name for cannabis), olive oil, and herbs.

1213 BC: Egyptian healers used cannabis for inflammation, glaucoma, abdominal problems, and enemas.

1000 BC: Indians drank "bhang" (cannabis and milk).

600 BC: Cannabis used as cure for leprosy in Indian medical literature.

440 BC: Written history use of cannabis by Greek historian Herodotus (Greeks and Romans used marijuana and hemp as did Muslims of North Africa); Arabic word hashish or hash refers to smoked marijuana/dry weed.

200 BC: Greeks used marijuana to cure edema, earache, and inflammation.

1 AD: Chinese text indicated cannabis as remedy for over 100 ailments such as gout, rheumatism, malaria, and improving memory.

30 AD: Jesus anointed followers with cannabis oil.

70 AD: Marijuana used by Roman doctors to cure earache, "suppress sexual longing."

200 AD: Chinese doctors use marijuana and wine (ma-yo) as anesthetic in surgery.

800 AD: Arabic doctors used cannabis as anesthetic and analgesic.

Current recorded history

1578: Medical treatise by Li Shizhen *Bencao Gangmu Materia Medica* indicated marijuana as cure for vomiting, bleeding, and parasites.

1600s: Pipes, bowls, and stems recovered from William Shakespeare's belongings.

1611–1762: Settlers in Jamestown brought hemp plants and cultivated it for fiber, oil, and recreational use. In 1762 in Virginia, colonists were charged penalties for *not* producing it.

1625: English herbalist Nichols Culpeper wrote thesis on use of hemp for gout pain, inflammation, and joint and muscle pain.

1745–1775: U.S. President George Washington grew hemp at Mount Vernon.

1774–1824: U.S. President Thomas Jefferson grew hemp.

1770s: French emperor Napoleon invaded Egypt and brought back cannabis to be studied for sedative and analgesic properties.

1842: William O'Shaughnessy re-introduced marijuana into British medicine upon his return from India.

1840s: Queen Victoria used marijuana as pain reliever for menstrual cramps (used as a tincture rather than smoked). English and French began using it for pain relief and medicine.

1850s: Cataloged in U.S. Pharmacopoeia as tincture effective for medical conditions for cholera, gout, convulsions, typhus, neuralgia, insanity, and opiate addiction.

1889: Medical journals report on effectiveness to replace opium use.

1900s: Squibb Company, Eli Lilly, and Parke-Davis manufactured drugs produced from cannabis as antispasmodics, sedatives, and analgesics.

1911: Massachusetts became first U.S. state to officially declare cannabis a dangerous drug and ban it.

1913–1917: Other states followed Massachusetts in banning use of cannabis.

1937: Marihuana Tax Act enacted by Federal Bureau of Narcotics, which criminalized use of the plant.

1964: Gaoni and Mechoulam isolated and defined THC.

1970: Schedule 1 controlled substance declaration along with heroin and cocaine, indicating it had no medical use and high potential for abuse and addiction plus medical research further restricted.

1980s: Synthetic THC (dronabinol) available.

1988: Discovery of CB1 receptor site by Allyn Howlett and William Devane.

1996: California became the first state to legalize use of medical cannabis.

2003: U.S. Department of Health & Human Services files patent on cannabinoids as useful antioxidants and neuroprotectants.

2011: U.S. National Cancer Institute acknowledges medical use of cannabis for cancer patients.

2014 U.S. President Obama signed Farm Bill of 2013 into law—Sec 7606 Legitimacy of Industrial Hemp Research of HR 2642—removing barriers to Cannabis sativa L. production in 31 states.

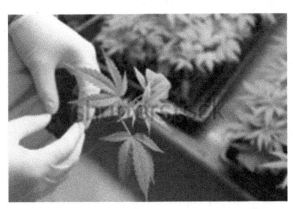

Contributors

Will Bankert
Shimadzu Scientific
    Instruments
Columbia, Maryland

David Berger MD, FAAP
Board Certified Pediatrician
and
Owner & Medical Director
Wholistic Pediatrics &
    Family Care
and
Assistant Professor
University of South Florida
    School of Nursing
Tampa, Florida

Vijay S. Choksi
Regulated Substance
    Attorney
Fort Lauderdale, Florida

Robert Clifford PhD
Shimadzu Scientific
    Instruments
Columbia, Maryland

Paul J. Daeninck MD, MSc, FRCPC
Attending Medical Oncologist
Cancer Care Manitoba
and
Assistant Professor
Department of Internal Medicine
University of Manitoba
and
Consultant Palliative Medicine
Winnipeg Regional Health
    Authority
Winnipeg, Manitoba, Canada

Scott Kuzdzal PhD
Shimadzu Scientific Instruments
Columbia, Maryland

Vincent Maida MD
Associate Professor
Division of Palliative Care
University of Toronto
Toronto, Ontario, Canada

and

Clinical Assistant Professor
Division of Palliative Care
McMaster University
Hamilton, Ontario, Canada

Robert W. Martin PhD
CEO CW Analytical
    Laboratories
Oakland, California

Chris D. Meletis ND
Naturopathic Physician

Joseph Pizzorno ND
Editor-In-Chief
Integrative Medicine
A Clinicians Journal
and
President
SaluGenecists, Inc.
and
Treasurer Board of Directors
Institute of Functional
    Medicine
and
Founding President
Bastyr University
Seattle, Washington

Lilach Power
Giving Tree Dispensary
Arizona

Amanda Reiman PhD, MSW
Alcohol Research Group
International Cannabis Farmer's
    Association
University of California
Berkeley, California

Rick Roos
CEO Nature's Best CBD
Littleton, Colorado

Juan Sanchez-Ramos PhD, MD
Professor of Neurology
University of South Florida
Tampa, Florida

George Scorsis
CEO and Director
Liberty Health Sciences, Inc.

Michelle Simon PhD, ND
President
Institute for Natural Medicine
Seattle, Washington

Jordan Tishler MD
President CMO
Inhale MD
Cambridge, Massachusetts

Ashley Vogel
Laboratory Manager
Alternative Medical Enterprises

Betty Wedman-St. Louis
Clinical Nutritionist
Private Practice
St. Petersburg, Florida

Paul Winkler
Shimadzu Scientific Instruments
Columbia, Maryland

Cannabis Science

chapter one

Cannabis 101

Betty Wedman-St. Louis

Contents

The term "marijuana" (sometimes spelled "marihuana") is Mexican in origin and usually refers to one of three distinctive subspecies of the cannabis plant called Cannabis sativa. If grown outdoors, it achieves maturity in 3–5 months compared to indoor cultivation with optimum heat and lighting reaching maturity in 60 days. Marijuana is the third most popular recreational drug in America behind alcohol and tobacco [1].

Two species of cannabis plants, Cannabis sativa and Cannabis indica, were assessed to identify genetic differences [2]. Using 14,031 single nucleotide polymorphisms (SNPs) genotyped in 81 marijuana and 43 hemp samples, research showed they were significantly different at a genome-wide level and THC content. Understanding and correctly identifying one of humanity's oldest crops remains poorly understood, which can further complicate medicinal use versus agricultural value [3,4].

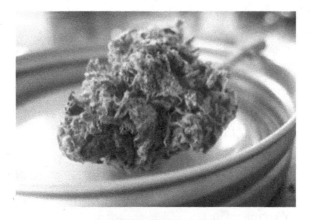

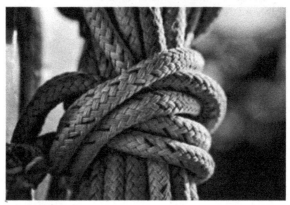

What is cannabis?

Many people consider cannabis as a recreational drug, while others have used it as medicine, but a plant that has been known at for least 4000 years will have gone through profound domestication and genetic diversity, as described by Gray et al. [5]. When modern civilization shifted from a hunter-gatherer lifestyle to an urbanized settlement of permanent dwellings to towns and cities, wild plants were domesticated into crops that were selected for genetic modification. Cannabis was among those wild plants with two distinct forms: hemp and medicinal species [6]. Fleming and Clarke describe how cannabis as a fiber crop/hemp became useful in a wide array of products. Medicinal forms of cannabis were domesticated by 3000 BC [7].

Today, there are hundreds of strains of cannabis grown around the world, many developed illegally and little studied. According to Nolan Kane, University of Colorado in Boulder, "Cannabis is the only multibillion dollar crop for which the genetic identities and origins of most varieties are unknown" [8]. The euphoric and other effects of drug varieties were due to the recognition of active ingredients on brain and immune receptors of animals, including humans [9,10].

Currently, the United States has feral cannabis plants still growing in the Midwest despite the criminalization of all hemp production in the 1960s due to safety concerns of the drug varieties [11]. Much information about its multiple uses remains to be discovered due to the last 50-plus years of research neglect.

Trends in use of cannabis

A poll cited in Marijuana as Medicine by the National Academies Press 2000 reported 1 in 3 Americans over the age of 12 had tried marijuana or hashish at least once, with only about 1 in 20 currently using these drugs [12].

Two eminent researchers describe why the use of cannabis has been forbidden and provide a compendium of its beneficial properties in Marijuana: The Forbidden Medicine [13]. They argue that only with legalization throughout the United States will all patients who need cannabis have access to it.

Participants in medical marijuana programs vary by state and over time. Participation in 13 U.S. states and the District of Columbia from 2001 to 2008 was less than 5 per 1000 adults but rose sharply in Colorado, Montana, and Michigan from 2009–2010. Higher rates are found in Colorado, Oregon, and Montana at 15–30 per 1000 adults. A national average is speculated as 7 to 8 per 1000 adults with two-thirds of the participation as male and over 50 years old. Colorado and Arizona are reporting larger numbers of young adults [21–30] in their patient registries [14].

Therapeutic potential

There is a growing interest in the therapeutic potential for using cannabis medicinally as the role of endocannabinoids in the central nervous system are elucidated. Over 60 neuroactive chemicals have been identified to date, which could influence disorders such as Parkinson's disease (PD), Huntington's disease (HD), multiple sclerosis (MS), dyskinesis, inflammatory bowel disease (IBD), and many others [15]. The endocannabinoid system has been shown to have a strong effect on the inflammatory, immune, cognitive, and motor systems of the body. Cannabidiol (CBD) and delta-9-tetrahydrocannabinol (THC) are the two main active compounds found in the cannabis plant.

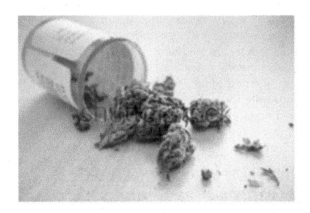

Cannabinoids

The cannabis plant contains more than 500 unique compounds with only slight awareness of how the cannabinoids, terpenoids, and flavonoids are synergistic in providing health benefits. Cannabinoids accumulate mainly in the trichomes of the plant (sticky outgrowths on the surface of the plant) [16]. Over 60 cannabinoids are known, but the most abundant ones studied to date are CBD and THC [17].

Other cannabinoids are cannabichromene (CBC), and cannabigerol (CBG) [18]. Cannabidivarin (CBDV), delta-9-tetrahydrocannabivan (THCV), and cannabichromevarin (CBCV) have also been identified [19].

The biosynthesis of cannabinoids occurs as a cannabinoid acid (e.g., cannabidiolic acid or CBDA) is decarboxylated into a neutral form (e.g., CBDA → CBD) when dried, stored, or heated [20]. Environmental factors influence the number of cannabinoids in different parts of the plant at different growth stages [21,22], whereas the CBD-to-THC ratio in cannabis plants is controlled by genetic profiles [23].

The important psychoactive component in cannabis is tetrahydrocannabinol (THC). It was the first phytocannabinoid discovered and has been more extensively researched than CBD. Its strong psychoactive effects can be intoxicating and alter behavior, which has made it a popular, illegal recreational drug, but THC has medicinal application as an effective analgesic for pain relief in HIV/AIDS and cancer.

CBD is separated and extracted from hemp varieties of cannabis and has no psychoactive component or recreational value. Cannabidiol works as an antioxidant on receptors to keep them in balance and functioning.

Terpenes or isoprenoids are another beneficial phytochemical found in cannabis that provides therapeutic effects. Two examples of terpene beneficial qualities are: Pinene acts as a bronchodilator, increasing THC absorption, and linalool imparts sedative effects [24]. Terpenoid metabolites have been shown to exhibit cytotoxicity against a variety of tumor cells in animal models [25], and other studies have shown anti-inflammatory and pain-relieving benefits [26].

Current research conflicts with U.S. government regulations

Research is showing the direct conflict of science with the U.S. federal government's stance that cannabis is a highly dangerous substance worthy of criminal prosecution. The February 11, 2010, University of California Center for Medicinal Cannabis Research (CMCR) Report to the Legislature and Governor of the State of California presented findings in four studies that cannabis has analgesic effects in pain conditions [27]:

- Secondary to injury (spinal cord injury)
- Disease of the nervous system (HIV)
- Muscle spasticity in multiple sclerosis (MS)

The creation of the CMCR was the passage by the people of California in 1996 of Proposition 215, the Compassionate Use Act, which approved the medical use of marijuana. By 1999, the California state legislature passed the Medical Marijuana Research Act (SB847] to create a three-year program for medical research at the University of California to "enhance understanding of the efficacy and adverse effects of marijuana as a pharmacological agent" [27].

Investigation of cannabis and cannabinoid compounds encompassed three primary research domains:

- Smoked cannabis, since it offered the most efficient delivery of cannabinoids for clinical assessment
- Non-smoked preparations for safety and effectiveness: vaporization, patches, suppositories, and alternative oral forms
- Molecules to target endocannabinoid system, natural and synthetic, to activate, modulate, or deactivate the body's native cannabinoid system

Overview of CMCR research

Chronic pain issues of neuropathic disorders are prevalent with limited treatment options, so four research studies focused on pain relief treatment from smoked and vaporized cannabis. All four studies demonstrated a significant decrease in pain after cannabis administration.

Multiple sclerosis (MS) is a chronic disabling disease of the nervous system caused from a loss of insulating sheath surrounding nerve fibers. Muscle spasms affect up to 70% of those with MS, which cause pain and difficulty walking. The study results found a significant improvement in muscle spasticity and pain intensity for those with MS.

"Results of the CMCR studies support the likelihood that cannabis may represent a possible adjunctive avenue of treatment for certain difficult-to-treat conditions such as neuropathic pain and spasticity" [27].

One of the primary researchers in the CMCR report was Donald Abrams, MD, oncologist at the University of California–San Francisco, who tried to initiate a clinical trial for medical marijuana as treatment for patients with HIV/AIDS because "Brownie Mary" (Mary Jane Rathbun) had supplied them with marijuana-laced brownies to alleviate their pain and wasting symptoms several years before the CMCR studies [28]. Later in a CMCR study, Abrams and colleagues [29] went on to report smoked cannabis was well tolerated and effective in relieving chronic neuropathic pain in HIV/AIDS. Mark Ware at McGill University, Montreal reported similar results in neuropathic pain relief from cannabis [30].

But Dr. Abrams advises that human studies should be conducted to address the numerous anecdotal reports about patients having remarkable responses to cannabis as an anticancer drug [31]. The 1993 discovery of the "Siberian Ice Maiden" unearthed after 2500 years revealed a pouch of cannabis among her possessions. Magnetic resonance images revealed she had a primary tumor in her right breast along with metastatic disease. It was speculated that she could have used cannabis to manage her pain or treat her malignant disease [32].

Safety of cannabis

Research continues to explore the use of cannabis as an alternative for chronic pain patients to lower opioid drug use. Cannabinoids possess a remarkable safety record compared to many other substances with regards to "no recorded cases of overdose fatalities or lethal dose for humans" [33].

But cannabis should not be viewed as harmless because its active components (i.e., THC) may produce a variety of physiological and euphoric effects that could result in loss of short-term memory, impaired linear thinking, panic attacks, or depersonalization events [34]. Patients with cardiovascular disorders could also experience adverse side effects [35]. As a recreational drug, cannabis poses dangers in social and emotional development during adolescence, according to Taylor [36], and deleterious effects while operating equipment [37,38].

Safety concerns are further elaborated by Borgelt et al. [39], which include:

- Increased risk of developing schizophrenia with adolescent use
- Impairments in memory and cognition
- Accidental pediatric ingestion
- Lack of safety packaging for medical cannabis formulations

Summary of health benefits from cannabis [40–42]

Many physicians and researchers agree that cannabis is safe enough to alleviate symptoms of diseases that are listed here. Further research is needed to access physiological function, dose recommendations, and delivery methods.

Alzheimer's disease	Reduces amyloid plaque formation
Appetite stimulation	Relieves nausea from drugs, improves food intake
Arthritis	Pain reduction, improved mobility
Brain trauma	Cerebral healing post stroke, brain injuries
Cancer	Antimetastatic effect/apoptosis
Epilepsy	Antiseizure effects
Glaucoma	Reduces intraocular pressure, reduces progression
Inflammatory bowel	Improves gut permeability, Crohn's disease, ulcerative colitis
Metabolic syndrome	Improves glucose tolerance
Multiple sclerosis	Reduces muscle spasms, contractions
Parkinson's disease	Reduces pain and tremors
PTSD (post-traumatic stress disorder)	Improves symptomsof anxiety, fear, nightmares

Future outlook

As cannabis becomes recognized as an important botanical, it is time to consign the term "marijuana" to the history books according to Duke Rodriguez, CEO and President of Ultra Health, Scottsdale, Arizona [43]. As the cannabis industry progresses, the terminology we use to describe the products made should represent the plant's scientific genus—Cannabis—instead of the racially charged, purgative term used since the 1900s in the United States—marijuana—Rodriguez wrote in the Analytical Scientist, February 2017. His commentary mentioned how supporters of prohibition called cannabis "devil's weed" and "marihuana," which was used to reinforce the connection between cannabis and the minorities who introduced the drug. Rodriguez capped off his comments by stating that researchers studying cannabis do not deserve to be derogatorily identified as "marijuana" scientists.

Mary Lynn Mathre, RN, MSN, CARN projects her outlook on cannabis use by recognizing that millions of people are suffering from various illnesses, and yet they lack the therapeutic benefits of the cannabis plant to ease their suffering [44]. Her book, *Cannabis in Medical Practice: A Legal, Historical, and Pharmacological Overview of the Therapeutic Use of Marijuana* published in 1997 includes her summation of the cannabis issue as "the illegal status of cannabis jeopardizes the health of the American people by denying them access to a remarkably safe and effective medicine." Mathre concludes her future outlook of cannabis with a quotation from Thomas Jefferson, the third president of the United States

"If people let government decide what foods they eat and medicines they take, their bodies will soon be in as sorry a state as are the souls of those who live under tyranny."

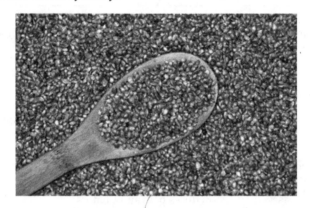

Since January 2014, Coloradoans have been using a variety of state legal cannabis products and cultivating their own plants for recreational purposes, reported Lawrence Downes in The New York Times [45]. "Cannabis sales from January through May brought the state about $23.6 million in revenue from taxes, licenses, and fees," Downes stated. The state is also developing and refining tools to deter drugged driving, which is more difficult to detect than drunk driving because THC can have a prolonged effect in the body. Further initiative has been launched to achieve clear labeling of edibles and discourage marketing to minors. Colorado is likely to serve as a national model for cannabis regulations, wrote Ash Lindstrom in HerbalGram [46].

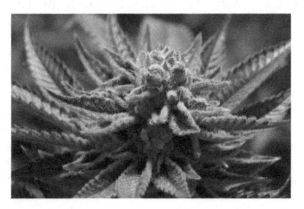

References

1. About marijuana. NORML—National Organization for the Reform of Marijuana Laws. www.norml.org.
2. Sawler J, Stout JM, Gardner KM et al. The genetic structure of marijuana and hemp. *PLOS* 2015;10(8):e0133292.
3. van Bakel H, Stout J, Cote A et al. The draft genome and transcriptiome of Cannabis sativa. *Genome Biol* 2011;12(10):R102.
4. Bostwick JM. Blurred boundaries: The therapeutics and politics of medical marijuana. *Mayo Clin Proc* 2012;87(2):172–186.
5. Gray DJ, Clarke RC, Trigiano RN. Introduction to the special issue on cannabis. *Crit Rev Plant Sci* 2017;35(5–6):289–292.
6. Fleming MP, Clarke RC. Physical evidence for the antiquity of Cannabis sativa L. *J Intl Hemp Assoc* 1998;(5):80–92.
7. Schultes RE. Man and marijuana. *Nat Hist* 1967;82:59–63.
8. Pennisi E. A new neglected crop: Cannabis. *Science* Apr 2017;356(6335):232–233.
9. Devane WA, Dysarz FA, Johnson MR et al. Determination and characterization of a cannabinoid receptor in rat brain. *Mol Pharmacol* 1988;(34):605–613.
10. Mackie K. Cannabinoid receptors as therapeutic targets. *Annu Rev Pharmacol Toxicol* 2005;(46):101–122.
11. Duvall C. *Cannabis*. Reakton, London 2014.
12. Medical Marijuana and Disease. *Marijuana As Medicine? The Science Beyond the Controversy*. The National Academies Press, Washington, DC, 2000.
13. Grinspoon L, Bakalar JB. *Marijuana: The Forbidden Medicine*. Yle University Press, New Haven, CT, 1997.
14. Fairman BJ. Trends in registered medical marijuana participation across 13 US states and the District of Columbia. *Drug Alcohol Depend* 2016;159:72–79.
15. Kluger B, Triolo P, Jones W, Jankovic J. The therapeutic potential of cannabinoids for movement disorders. *Mov Disord* 2015 Mar;30(3):313–327.
16. Mechoulam R. Marijuana chemistry. *Science* 1970;168:1159–1166.
17. de Zeeuw RA, Malingre THM, Merkus FWHM. Tetrahydrocannabinolic acid, an important component in the evaluation of cannabis products. *J Pharm Pharmacol* 1972;24:1–6.
18. Holley JH, Hadley KW, Turner CE. Constituents of Cannabis sativa L.XI. Cannabidiol and cannabichromene in samples of known geographic origin. *J Pharm Sci* 1975;64:892–894.
19. de Zeeuw RA, Wijsbek J, Breimer DD et al. Cannabinoids with propyl side chain in Cannabis. Occurence and Chromatographic behavior. *Science* 1972;175:778–779.
20. Taura F, Morimoto S, Shoyama Y. First direct evidence for the mechanism of delta-1-tetrahydrocannabinolic acid biosynthesis. *J Am Chem Soc* 1995;38:9766–9767.
21. Lydon J, Teramura AH, Coffman CB. UV-B radiation effects on photosynthesis, growth and cannabinooid production of two cannabis sativa chemotypes. *Photochem Photobiol* 1987;46:201–206.
22. Bocsa I, Mathe P, Hangyel L. Effect of nitrogen on tetrahydrocannabinol (THC) content in hemp (Cannabis sativa L.) leaves at different positions. *J Int Hemp Assoc* 1997;4:80–81.

23. Fournier G, Richez-Dumanois C, Duvezin J et al. Identification of a new chemotype in Cannabis sativa: Cannabigerol-dominant plants, biogenetic and agronomic prospects. *Plant Med* 1987;53:277–280.

24. Kuzdzal S, Lipps W. Unraveling the cannabinoid. http://the analyticalscientist. com/issue/0915.

25. Sharma SH, Thulasingam S, Nagarajan S. Terpenoids as anti-colon cancer agents—a comprehensive review on its mechanistic perspectives. *Eur J Pharmacol* 2017;795:169–178.

26. Sulsen V, Lizarraga E et al. Potential of terpenoids and flavonoids from asteraceae as anti-inflammatory, anti-tumor, and antiparasitic agents. *Evid Based Complement Altern Med* 2017 July 12: 6196198.

27. Center for Medicinal Cannabis Research. Feb 11, 2010. University of California. www.cmcr.ucsd.edu.

28. Eisenstein M. Medical marijuana: Showdown at the cannabis corral. *Nature* 2015 Sept 24;525:S15–S17.

29. Abrams D, Jay CA, Shade SB et al. Cannabis in painful HN-associated sensory neuropathy: A randomized placebo-controlled trial. *Neurology* 2007;68(7):515–521.

30. Ware MA, Wang T, Shapiro S et al. Smoked cannnabis for chronic neuropathic pain: A randomized controlled trial. *CMAJ* 2010;182(14):E694–E701.

31. Abrams DI. Integrating cannabis into clinical cancer care. *Curr Oncol* 2016 Mar;23(Suppl 2):S8–S14.

32. Mosbergen D. *Now We Know What Killed the Ancient "Ice Princess" and Why She Had That Marijuana.* The Huffington Post, NY. 2014. www.huffingtonpost. com/2014/10/16/siberian-ice-princess-cancer-cannabis.

33. Hall W, Room R, Bondy S. WHO Project on Health Implications of Cannabis Use: a comparative appraisal of the health and psychological consequences of alcohol, cannabis, nicotine and opiate use. Schaffer Library of Drug Policy Aug 28, 1995. www.druglibrary.org.

34. Taylor HG. Analysis of the medical use of marijuana and its societal implications. *J Am Pharm Assoc (Wash)* 1998 Mar–Apr;38(2):220–7.

35. Mukamal KJ, Maclure M, Muller JE, Muttleman MA. An exploratory prospective study of marijuana use and mortality following acute myocardial infarction. *Am Heart J.* 2008 Mar;155(3):465–470.

36. Taylor HG. Analysis of the medical use of marijuana and its societal implications. *J Am Pharm Assoc (Wash)* 1998 Mar–Apr;38(2):220–7.

37. Hollister LE. Health aspects of cannabis. *Pharmacol Rev* 1986 Mar;38(1):1–20.

38. Albertson TE, Chenoweth JA, Colby DK, Sutter ME. The changing drug culture: Medical and recreational marijuana. *FP Essent* 2016 Feb;441:11–17.

39. Borgelt LM, Franson KL, Nussabaum AM et al. The pharmacologic and clinical effects of medical cannabis. *Pharmacotherapy* 2013;33(2):195–209.

40. Pertwee RG. Emerging strategies for exploiting cannabinoid receptor agonists as medicine. *Br J Pharmacol* 2009;156:397–411.

41. Russo EB. Taming THC: Potential cannabis synergy and phytocannabinoid-terpenoid entourage effects. *Br J Pharmacol* 2011;163:1344–1364.

42. Ware MA, Adams H, Guy GW. The medical use of cannabis in the UK: Results of a nationwide survey. *Int J Clin Pract* 2005 Mar;59(3):291–295.

43. Rodriguez D. What's in a name. Feb 2017. www.theanalyticalscsientist.com.

44. Mathre ML. *Cannabis in Medical Practice: A Legal, Historical, and Pharmacological Overview of the Therapeutic Use of Marijuana.* Mc Farland & Co., Jefferson, NC, 1997.
45. Downes L. The great Colorado weed experiment. *New York Times.* 2014 Aug 2, www.nytimes.com/2014/08/03/opinion/sunday/high-time-the-great-colorado-weed-experiment.html.
46. Lindstrom A. An overview of the New York Times "High time: An editorial series on marijuana legalization". *Herbal Gram* 104, 2014. www.herbalgram. org.

chapter two

Endocannabinoid system

Master of homeostasis, pain control, & so much more

Jordan Tishler and Betty Wedman-St. Louis

Contents

Cannabinoids are a diverse group of chemical compounds that bind to receptors throughout the human body and are collectively known as the endocannabinoid system. Scientists have come to believe that the endocannabinoid system may be the most widely distributed receptor system in the human body [1]. Cannabinoid receptors in the brain, lungs, liver, kidneys, and immune system are activated by the therapeutic and psychoactive properties in cannabis [2].

The endocannabinoid system (ECS) is found in every mammal and regulates many biological functions through a biochemical modulation of receptor-mediated regulation of intercellular calcium. When a cannabinoid or combination of cannabinoids bind to a receptor, an event is triggered in the cell resulting in a change of cell activity [3].

Kinds of cannabinoids

Cannabinoids are found predominately in three places [4]:

Endocannabinoids are fatty-acid cannabinoids produced naturally in the body (anandamide and 2-AG).

Phytocannabinoids are concentrated in the oil resin of cannabis buds and leaves (THC and CBD) with over 100 identified in the cannabis plant.

Synthetic cannabinoids are manufactured artificially in a laboratory to mimic the effects of natural cannabinoids.

Cannabinoid receptors

Cannabinoid receptors are found in the central nervous system and peripheral tissues. Two primary receptors have been identified: Cannabinoid type 1 receptors (CB1) and cannabinoid type 2 (CB2). These receptors can be unlocked by any of the three kinds of cannabinoids previously mentioned.

CB1 functions to modulate neurotransmitter activity in the brain, which can influence nausea, muscle spasticity, and seizures, and are found throughout the body [5].

CB2 functions are associated with the immune system found outside the brain in splenocytes, macrophages, monocytes, microglia, and B and T cells [5].

Functions of the ECS

The endocannabinoid system is the master of homeostasis by modulating neuronal activity, which is a factor in mood, anxiety, appetite, reward stimulation, and stress management [6–9]. Pain control is another function of cannabinoids, with the National Academies of Sciences, Engineering, and Medicine presenting substantial evidence that cannabis can be an effective treatment [10]. In 2010, the Center for Medical Cannabis Research (CMCR) described the many types of pain caused by stimulation of specialized pain receptors on nerve endings, with studies demonstrating significant decrease in pain after cannabis administration [11]. Since pain is the number one complaint for patients, the endocannabinoid system is a primary target for remediation [12].

Phytocannabinoids in clinical practice

The pharmacology of the endocannabinoid system is characterized by two phenomena that need to be considered in the clinical use of cannabis. Most of the effects are due to the THC—tetrahydrocannabinol—and its exerted influence on the central nervous system. The high-lipid solubility of cannabinoids greatly influences side effects throughout the brain. The second phenomena is the low toxicity in phytocannabinoids, with research showing very little negative effect on long-term use at moderate doses. Emerging data suggests that high doses may be harmful [13].

Chronic use may have direct effects on neuronal signaling or on the organ itself, but research is needed to clarify the state of knowledge regarding high doses of cannabinoids used for extended periods [14]. Research conducted during the 1970s indicated tolerance can develop to the psychoactive properties of THC [15], so tolerance can best be managed by maintaining a consistent low dose of cannabinoid use [16].

Repeated use of phytocannabinoids can produce an abstinence syndrome if either THC or CBD administration is abruptly withdrawn [17]. Due to its lipophilic nature, this symptom can slowly occur, and clinicians need to be aware. Another clinician concern is tolerance to a dose which manifests as needing a higher dose for symptom management. Clinicians can recommend a "cannabis holiday" of several days to a week to enhance effectiveness of the cannabinoid receptor activity [18].

Evidence has emerged that phytocannabinoids can be effective in treating a range of disorders [19]:

Multiple sclerosis
Numerous pain syndromes
Cancer
Schizophrenia
Post-traumatic stress disorder
Intestinal disease
Traumatic head injury

Entourage effect

Cannabis is an herbal plant containing more than 400 chemicals and over 100 identified cannabinoid compounds. Herbal medicine specialists state that all the healing elements in the plant are in balance, and best results come from using a whole plant. This is called the "entourage effect," which was introduced in 1998 by Israeli scientists Shimon Ben-Shabat and Raphael Mechoulam [20].

Routes of administration

Cannabis in the raw plant exists in an acid form—THCA, CBDA—which are not psychoactive. THCA and CBDA must be heated to decarboxylate the acid to THC and CBD. Decarboxylation is a heating and drying process that activates the chemical compounds in cannabis, making them available for use in the human body [21].

The THC effects include psychoactive, euphoric, analgesic, antibacterial, antiemetic, antitumoral (high doses), bronchodilator, appetite stimulant, neuroprotective, sleep-inducing, anticonvulsant, muscle relaxant, and immunomodulating.

CBD effects on the body include: nonpsychoactive, anti-inflammatory, antianxiety, antibacterial, anticonvulsant, antitumoral (high doses), anti-ischemic, neuroprotective, muscle relaxant, antipsychotic, and immunomodulating [22].

Smoking

Smoking cannabis has been the classic method of delivery. Typically, the dried flower of the plant is the usual source. More concentrated forms—kief or kif (powdered hashish) and hash (trichomes of cannabis plant compressed into a resin)—are also available on the recreational market. Smoking provides a rapid onset of effects over a short onset of 10 to 15 minutes, and it is the cheapest, delivery system.

Cannabis smoke is irritating to the throat and lungs and frequently causes bronchial inflammation and a cough. Research is suggestive that smoking cannabis does not cause lung cancer or COPD.

One joint usually contains 0.5 to 1 g of cannabis. The THC absorbed from smoking 1 g of cannabis (15% THC) would be ~20 mg with effects lasting two to four hours [23].

Vaporizing

Vaporizing devices heat cannabis to 180–200 degrees C (356–392 degrees F), which releases cannabinoids as a vapor without smoke. Concentrates used in the vapor devices usually do not contain terpenes, which give off the characteristic cannabis aroma. Delivery of THC in some studies showed similar efficiency to smoking and is considered better for respiratory patients [24].

Oral intake

Ingestion of cannabis results in a delayed onset of effects by about an hour or more, with peak concentration in four to six hours. The THC is converted by the liver, which can result in psychoactive and sedative effects. The bioavailability of the THC varies based on the fat content of the food, gut motility, and other components of the preparation.

A food with 20 mg cannabis (10% THC) will provide ~2 mg THC [23]. It is easy to overdose on edibles because of the delayed onset of effects.

Capsules usually contain cannabinoids in various amounts from 10–50 mg THC, which can be used two to three times per day [23].

Suppositories

Rectal suppositories can also be used to provide therapeutic effects. Most suppositories are made from cannabis-infused coconut oil or cocoa butter. Rectal delivery is absorbed directly into the bloodstream. Suppositories are frequently used for sedation and pain relief overnight.

Raw cannabis

Raw cannabis has medicinal activity from cannabinoid acids, which are nonpsychoactive. Tender, young leaves can be eaten in a salad or juiced for consumption three to four times a day. Recipes are provided in the nutrition section. Only organically grown cannabis is recommended to ensure pesticides and heavy metals are not compromising the plant quality.

Clinical challenges

- Cannabis plants vary greatly based on strain, cultivation techniques, and processing. To assist patients with proper titration of their cannabis medication, products need to be secured from a source that provides standardized and tested material.
- Frequency of use and dose needed for maximum benefit should be individualized.
- Cannabis is an herbal medicine and not a pharmaceutical drug, so effects can take days or months to show benefits. Patience is needed to find thee must effective treatment regime.

Terpenes

While there are over 100 known phytocannabinoids in cannabis, more than 200 terpenes have been identified as the source of flavor and fragrance in the cannabis plant [25]. Terpenes are thought to work synergistically with the cannabinoids to produce therapeutic responses ranging from lowering inflammation and regulating blood glucose to protection of neurons and gastric cells [26]. Terpenoid properties even include cancer chemoprotective effects [27].

Terpenes are fragrant oils that are secreted in the flower's sticky resin glands, the same ones that produce THC, CBD, and other cannabinoids. Terpenes are not unique to cannabis and can be found in many other herbs, fruits, and plants. Cannabis is unique in that each strain has a unique profile of terpenes that exhibit medicinal properties independent from cannabinoids [28].

Terpene profile differences can be used to distinguish between cannabis strains, according to Casano et al. [29]. Biotype "mostly indica" strains have high levels of β-myrcene, while "mostly sativa" strains have more complex terpene profiles, which include α-pinene as the dominant terpenoid. Further research is needed to assess the potential medical value of these terpenoid biotypes and analyze their biological activity.

Horticulturalists believe that plants developed terpenes to repel predators and lure pollinators. Many factors influence a plant's terpene production—climate, weather, age, fertilizers used in production, and even soil content. Terpenes are volatile aromatic molecules that evaporate easily and makeup the odorous, oily substance that repels insects and prevents fungal growth.

Importance in health

Terpenes are healthy for humans as well as plants, according to Ethan Russo, MD, of GW Pharmaceuticals, Salisbury, Wiltshire UK [30]. Monoterpenes usually predominate (limonene, β-myrcene, α-pinene) but can be diminished with drying, irradiation, and storage of cannabis [31]. Lower leaves of Cannabis sativa have higher concentrations of bitter sesquiterpenoids that repel grazing animals, according to Potter [32], and give terpenoid balance to the mixture.

The European Pharmacopeia Sixth Edition in 2007 [33] listed 28 essential oils that are lipophilic with activity in cell membranes, neuronal and muscle ion channels, neurotransmitter receptors, and messenger systems, which included cannabis terpenoids. Animal studies by Buchbauer [34] show support for cannabis terpenes having a pharmacological effect on the brain. Russo [35] and Huestis [36] yield insight into human pain therapeutic effects provided by terpenes.

Most common cannabis terpenes

Limonene [37]
  Aroma: Lemon, citrus
  Effects: Elevated mood, stress relief
  Medical value: Antifungal, antibacterial, gastrointestinal issues, apoptosis of breast cancer cells, antidepressant

β-Myrcene [37]
  Aroma: Cloves, musky, earthy
  Effects: Sedating, relaxing
  Medical value: Antioxidant, anticarcinogenic, muscle relaxant, sedative, pain, inflammation

α-Pinene [37]
  Aroma: Pine
  Effects: Alertness, memory
  Medical value: Antibiotic, bronchodilator, insect repellant, anti-inflammatory, acetylcholinesterase inhibitor

β-Caryophyllene [37]
  Aroma: Black pepper, spicy, cloves, cinnamon leaves
  Effects: Binds to CB2 receptor as agonist
  Medical value: Gastroprotective, anti-inflammatory, dermatitis, chronic pain

D-Linalool [37]
  Aroma: Floral, lavender
  Effects: Anxiety relief, sedation
  Medical value: Anticonvulsant, antidepressant, antiglutamatergic, seizure reduction

Humulene [38]
  Aroma: Hops (beer)
  Effects: Used in Chinese medicine for thousands of years
  Medical value: Antitumor, antibacterial, anti-inflammatory, anorectic/suppresses appetite

Terpenes & cannabinoids

Terpenes, like cannabinoids, can increase blood flow, enhance cortical activity, and kill respiratory pathogens along with modulating pain and inflammation [39]. Terpenoid profiles of cannabis plants vary from strain to strain, but studies have shown that the cannabinoid-terpenoid interactions improve the beneficial effects of cannabis. A validated method for analysis of both terpenes and cannabinoids in cannabis is critical to ensure quality of active compounds. Since the requirements for an acceptable cannabis assay have changed over the years, Giese, Lewis et al. in the Journal of AOAC International [40] provide guidance in this analysis so that patients can be assured of the benefits in their product.

Terpene odor & law enforcement

The distinct odor of cannabis terpenes has allowed law enforcement agencies to incarcerate millions of people, according to Small [41]. Drug enforcement personnel recognize the odor with the help of devices and "sniffer dogs" to detect the volatile terpene odor. As more patients are approved for medical cannabis use, regulatory restrictions need to be modified to avoid unreasonable search and seizure.

Synthetic cannabinoids

Synthetic cannabinoids are man-made molecules and compounds that are legal under U.S. federal law and are designed to mimic the effects of phytocannabinoids. As Ethan Russo describes in *Cannabis: From Pariah to Prescription*, synthetic derivatives are moving into the U.S. pharmacopeia following the marketing potential of synthetic THC: dronabinol from Solvay Pharmaceuticals marketed as Marinol [42].

The U.S. Food and Drug Administration (FDA) is aware that cannabis and cannabis-derived products are being used for patient management in AIDS wasting syndrome, epilepsy, neuropathic pain, spasticity associated with multiple sclerosis, and cancer chemotherapy-induced nausea [43], but no approval has been given to any product containing or derived from the whole cannabis plant.

As Dr. Sanjay Gupta's WEED documentary discussed, cannabis is a Schedule I drug with "no medicinal value and a high potential for abuse" [44]. Even though the American Medical Association (AMA) and the Institute of Medicine have recognized the medicinal potential of cannabis, no further review of the Schedule I status has been forthcoming. The documentary explained how the U.S. government recognized cannabis as medicine in 2003 when scientists at the U.S. Department of Health and Human Services wrote a patent describing cannabinoids as useful antioxidants and neuroprotectants [45].

In 2011, the U.S. National Cancer Institute PDQ Complementary and Alternative Medicine (CAM) Editorial Board acknowledged medicinal uses of cannabis by publishing an online summary of cannabis and cannabinoids as CAM treatment for cancer patients [46].

Synthetic isolates approved

The FDA has approved three cannabinoid-based medicines derived from isolated synthetics: Marinol, Syndros, and Cesamet. Marinol and Syndros contain dronabinol. Cesamet has the active ingredient nabilone, which has a chemical structure similar to THC [47]. While these synthetic drugs have been afforded medical approval from FDA, cannabis users and manufacturers of cannabis-based products still risk incarceration until federal laws are changed.

Dronabinol

Dronabinol is a yellow, sticky man-made resin formulated from sesame oil that requires liver metabolism, which can result in an estimated 10 to 20% effectiveness for each capsule.

Marinol is the brand name for an oral form of dronabinol that has been approved for use in treating anorexia in AIDS and nausea from chemotherapy. Capsules are available in 2.5, 5, and 10 mg of dronabinol. Patients intolerant/allergic to sesame oil should not be given Marinol [48]. Patients prescribed Marinol may have **more** psychoactive effects than from natural cannabis—feeling "high," drowsiness, and confusion—which can last four to six hours and may result in them discontinuing the use of Marinol. The cost of Marinol varies depending on insurance coverage.

Syndros is a liquid formulation of dronabinol and used for the same conditions as Marinol.

Nabilone

The brand-name product of nabilone is Cesamet, and it claims to activate CB1 cannabinoid receptors that reduce nausea and vomiting. A 1 mg capsule of Cesamet contains 1 mg nabilone plus povidone (polyvinylpyrrolidone or PVP) and cornstarch [49]. PVP is used in the pharmaceutical industry as a synthetic polymer for aiding absorption in the human gastrointestinal tract. Cesamet can have significant effects on the nervous system with changes in mood, confusion, and hallucinations when large doses are given. The cost of Cesamet varies depending on insurance coverage and possible patient assistance programs offered.

Drug testing: Synthetic vs. natural cannabis

A basic drug test does not differentiate between THC from dronabinol products and the THC from natural cannabis, according to a clinical study by ElSohly et al. [50]. Synthetic THC is chemically the same as naturally occurring THC, so a urine test will be positive for either. A drug test that uses THCV (delta-9-tetrahydrocannabivin) as a marker could identify the natural component in cannabis compared to THC in the synthetic dronabinol, according to ElSohly.

References

1. Meijerink J, Balvers M et al. Omega-3 polyunsaturated N-acylethanolamines: A link between diet and cellular biology. In: Di Marzo, V., and Wang, J., (eds.). *The Endocannabinoidome*. Elsevier, London, 2015, 16–17.
2. Di Marzo V, Melck D et al. Endocannabinoids: endogenous cannabinoid receptor ligands with neuromodulatory action. *Trends Neurosci* 1998; 21, 521–528.
3. Lutz B. Genetic dissection of the endocannabinoid system and how it changed our knowledge of cannabinoid pharmacology and mammalian physiology. In: Di Marzo V. (ed.). *Cannabinoids*. Wiley, Oxford, 2014, 95–137.
4. Sulak D. Introduction to the endocannabinoid system. NORML website. www.norml.org/library.
5. Mc Partland JM, Duncan M et al. Are Cannabidiol and Δ^9-tetrahydrocannabivan negative modulators of the endocannabidoid system? A systemic review. *British J Pharm* 2015; (172), 737–753.
6. Haller J, Bakos V, Szermay M et al. The effects of genetic and pharmacological blockade of the CB1 cannabinoid receptor on anxiety. *Eur J Neurosci* 2002; 16 (7), 1395–1398.
7. Fride E, Ginzburg Y et al. Critical role of endogenous cannabinoid system in mouse pup suckling and growth. *Eur J Phamacol* 2001; 419 (2–3), 207–214.
8. Kirilly E, Gonda X, Bagdy G. CB1 receptor antagonists: New discoveries leading to new perspectives. *Acta Physiol (Oxf)* 2012; 205 (1), 41–60.
9. Carai MAM, Colombo G et al. Efficacy of rimonabant and other cannabinoid CB1 receptor antagonists in reducing food intake and body weight: Preclinical and clinical data. *CNS Drug Rev* 2006; 12(2), 91–99.
10. The Health Effects of Cannabis and Cannabinoids. *The Current State of Evidence and Recommendations for Research*. NA Press, Wash D.C., 2017, 85–90.
11. Center for Medical Cannabis Research- report to the legislature and governor of the State of California. Feb 2010. UCSD www.cmcr.ucsd.edu.
12. Pacher et al. The endocannabinoid system as an emerging target of pharmacotherapy. *Pharmaceutical Reviews* 2006; 58, 389–462.
13. Dewey WL. Cannabinoid pharmacology. *Pharm Rev* June 1986; 38(2), 151–178.
14. Robson P. Human studies of cannabinoids and medical cannabis. *Cannabinoids—Handbook of Experimental Pharmacology*. Springer-Verlag 2005; (168), 719–756.
15. Tanda G, Goldberg SR. Cannabinoids: Reward, dependence, and underlying neurochemical mechanisms—a review of recent preclinical data. *Psychopharmacology* 2003; 169, 115–134.
16. Pertwee RG. Cannabinoid pharmacology: The first 66 years. *British J Pharmacol* Jan 2006; 147 (Supp 1), S163–S171.
17. Pertwee RG. Tolerance to and Dependence on Psychotropic Cannabinoids. In: Pratt, J.A. (ed.). *The Biological Bases of Drug Tolerance and Dependence*. Academic Press, Cambridge, MA, 1991, 231–263.

18. De Petrocellis L, Di Marzo V. An introduction to the endocannabinoid system: From the early to the latest concepts. *Best Pract Res Clin Endocrinol Metab* 2009; 23 (1), 1–15.
19. Pertwee RG. Cannabinoid pharmacology: The first 66 years. *British J Pharmacol* Jan 2006; 147 (Supp 1), S163–S171.
20. Russo EB. Taming THC. potential cannabis synergy and phytocannabinoid-terpenoid entourage effects. *British J Pharmacol* 2011; 163 (7), 1344–1364.
21. Doorenbos NJ, Fetterman PS, Quimby MV et al. *Cultivation, Extraction, and Analysis of Cannabis Sativa L.* Annuals of NY Academy of Sciences, Dec 1971.
22. Pertwee RG. Cannabinoid pharmacology: The first 66 years. *British J Pharmacol* Jan 2006; 147 (Supp 1), S163–S171.
23. Malka D. Delivery and Dosage of cannabis medicine. www.CannaHoldings/ delivery-and-dosagesofcannabis medicine-bydeborah-malka-md-phd.
24. Pletcher et al. Association between marijuana exposure and pulmonary function over 20 years. *JAMA* 2012; 307, 173–181.
25. Hendriks H et al. Mono-terpene and sesqui-terpene hydrocarbons of the essential oil of Cannabis sativa. *Phytochem* 1975; 14, 814–815.
26. Schug KA. Into the Cannabinome. *The Analytical Scientist*, Feb 2017. www.theanalyticalscientist.com.
27. Paduch R, Kanderfer-Szerszen M et al. Terpenes:substances useful in human healthcare. *Archivum Immunologiae et Therapiae Experimentalis* 2007; 55, 315–327.
28. Cannabinoid and Terpenoid Reference Guide (n.d.) www.Steephilllab.com/ science/terpenes.
29. Casano S, Grassi G et al. Variations in terpene profiles of different strains of cannabis sativa L. *Acta Hortic. Acta Horticulturae* 2011; 115–121.
30. Russo EB. Taming THC: Potential cannabis synergy and phytocannabinoid-terpenoid entourage effects. *British Journal of Pharmacology.* Aug 2001; 163 (7), 1344–1364.
31. Ross SA, El Sohly MA. The volatile oil composition of fresh and air-dried buds of Cannabis sativa. *J Nat Prod* 1996; 59, 49–51.
32. Potter DJ. *The Propagation, Characturisation and Optimisation of Cannabis Sativia L. as a Phytopharmaceutical.* 2009. PhD King's College, London.
33. Pauli A, Schilcher H. In vitro antimicrobial activities of essential oils monographed in the European Pharmacopoeia 6th ed. In Baser KHC, Buchbauer G ed. *Handbook of Essential Oils: Science, Technology and Applications.* CRC Press, Boca Raton, FL, 2010, 353–548.
34. Buchbauer G, Jirovetz L et al. Fragrance compounds and essential oils with sedative effects on inhalation. *J Pharm Sci* 1993; 82, 660–664.
35. Russo EB, The solution to the medicinal cannabis problem. In: Schatman EM, ed. *Ethical Issues in Chronic Pain Management.* Taylor Francis, Boca Raton, FL, 2006, 165–194.
36. Huestis MA. Human Cannabinoid Pharmacokinetics. *Chem Biodivers* 2007; 4, 1770–1804.
37. Russo EB. Taming THC: Potential cannabis synergy and phytocannabinoid-terpenoid entourage effects. *British Journal of Pharmacology.* Aug 2001; 163 (7), 1344–1364.
38. Casano S, Grassi G et al. Variations in terpene profiles of different strains of cannabis sativa L. *Acta Hortic. Acta Horticulturae* 2011; 115–121.

39. McPartland JM, Russo EB. Cannabis and cannabis extracts: Greater than the sum od their parts? *Journal of Cannabis Therapeutics* 2001;1, 103–132.
40. Geise MW, Lewis MA et al. Development and validation of a relaible and robust method for the analysis of cannabinoids and terpenes in cannabis. *J of AOAC International* 2015; 98 (6), 1503–1522.
41. Small E. *Cannabis—A Complete Guide.* CRC Press, Boca Raton, FL, 2007, 179–189.
42. Russo E ed. *Cannabis: From Pariah to Prescription.* Haworth Press, Binghamton, NY, 2004.
43. Davis M, Maide V, Daeninck P et al. The emerging role of cannabinoid neuromodulators in symptom management. *Supportive Care in Cancer.* 2006; 15 (1), 63–71.
44. WEED. A Dr. Sanjay Gupta Special. CNN. Originally aired August 11, 2013.
45. United States Patent 6,630,507. Hampson et al. Oct 7, 2003. Cannabinoids as antioxidants and neuroprotectants. USPTO Patent Full-Text and Image Database.
46. Stafford L. Update: US government institution acknowledges medical uses of cannabis. *Herbal Gram* 2011; 91, 20–23.
47. Mack A, Joy J. *Marijuana as Medicine? The Science Beyond the Controversy. Pharmaceuticals from Marijuana.* National Academies Press 2000. www.ncbi. nlm.nih.gov.
48. Armentano P. Marinol vs Natural Plant. www.norml.org/pdf_files/ NORML_Marinol_vs_Natural_Cannabis.pdf.
49. Davis MP. Oral nabilone capsules in the treatment of chemotherapy-induced nausea and vomiting and pain. *Expert Opin Investig Drugs* Jan 2008; 17 (1), 85–95.
50. El Sohly MA, Dewit H, Wachtel SR et al. Delta-tetrahydrocannabivarin as a marker for the ingestion of marijuana versus Marinol (R): Results of a clinical study. *J of Analytical Toxicology* 2001; 25 (7), 565–71.

Additional references

Bonamin F, Moraes TM et al. The effect of a minor constituent of essential oil from Citrus aurantium: The role of β-myrcene in preventing peptic ulcer disease. *Chemico-Biological Interactions* 212, 11–19.

Chen W, Liu Y et al. Anti-tumor effect of α-pinene on human hepatoma cell lines through inducing G2/M cell cycle arrest. *Journal of Pharmacological Sciences* 2015; 127(3), 332–338.

Earley A. *Understanding Marijuana: A New Look at the Scientific Evidence.* Oxford Press, Oxford, 2002.

Horvath B, Mukhopadhyay P et al. β-Caryophyllene ameliorates cisplatin-induced nephrotoxicity in a cannabinoid 2 receptor-dependent manner. *Free Radical Biology and Medicine* 2012; 52(8), 1325–1333.

Leishman E, Bradshaw HB. N-acyl amides: Ubiquitous endogenous cannabimimetric lipids that are in the right place at the right time. In: Di Marzo, V., and Wang, J. (ed.). *The Endocannabinoidome- the World of Endocannabinoids and Related Mediators.* Elsevier, Amsterdam, 2015, 33–48.

Ma J, Xu H, Wu J et al. Linalool inhibits cigarette smoke-induced lung inflammation by inhibiting NF-χB activation. *International Immunopharmacology* 29(2), 708–713.

Onaivi E, Sugiura T, Di Marzo (eds.). *Endocannoidinoids: The Brain and Body's Marijuana and Beyond.* CRC Press, Boca Raton, FL, 2005.

Rohr AC, Wilkins CK et al. Upper airway and pulmonary effects of oxidation products of (+) alpha-pinene, d-limonene, and isoprene in BALB/c mice. *Inhalation Toxicology* 2002; 14(7), 663–684.

Sabogal-Guaqueta AM, Osorio E, Cardona-Gomez GP. Linalool reverses neuropathological and behavioral impairments in old triple transgenic Alzheimer's mice. *Neuropharmacology* 2016; 102, 111–120.

Wade D et al. A preliminary controlled study to determine whether whole plant cannabis extracts can improve intractable neurogenic symptoms. *J Clin Rehab* 2003; 17(1), 21–29.

Ware M, Wang T, Shapiro S et al. Smoked cannabis for chronic neuropathic pain: A randomized controlled trial. *Canadian Med Assn J* 2010; 182(14), 694–701.

Williamson EM, Evans FJ. Cannabinoids in clinical practice. *Drugs* Dec 2000; 60(6), 1303–1314.

chapter three

Endocannabinoid system
Regulatory function in health & disease

Betty Wedman-St. Louis

Contents

The first Western physician to be interested in cannabis was W.B. O'Shaughnessey, a young professor at the Medical College of Calcutta who learned of its multiple uses throughout India. When he returned to England in 1842, he brought with him how to make hemp solutions as an analgesic, along with knowledge of its use in epilepsy, tetanus, and rheumatism [1]. Cannabis was given to Queen Victoria by her physician for menstrual cramps, and it was listed in the U.S. Dispensatory in 1854 with cannabis preparations purchased in drug stores. By 1860, Dr. R.R. McMeens reported on the findings of cannabis use to the Ohio State Medical Society, and in 1887, H.A. Hare stated that he believed "cannabis to be as effective a pain reliever as opium" [2].

But cannabis use declined by the end of the nineteenth century as synthetic drugs such as aspirin, chloral hydrate, and barbiturates offered a standardized dose at a time when cannabis preparations varied significantly and individual responses to oral consumption was unpredictable [3].

Knowledge about the therapeutic potential of cannabis has become an intense area of study since the endogenous cannabinoid system was discovered over 20 years ago. The endocannabinoid system (ECS) is a natively produced biological system for regulating cell function through paracrine (cell-to-cell) and autocrine (within a cell) activity. Endocannabinoids are lipophilic with a brief lifespan and the ability to be synthesized as needed. The two major endocannabinoids produced by the human body are 2-AG and anandamide (AEA). Anandamide was discovered in 1992, and 2-AG followed in 1995.

Two G-protein receptors CB1 (predominately in the nervous system—brain and spinal cord) and CB2 (in the immune system with high density in the liver) are the key players in the ECS [4]. CB1 receptors have also been found in reproductive tissues and adipose tissues as well as other glands and organs. CB2 receptors have also been located in injury sites and inflamed body tissues. G-protein-coupled receptors open and close ion channels to inhibit or stimulate the adenylate cyclase reaction for cell metabolism.

Each receptor responds to different cannabinoids, but 2-AG and anandamide can interact with both the CB1 and CB2 receptors. CB1 receptors are involved in appetite regulation and pain sensations, while CB2 receptors in the peripheral nervous system are activated by immune disorders or inflammation.

The endocannabinoid system regulates a broad range of basic functions in the human body: appetite, metabolism, sleep, mood, body movement, temperature, immune function, inflammation, neuronal development and protection, digestion, reproduction, memory, and learning. Endocannabinoids and their receptors are present in every animal, including fish, reptiles, earthworms, leeches, amphibians, birds, and mammals, except insects [5]. Endocannabinoids and their receptors are the major focus of the International Cannabinoid Research Society (ICRS) formed in 1992 to advance research into treatments for cancer, diabetes, neuropathic pain, arthritis, obesity, Alzheimer's disease, multiple sclerosis, depression, and other diseases that cannabinoids may affect.

An example of how the ECS works can be explained in a human immune system example. The immune system "kicks on like a furnace when a fever is required to fry a virus or bacterial invader. And when the job is done, endocannabinoid signaling turns down the flame, cools the fever, and restores homeostasis" [6]. Cannabinoids are anti-inflammatory, but if the immune system overreacts to chronic stress or creates antibodies against one's own body, the stage is set for an autoimmune disease or an inflammatory disorder to develop.

Pope, Mechoulam, and Parsons describe the beneficial effects of CB1 and CB2 receptors and their endocannabinoids—2-AG and AEA—in traumatic brain injury, organophosphate toxicity, and hepatic encephalopathy [7]. Scientists have learned that CB 1 receptor signaling can also regulate neurogenesis or brain cell growth along with stem cell migration.

The endocannabinoid system has significant implications in mammalian reproduction. Mauro Maccarrone, PhD, at the University of Teramo, Italy reports the ECS is a "gatekeeper" for reproduction. It affects the entire reproductive process from spermatogenesis to fertilization, oviductal transport of the zygote, embryo implantation, and fetal development [8]. Inadequate anandamide (2-AG) could lead to ectopic pregnancy and miscarriage or spontaneous abortion.

High levels of endocannabinoids in maternal milk are critical in developing suckling in the newborn and offsetting infant colic. Israeli neuroscientist Ester Fride, PhD, observed that infants who suffer from failure to thrive syndrome needed CB1 receptors to survive [9]. Her work suggests that the endocannabinoid CB1 receptor system is unique in its absolute control over the initiation of the neonatal milk suckling response. In addition, cannabis is a known appetite stimulant and may have the undesirable side effect in weight gain versus reducing wasting syndrome in AIDS and cancer due to inadequate CB1 [10].

Endocannabinoid deficits are associated with a reduced ability to adapt to chronic stress. Prolonged exposure to stress depletes endocannabinoid vigor whether from poor diet, environmental toxins, drug abuse, lack of exercise, or genetic factors [11]. Ethan Russo MD, senior medical adviser to GW Pharmaceuticals, examined clinical endocannabinoid deficiency (CECD) as the underlying pathophysiology of migraine, fibromyalgia, irritable bowel syndrome, and other conditions known to be alleviated by cannabis use [12]. He concluded that an underlying CECD needs to be considered and treatment with cannabinoid medicines recommended. Similar deficiencies have been reported in post-traumatic stress disorder (PTSD), neuropathic pain, intractable depression, interstitial cystitis, and complex pain syndrome [13].

Many cancer patients have increased amounts of CB1 and/or CB2, which researchers believe is the body's effort to combat the disease. Cancer arises due to malignant cells not undergoing apoptosis or cell death. These cells become immortalized, divide, and grow into invasive tissues with their own blood supply and can metastasize to distant areas of the body [14]. The phytocannabinoid CBD has been reported to reverse or prevent many of the cancer cell growths in experiments. In addition to cell growth management, cannabinoid treatment may have additional benefits in pain, nausea, sleep, depression, and anxiety associated with cancer.

A third cannabinoid receptor, TRPV1 (transient receptor potential vanilloid-one) is considered part of the ECS. It is best known for its action with capsaicin, the active ingredient in chili peppers, with implications for use in pain, inflammation, respiratory, and cardiovascular disorders. TRPV1 mediates pain signals through a different mechanism than endogenous cannabinoids and opioids, but the receptor is subject to desensitization whereby continuous stimulation causes the pathway to slow down or stop, thus reducing pain [15].

The three cannabinoid receptors of the ECS, the endocannabinoids and their regulatory enzymes, are considered the mediators of physiological homeostasis to ensure the human body functions within tight parameters of neither deficiency or excess [16]. Professor Raphael Mechoulam has hypothesized that the endocannabinoid system serves an analogous role in the body as the immune system. The immune system deals with invasive proteins from bacteria and viruses, while the ECS neutralizes non-protein insults such as trauma or lack of oxygen.

Normal ECS: Normal mental function
   No pain
   Good digestion
Imbalanced ECS: Obesity or wasting syndrome
   Metabolic syndrome
   Diabetes
   Liver fibrosis
   Idiopathic bowel syndrome
   Chronic pain
   Fibromyalgia
   Neurodegenerative diseases

ECS and neurodegenerative disorders

Cannabinoid receptors anandamide and 2-AG are endogenous neuroprotective agents produced by the nervous system in response to chemical and mechanical trauma [17]. When neurons are injured, they release their contents, and excitatory neurons release glutamate that becomes toxic to surrounding cells, producing excitotoxicity. Cannabinoids halt that process, as evidenced by the U.S. Department of Health and Human Services patent on the use of cannabinoids as antioxidants and neuroprotectants. This beneficial effect of cannabinoids has implications in treating neurodegenerative conditions such as multiple sclerosis, Alzheimer's disease, Parkinson's, and Huntington's cholera.

Multiple sclerosis

Many human and animal studies suggest multiple sclerosis is a disorder associated with changes in the ECS [18,19]. The CB1 receptor is important to control tremor and spasticity, while the exact function of the CB2 receptor seems to be regulation of the inflammatory process [20]. Research has shown cannabinoids have potential for symptomatic benefit in MS pain, spasticity, tremor, and urinary dysfunction [21].

Parkinson's disease

In Sir William Gowers textbook on neurology in 1888, cannabis was recommended for Parkinson's disease and other movement disorders [22]. The involuntary choreiform movements are associated with overactivity of the globus pallidus and glutamatergic striatal excitation, which cannabinoid receptors on GABA terminals can improve [23,24].

Alzheimer's disease

Alzheimer's disease is a form of dementia affecting 30 to 50% of those over 85 years old. Accumulation of plaque consisting of amyloid-β and neurofibrillary tangles leads to inflammation from hyperphosphorylation of tau proteins. Abnormalities in the endogenous cannabinoid system have been noted, and cannabinoids have been demonstrated to inhibit tau hyperphosphorylation and inhibit acetylcholinesterase [25]. THC has been shown to have neuroprotective antioxidant effects [26], while CB2 receptors stimulate decreases in microglial activation and lower amyloid-β levels in mice [27].

Huntington's disease

Huntington's disease (HD) is a hereditary neurodegenerative disease affecting mood, mentality, and movement [28]. Studies with cannabinoids have been performed in HD animal models, with several demonstrating preservation of striatal neurons [29]. Anecdotal reports indicate cannabis benefits painful dystonia, chorea, and acts as a mood enhancer, but no clinical trials have been done [30].

Tourette's syndrome

Tourette's syndrome, with its characteristic motor and vocal tics, has shown improvement with THC in a small, single-dose trial using an examiner and self-rating scale to report outcome [31].

Amyotrophic lateral sclerosis

Neuroinflammation plays a role in the pathogenesis of ALS, and cannabis may participate in the immune system regulation through its action on CB2 receptors. Cannabinoids downregulate the proinflammatory cytokine and chemokine production [32]. ALS symptoms of pain, spasticity, weight loss, dyspnea, and depression can be ameliorated by cannabis, although more research is needed on routes of administration and dosing [33].

Stroke

Ischemic stroke is the most common form of stroke and is caused by a transient interruption of blood supply to the brain via a thrombotic occlusion of blood vessels. It can be a cause of death and disability. Cannabinoids can provide neuroprotective benefits by protecting against hypoxia and glucose deprivation after the occlusion, but their usefulness in treatment after the stroke warrants future research [34,35].

Epilepsy

The ECS is associated with neuronal tone and excitability, which influences epileptic activity. Human and animal studies show changes in CB1 receptor activity in the hippocampus with CB1 receptor agonists having the potential to suppress epileptic activity [36]. Cannabis can reduce seizure frequency but can provoke seizures in others. Cannabidiol (CBD) has been examined as a potential antiepileptic in humans with a dose of 200 to 300 mg of CBD safely administered [37].

ECS and pain

The ECS plays a significant role in pain management whether it is acute pain, persistent inflammation pain, or neuropathic pain. Cannabinoids have antinociceptive effects that decrease the perception of pain, especially when associated with injury. CB1 receptors open potassium channels and cause the nociceptor to hyperpolarize and reduce their response. CB2 receptors reduce the signaling from area immune cells [38].

Neuropathic pain is defined as pain arising because of a disorder affecting the somatosensory system [39]. Interest in using cannabis for pain began in the 1800s when dogs were administered smoked cannabis to assess their response to pain [40]. Cannabis was recommended not only to improve pain but relieve nausea, depressed mood, anxiety, and disturbed sleep [41].

The analgesic response to exogenous cannabinoids indicates a ECS role in nociceptive pain sensitivity. Increased anandamide levels in some brain areas involved in nociceptive pain were identified in a rat study, which supported the CB1 mediated analgesic activity of THC [42].

ECS and cancer

Cannabinoids also have a direct effect on cancer and the side effects of chemotherapy. They have been shown to inhibit tumor growth in multiple cell lines [43]. Animals treated with cannabinoids had a slower tumor growth than control animals, and cannabinoids do not harm healthy cells at the same dose that is needed to kill cancer cells.

Chemotherapy-induced nausea and vomiting are very distressing and all too common an event associated with cancer treatment. The use of cannabis/cannabinoids has been shown to provide benefit [44]. CB1 and CB2 receptors have been found in areas of the brainstem associated with emetogenic control [45]. Studies have shown delta-8-THC to be more potent antiemetic than delta-9-THC [46].

ECS: Gastrointestinal disorders and Crohn's disease

Cannabinoids have many functions in the digestive tract, including inhibition of gastric acid production, gastrointestinal motility, secretion transport as well as inflammation [47]. Irritable bowel syndrome (IBS) is the most common gastrointestinal disorder and is characterized by chronic abdominal pain and alterations in bowel function. CB1 receptor expression is found in human colonic epithelium and stomach parietal cells [48], while CB2 receptors are located throughout the gastrointestinal system from the lamina propria to the macrophages and myenteric and submucosal plexus ganglia of the ilium [49]. CB2 receptors likely involve inflammation control, visceral pain, and intestinal motility within the inflamed gut. Ni et al. [50] describes how gut dysbiosis and Crohn's disease may respond to therapeutic cannabinoid use. Cannabis improvement has been noted in relief of abdominal pain, improved appetite, and reduction of diarrheal symptoms [51].

ECS and liver

The liver has both CB1 and CB2 receptors with CB1 found in endothelial cells and hepatocytes, while CB2 receptors are in Kupffer cells [52]. CB1 and CB2 receptors have different effects on the liver fibrosis, with early injury causing steatosis leading to CB1 activation. Prolonged injury and inflammation signals both CB1 and CB2 to promote liver regeneration unless the inflammation is so prolonged that fibrosis overcomes [53]. The opposing roles of CB1 and CB2 are highlighted in this example. Activation of CB1 receptors is implicated in the progression and worsening of alcoholic steatosis, while CB2 confers beneficial effects in alcoholic fatty liver [54,55].

ECS and appetite

The ECS is also responsible for controlling hunger and the desire to eat through modulating cell metabolism via hormones ghrelin, leptin, orexin, and adiponectin. Hollister identified the appetite-promoting effect of smoked marijuana before the identification of specific cannabinoid receptors [56]. Animal studies documented that THC promoted food intake, which has been linked to CB1 receptor activity [57]. In obesity, adipocytes produce excessive endocannabinoids that drive CB1 receptors into dysfunction, leading to metabolic syndrome [58]. Kim et al. [59,60] explain the components of the ECS and its role in adipose and muscle metabolism. Dietary modifications of essential fatty acids and use of omega-3 polyunsaturated fatty acids, like those found in cannabis, may improve insulin sensitivity and reduce body fat.

Another factor is the absence of leptin related to increased endocannabinoid activity, which reduces anandamide levels needed for appetite control [61]. Cannabinoids can increase the intake of food related to reward-seeking behavior [62]. A synergism between the endogenous opioid and cannabinoid systems in mediating food intake has been proposed [63]. Endocannabinoids may also be involved in ghrelin release, which is the gut hormone to stimulate food intake, but more research is needed to define the downstream mediators of appetite control.

Cachexia and anorexia are negative energy balance states that result in decreased appetite and weight loss. It can be the consequence of wasting diseases such as AIDS and metastatic cancer, but it could also be associated with neuropsychiatric conditions such as anorexia nervosa and dementia. The therapeutic effectiveness of THC as an appetite boost is shown in numerous studies [64–66].

ECS and lifestyle

Chronic stress has been shown to impair the ECS by decreasing anandamide and 2-AG. Rat studies showed that social play increased CB1 phosphorylation, which is a marker of CB1 activation in the amygdala [67].

ECS and glaucoma

Glaucoma is a leading cause of blindness within the Unites States and is characterized by abnormally high intraocular pressure that damages the optic nerve and results in vision loss [68]. Research indicates cannabinoids may have the potential to be an effective treatment for reducing pressure in the eye. Robert S. Hepler, MD, of the Jules Stein Eye Institute at UCLA conducted studies in the 1970s on marijuana's effect on pupillary dilation when smoking marijuana and checked intraocular pressure (IOP) of the research subjects [69]. He found marijuana rapidly reduced IOP in both normal and glaucomatous eyes. According to Hepler, the IOP lowering effect of marijuana occurs about 45 minutes after smoking and lasts from three to five hours. Research suggests that cannabinoids have potential as an effective treatment for reducing eye pressure [70] when administered orally, intravenously, or by inhalation but not when applied directly to the eye [71].

The first reports of marijuana effects on IOP were published in the 1970s at a time when there were no drugs available to treat the condition, but it took over 30 years to even reconsider marijuana as a treatment option.

Marijuana: The forbidden medicine

Lester Grinspoon, MD, associate professor of psychiatry at Harvard Medical School, and James B. Bakalar, associate editor of the Harvard Mental Health Letter, wrote *Marijuana: The Forbidden Medicine* [72], which compiles the medical benefits of cannabis before the endocannabinoid system was discovered. It explains why cannabis is not the harmful substance reported over the past 50 years. The authors report contributions by users of marijuana who declare its therapeutic value. A highlight of the book is the historical perspective about how cannabis was reported in the medical literature as a therapy for numerous medical disorders but never used as a treatment option. As you read through this summary, think of how many patients were deprived of a therapeutic benefit since cannabis was declared a Schedule I drug.

Cancer	1975 Chemotherapy nausea and vomiting in acute lymphatic leukemia [73]
	1979 High-dose methotrexate, nausea and vomiting [74]
	1991 Oncologists consider smoking marijuana more effective and safer than oral synthetic [75]
	1976 Antitumor effects in animal studies [76]
Glaucoma	1971 and 1976 Lowers eye pressure up to four to five hours [77,78]
Epilepsy	1949 Antiepileptic action of marijuana [79]
	1975 Anticonvulsant drugs = serious side effects compared to marijuana [80,81]
	1975 Anticonvulsant effects from smoking marijuana [82]
	1980 CBD = improvement in seizures [83]

(Continued)

Multiple sclerosis	1983 THC used [84]
	1989 Marijuana reduces muscle spasms [85]
AIDS	1971 Improved appetite from marijuana [86]
	1976 Marijuana smokers ate more and gained weight [87]
Chronic pain	1975 THC relieves pain at 5 to 10 mg [88]
	1975 Pain tolerance greater in regular marijuana users [89]
Migraine	1985 Cannabinoids block serotonin [90]
Depression and mood	1973 THC reduces symptoms [91]

References

1. Grinspoon L, Bakalar JB. *Marijuana the Forbidden Medicine*. Yale University Press, New Haven, CT., 1993 p 4.
2. Hare HA. Clinical and physiological notes on the action of cannabis indica. *Therapeutic Gazette* 1887;11:225–226.
3. Grinspoon L, Bakalar JB. *Marijuana the Forbidden Medicine*. Yale University Press, New Haven, CT. 1993 p 4.
4. Pacher P, Batkai S, Kunos G. The endocannabinoid system as an emerging target of pharmacotherapy. *Pharmacol Rev*. 2006;58(3):389–462.
5. Lee MA. The discovery of the endocannabinoid system. *O'Shaughnessy's*. 2010. www.beyondthc/com/wp-content/uploads/2012/07/eCBSsystemLee.pdf.
6. Lee MA. The discovery of the endocannabinoid system. *O'Shaughnessy's*. 2010. www.beyondthc/com/wp-content/uploads/2012/07/eCBSsystemLee.pdf.
7. Pope C, Mechoulam R, Parsons L. Endocannabinoid signaling in neurotoxicity and neuroprotection. *Neurotoxicology* 2010;31(5):562–571.
8. Maccarrone M. Endocannabinoids: Friends and foes of reproduction. *Progress in Lipid Research* 2009;48(6):344–354.
9. Fride E. Cannabinoids and feeding: the role of the endogenous cannabinoid system as a trigger for newborn suckling. In: *Women and Cannabis: Medicine, Science, and Sociology*. Haworth Press, 2002, p 51–62.
10. Mechoulam R, Hanus L, Fride E. Towards cannabinoid drugs-revisited. *Prog Med Chem*. 1998;35:199–243.
11. Lee MA. Smoke Signals: A Social History of Marijuana-medical, recreational and scientific. 2013;35:199–243.
12. Russo EB. Clincal Endocannabinoid Deficiency (CECD): Can this concept explain therapeutic benefits of cannabis in migraine, fibromyalgia, irritable bowel syndrome and other treatment-resistant conditions? *Neuroendocrinology Letters* 2004;25(1/2):11–20.
13. Russo EB, Hohmann AG. Role of cannabinoids in pain management. In: *Comprehensive Treatment of Chronic Pain by Medical Interventional and Behavioral Approaches*, Deer T, Gordon V, eds, 2013, Springer, NY.
14. Ligresli A, Moriello AS, Starowicz K et al. Anti-tumor activity of plant cannabinoids with emphasis on the effect of cannabidiol on human breast carcinoma. *J Pharmacol Exp Ther*. 2006;318(3):1375–1387.

15. Russo EB, Hohmann AG. Role of cannabinoids in pain management. In: *Comprehensive Treatment of Chronic Pain by Medical Interventional and Behavioral Approaches,* Deer T, Gordon V, eds, 2013, Springer, NY.
16. Pope C, Mechoulam R, Parsons L. Endocannabinoid signaling in neurotoxicity and neuroprotection. *Neurotoxicology* 2010;31(5):562–571.
17. Sulak D. An introduction to the endocannnabinoid system—a description of the lipid signaling system to health, healing, and homeostasis, long excluded from the medical school curriculum. *Society of Cannabis Clinicians' CME course.* www.cannabisclinicians.org.
18. Baker D, Pryce G, Crawford JL et al. Cannabinoids control spasticity and tremors in a multiple sclerosis model. *Nature* 2000;404:84–87.
19. Pertwee RG. Cannabinoids and multiple sclerosis. *Mol Neurobiol.* 2007;36:45–49.
20. Maresz K, Pryce G, Ponomarev ED et al. Direct suppression of CNS autoimmune inflammation via the cannabinoid receptor CB1 on neurons and CB2 on autoreactive T cells. *Nat Med.* 2007;13:492–497.
21. Koppel BS, Brust JCM, Fife T et al. Systemic review: Efficacy and safety of medical marijuana in selected neurological disorders. Report of the Guideline Development Subcommittee of the American Academy of Neurology. *Neurology* 2014;82(17):1556–1563.
22. Gowers W. *A Manual of Diseases of the Nervous System.* P. Blakiston Son and Co., Philadelphia PA. 1888.
23. Lotan I, Trevest A, Roditi Y et al. Cannabis (medical marijuana) treatment for motor and non-motor symptoms of Parkinson's disease: An open-label observational study. *Clin Neuropharmacol.* 2014;37:42–44.
24. Fox SH, Henry B, Hill M et al. Stimulation of cannabinoid receptors reduced levodopa-induced dyskinesia in the MPTP-lesioned non-human primate model of Parkinson's disease. *Mov Disord.* 2002;17:1180–1187.
25. Esposito G, De Filippis D, Carnuccio R et al. The marijuana component cannabidiol inhibits beta-amyyloid-induced tau protein hyperphosphorylation through Wnt/beta-catenin pathway rescue in PC12 cells. *J Mol Med.* 2006;84:253–258.
26. Hampson AJ, Grimaldi M, Lolic M et al. Neuroprotective antioxidants from marijuana. *Ann NY Acad Sci* 2000;899:274–282.
27. Martin-Moreno AM, Brera B, Spuch C et al. Prolonged oral cannabinoid administration prevents neuroinflammation, lowers beta-amyloid levels and improves cognitive performance in TgAPP25776 mice. *J Neuroinflamm.* 2012;9:8.
28. Benbadis SR, Sanchez-Ramos J, Bozorg A et al. Medical marijuana in neurology. *Expert Rev Neurother.* 2014;14(12):1453–1465.
29. Sagredo O, Pazos MR, Valdoelivas E et al. Cannabinoids:normal medicines for the treatment of Huntington's disease. *Recent Pat CNS Drug Discov.* 2012;7(1):41–48.
30. Benbadis SR, Sanchez-Ramos J, Bozorg A et al. Medical marijuana in neurology. *Expert Rev Neurother.* 2014;14(12):1453–1465.
31. Muller-Vahl KR, Schneider U, Koblenz A et al. Treatment of Tourette's syndrome with Δ-9-tetrahydrocannabinol (THC): A randomized crossover trial. *Pharmacopsychiatry* 2002;35:57–61.
32. The ALS Untangled Group. ALS Untangled No.16:Cannabis. *Amyotrophic Lateral Sclerosis* 2012;13:400–404.

33. McAllister SD, Rizvi G et al. Amyotropic lateral sclerosis:delayed disease progression in mice by treatment with a cannabinoid. *Amyotroph Lateral Scler Other Motor Neuron Disord.* 2004;5(1):33–39.

34. Begg M, Pacher P, Batkai S et al. Evidence for novel cannabinoiod receptors. *Pharmacol Ther.* 2005;106:133–145.

35. Pertwee RG. Pharmacological actions of cannabinoids. In: Pertwee R, ed. *Cannabinoids.* Springer, NY, 2005, p1–53.

36. Smith PF. Cannabinoids as potential anti-epileptic drugs. *Curr Opin Investig Drugs.* 2005;6:680–685.

37. Lutz B. On-demand activation of the endocannabinoid system in the control of neuronal excitability and epileptiform seizures. *Biochem Pharmacol.* 2004;68:1691–1698.

38. Sulak D. An introduction to the endocannnabinoid system—a description of the lipid signaling system to health, healing, and homeostasis, long excluded from the medical school curriculum. Society of Cannabis Clinicians' CME course. www.cannabisclinicians.org.

39. Dworkin RH, O'Connor AB, Audette J et al. Recommendations for the pharmacological management of neuropathic pain: An overview and literature update. *Mlin Proc* 2010;85:s3–14.

40. Dixon WE. The pharmacology of Cannabis indica. *Br Med J.* 1899;2: 1354–1357.

41. Rahn EJ, Hofmann AG. Cannabinoids as pharmacotherapies for neuropathic pain: From the bench to the bedside. *Neurotherapeutics* 2009;6(4):713–737.

42. Walter JM, Huang SM, Strangman NM et al. Pain modulation by release of the endogenous cannabiploid anandamide. *Proc Natl Acad Sci USA.* 199;96:12198–12203.

43. Chakravarti B, Ravi J, Ganju RK. Cannabinoids as therapeutic agents in cancer: Current status and future implications. *Oncotarget* 2014;5(15): 5852–5872.

44. Parker LA, Rock E, Limebeer C. Regulation of nausea and vomiting by cannabinoids. *Br J Pharmacol.* 2010;163:1411–1422.

45. Hornby PJ. Central neurocircuitory assocciated with emesis. *Am J Med.* 2001;111, Suppl 8A:106s–112s.

46. Darmani NA, Janoyan JJ, Crim J et al. Receptor mechanism and antiemetic activity of structurally-deverse cannabinoids against radiation-induced emesis in the least shrew. *Eur J Pharmacol.* 2007;53:187–1196.

47. Izzo AA, Sharkey KA. Cannabinoids and the gut: New developments and emerging concepts. *Pharmacol Ther.* 2010;126:21–38.

48. Wright K, Rooney N, Feeney M et al. Differential exxpression of cannabinoid receptors in the human colon: Cannabinoids promote epithelial wound healing. *Gastroenterology* 2005;129:437–453.

49. Ros J, Claria J, To-Figueras J et al. Endogenous cannabinoids: A new system involved in the homeostasis of arterial pressure in experimental cirrhosis in the rat. *Gastroenterolgy* 2002;122:85–93.

50. Ni J, Shen T-CD, Chen EZ et al. A role for bacterial urease in gut dysbiosis and Crohn's disease. *Sci Translational Med.* 2017;9(416):ea ah6888.

51. Lal S, Prasad N, Ryan M et al. Cannabis use amongst patients with inflammatory bowel disease. *Eur J Gastroenterol Hepatol.* 2011;23:891–896.

52. Tam J, Liu J, Mukhopadhyay B et al. Endocannabinoids in liver disease. *Hepatology* 2011;53:346–355.

53. Lim MP, Devi LA, Rozenfeld R. Cannabidiol causes activated hepatic stellate cell death through a mechanism of endoplasmic reticulum stress-induced apoptosis. *Cell Death Dis* 2011;2:e170.

54. Patsenker E, Stoll M, Millonig G et al. Cannabinoid receptor type 1 modulates alcohol-induced liver fibrosis. *Mol Med.* 2011;17:1285–1294.

55. Trebicka T, Racz I, Siegmund S et al. Role of cannabinoid receptors in alcoholic hepatic injury: Steatosis and fibrogenesis are increased in CB2 receptor-deficient mice and decreased in CB1 receptor knockouts. *Liver Int.* 2011;31:860–870.

56. Hollister LE. Hunger and appetite after single doses of marijuana, alcohol and detroamphetamine. *Clin Pharmacol Ther.* 1971;12:45–49.

57. Williams CM, Kirkham TC. Anandamide induces overeating: Mediation by central cannabinoid (CB1) receptors. *Psychppharmacology (Berl)* 1999;143:315–317.

58. Di Marzo V, Matias I. Endocannabinoid control of food intake and energy balance. *Nat Neurosci 2005*;8(5):585–589.

59. Kim J, Li Y, Watkins BA. Endocannabinoid signaling and energy metabolism: A target for dietary intervention. *Nutr.* 2011;27(6):624–632.

60. Watkins BA, Kim J. Endocannabinoid system: Directing eating behavior and macronutrient metabolism. *Front Psychol.* 2014;5:1506–1521.

61. Di Marzo V, Goparaju SK, Wang L et al. Leptin-regulated endocannabinoids are involved in maintaining food intake. *Nature (Lond)* 2001;410:822–825.

62. Harris GC, Wimmer M, Aston-Jones G. A role for lateral hypothalamic orexin in neurons in reward seeking. *Nature (LOND)* 2005;437:556–559.

63. Solinas M, Goldberg SR. Motivational effects of cannabinoids and opioids on food reinforcement depend on simultaneous activation of cannabinoids and opioids system. *Neuropsychopharmacology* 2005;30:2035–2045.

64. Regelson W, Butler JR, Schultz J et al. Δ-9-THC as an effective antidepressant and appetite-stimulating agent in advanced cancer patients. In: Braude MC, Szara S, eds. *The Pharmacology of Marijuana.* Raven Press, NY. 1976, p763–776.

65. Gorter R, Seefried M, Volberding P. Dronabinol effects on weight in patients with HIV infection. *AIDS* 1992;6:127.

66. Beal JE, Olson R, Laubenstein L et al. Dronabinol as a treatment for anorexia associated with weight loss in patients with AIDS. *J Pain Symptom Manage.* 1995;10:89–97.

67. Sulak D. An introduction to the endocannnabinoid system—a description of the lipid signaling system to health, healing, and homeostasis, long excluded from the medical school curriculum. *Society of Cannabis Clinicians' CME course.* www.cannabisclinicians.org.

68. Randall RC. Glaucoma: a patient's view. In: Mathre ML (ed). *Cannabis in Medical Practice.* 1997 McFarland & Company, Jefferson NC. p94–102.

69. Hepler RS, Frank IM. Marijuana smoking and intraocular pressure. *JAMA* 1971;27(10):1392.

70. Tomida I, Azura-Blanco A, House H et al. Effect of sublingual application of cannabinoids on intraocular pressure: A pilot study. *J Glauccoma* 2006;15:349–353.

71. Institute of Medicine. *Marijuana and Medicine: Assessing the Science Base.* National Academy Press, Wash. D.C. 1999, p203–204.

72. Grinspoon L, Bakalar JB. *Marijuana the Forbidden Medicine.* Yale University Press, New Haven, CT., 1993.

73. Sallan SE, Zinberg NE, Frei III E. Antiemetic effect of delta-9-tetrahydrocannabinol in patients receiving cancer chemotherapy. *New Eng J Med.* 1975;293:795–797.

74. Chang AE et al. Delta-9-tetrahydrocannabinol as an antiemetic in cancer patients receiving high dose methotrexate: A prospective, randomized evaluation. *Annuals of Internal Med* 1979;91:819–824.

75. Doblin R, Kleiman MAR. Marijuana as anti-emetic medicine: A survey of oncologists' attitudes and experiences. *J of Clin Oncology* 1991;9:1275–1280.

76. Harris LS, Munson AE, Carchmaan RA. Antitumor properties of cannabinoids. In: *The Pharmacology of Marijuana*, Braude MC & Szara S (eds). Raven NY., 1976;2:773–776.

77. Hepler RS, Frank IM. Marijuana ssmoking and intraocular pressure. *JAMA* 1971;217:1392.

78. Hepler RS, Frank IM, Petrus R. Ocular effects of marijuana smoking. In: *The Pharmacology of Marijuana*, Braaude MC & Szara S (eds). Raven, NY., 1976;2:815–824.

79. Davis JP, Ramsey HH. Antiepileptic action of marijuana-active substances. *Federation Proceedings* 1949;8:2284–285.

80. Robb P. Focal epilepsy: The problem, prevalence and contributing factors. *Advance Neurology* 1975;8:11–22.

81. Kutt H, Louis S. Untoward effcets of anticonvulsants. *NEJM* 1972;286:1316–1317.

82. Consroe PF, Wood GC, Buchsbawm H. Anticonv ulsant nature of marijuana smoking. *JAMA* 1975;234:306–307.

83. Cunha JM, Carlin EA, Pereira AE et al. Chronic administration of cannabidiol to healthy volunteers and epileptic patients. *Pharmacology* 1980;21:175–185.

84. Clifford DB. Tetrahydrocannabinol for tremors in multiple sclerosis. *Annuals of Neurology* 1983;13:669–671.

85. Meinak HM, Shonle PW, Conrad B. Effect of cannabinoids on spastisity and ataxia in multiple sclerosis. *J Neurology* 1989;236:120–122.

86. Hollister LE. Hunger and appetite after single doses of marijuana, alcohol and dextroamphetamine. *Clin Pharmacol Ther.* 1971;12:45–49.

87. Greenberg I, Kuehnle J, Mendelson JH et al. Effects of marihuana use on body weight and calorie intake in humans. *J Psychopharmacology (Berlin)* 1976;49:79–84.

88. Noyes Jr R, Brunk SF, Baram DA et al. Analgesic effect of delta-9-tetrahydrocannabinol. *J Clin Pharmacology* 1975;18:84–89.

89. Milstein SL, Mac Cannell K, Karr G et al. Marijuana-produced changes in pain tolerance: Experienced and non-experienced subjects. *Int Pharmacopsychiatry* 1975;10:177–182.

90. Volfe Z, Dvilansky A, Nathan I. Cannabinoids block release of serotonin from platelets induced by plasma from migraine patients. *Int J Clin and Pharmacological Research* 1985;5:243–246.

91. Kotin J, Post RM, Goodwin FK. Delta-9-tetrahydrocannabinol in depressed patients. *Archives of General Psychiatry* 1973;28:345–348.

chapter four

Cannabinoid medications for treatment of neurological disorders

Juan Sanchez-Ramos and Betty Wedman-St. Louis

Contents

Cannabis has a long history as a medical substance, but legal restrictions have limited research and well-controlled clinical trials. As legal restrictions on medical use of cannabis are being lifted, cannabinoid drug research has begun to increase in relation to neurological disorders.

Neuropharmacologists have also begun to recognize that phytocannabinoids tetrahydrocannabinol (THC) and cannabidiol (CBD) provide greater therapeutic effects when given together than in isolation. The combination is called the "entourage effect" [1]. Mechoulam [2] defined the entourage effect as the synergism found in plants such as phytocannabinoids that create a better therapeutic response than an isolated component produced as a drug [3]. The entourage effect is not unique to phytocannabinoids, as pharmaceutical companies have learned from other monotherapies [4].

The cannabis plant is a highly variable and versatile botanical with many strains [5]. The two primary species for medical use are Cannabis sativa and Cannabis indica, which contain over 100 compounds and greater than 200 terpenoids [6]. What purpose these compounds offer to the plant has yet to be elucidated, but the activity of these phytocannabinoids in the human brain is gaining neurological attention [7].

Administration of delta-9-THC either orally, intravenously, or inhaled as smoke resulted in psychological changes similar to those of recreational plant material effects, and the THC metabolite could be detected in human urine for several weeks post use [8].

Cannabinoid receptors

In the 1980s, brain receptors that interact with natural and synthetic cannabinoids were identified. After many years of research, endogenous cannabinoid receptors were identified and named anandamide [9]. The molecule is found in nearly all tissues in many animals, with anandamide binding to both CB1 receptors (found in the central nervous system) and CB2 receptors (found in peripheral tissues, immune cells, and some brainstem neurons).

The cannabinoid receptor CB1 is primarily distributed in the basal ganglia of the human and rodent brain [10,11]. The basal ganglia refer to the interconnected deep gray structures in the brain: substantia nigra, subthalamic nucleus, putamen, caudate, and globus pallidus. These brain areas are responsible for automatic execution of learned motor skills. Dysfunction in this circuitry results in disorders characterized by involuntary movements or difficulty starting or stopping, a movement characteristic of Parkinson's disease, Huntington's disease, and Tourette syndrome tics [12].

Most of the CB2 receptors are abundant in the immune tissues, and most of the brain's CB2 receptors are expressed as glial cells [13,14]. Astrocytes and microglia in Parkinson's disease and Huntington's disease are associated with increased CB2 receptor activity for neuroprotection, according to Fernandez-Ruiz [14].

As research increases on endogenous cannabinoid signaling of the CB1 and CB2 receptors, patients may benefit from compassionate use of cannabinoid preparations to mitigate the progression of their disease.

Cannabinoids and neurotransmission

Szabo and Schlicker describe the effects of cannabinoids on neurotransmission [15]. Dopamine is the major neurotransmitter produced by neurons in the substania nigra. As dopamine is reduced, symptom manifestation leads to progressive slowness, rigidity, and tremors. GABA is the major inhibitory neurotransmitter and serves as a "brake" in the control of movement, while cannabinoids can produce a trance-like state or catalepsy [16]. Glutamate is the dominate excitatory transmitter whereby they may contribute to neuronal degeneration through excitotoxicity. Cannabinoids can inhibit glutamate activity to reduce some symptoms of Parkinson's disease and slow the progression of the disease [17].

Due to the high quantity of cannabinoid receptors in the basal ganglia, cannabinoids can have significant effect on motor activity throughout life. They are neuroprotective and have reduced neurodegeneration in animal studies while showing antioxidant benefits [18].

Cannabinoids and Parkinson's disease

Parkinson's disease (PD) is a neurodegenerative disease characteristically identified by slow movement, rigid muscles, and a loss of usual muscle reflexes [19]. Symptoms can range from mild to severe and can include trembling in the hands, arms, legs, jaw, or face. The stiffness in the limbs and postural instability make completing simple tasks increasingly difficult.

Currently there is no cure for PD, but medications can reduce the severity of the symptoms. Levodopa and carbidopa are the medications usually prescribed for PD. Levodopa side effects include nausea, vomiting, and loss of appetite. Because levodopa competes with dietary amino acids for absorption, a low-protein diet can be used during the day to improve medication effectiveness followed by a high-protein evening meal to provide adequate amino acids for metabolism.

Studies have shown that treatment with levodopa can result in elevated homocysteine levels, a known risk factor in cardiovascular disease and indicator of inflammation. Dietary supplementation with folate, pyridoxine (vitamin B6), and methylcobalamin (vitamin B12) should be recommended to reduce homocysteine levels in these patients [20].

It is estimated that at least 40% of the PD patients in the United States use some type of complimentary or alternative medicine (CAM) for management of their disease [21]. Research by Wang et al. reported that many have high levodopa intake and embrace cannabis as a treatment adjunct for relief of motor symptoms. Cannabis has been reported to significantly relieve tremor, rigidity, and bradykinesia 30 minutes after smoking. Reducing pain and improved sleep was also cited by Lotan et al. [22].

Venderova et al. [23] surveyed PD patients in a European country via mailed questionnaire to ascertain their use of marijuana. Out of 630 questionnaires, 53.8% were returned confirming most of the respondents consumed one-half teaspoon fresh or dried cannabis leaves orally, with only one patient smoking the cannabis. All reported continuing their prescribed medications while using cannabis. A substantial number of patients reported improvement in their symptoms, and only four claimed cannabis worsened their symptoms [24].

Parkinson's disease is the second most common neurodegenerative disorder, following Alzheimer's disease, and the fourteenth leading cause of death in all age groups in the United States [25]. The diagnosis of PD increases with age and currently indicates a higher male-to-female ratio in the same age group. Dorsey [26] and Tan [27] project at least 9 million cases of PD throughout the world by 2030.

Cannabidiol (CBD) has been shown to be effective in the treatment of psychosis and sleep disorders in PD patients [28–30]. Garcia et al. [31] studied the effect of delta-9-THCV (tetrahydrocannabivarin) in an animal disease model that provided neuroprotective and symptom-relief effects. Numerous states within the United States have allowed cannabidiol use as an alternative or add-on therapy for Parkinson's disease.

Cannabinoids have also demonstrated neuroprotective antioxidative and anti-inflammatory benefits for PD patients. Studies found CBD could upregulate superoxide dismutase to decrease oxidative stress and inflammation, thereby reducing damage on dopaminergic neurons in the PD brain [32–34]. The combination of CBD and THC to provide anti-inflammatory properties in the PD brain has been shown benefit in several studies [35–38].

Depression is another common symptom experienced by PD patients. Studies have shown that the endocannabinoid system is important in mood, anxiety, and depressive symptoms. Studies by Hoogendijk et al. [39], Yamamoto [40], and Reijnders et al. [41] indicate that cannabinoids need to be considered for alleviating these symptoms since some regular cannabis users have exhibited less depressed mood and a more positive outlook than non-users [42]. Another study has shown that heavy cannabis use can increase the risk of depression [43], so moderate use in PD patients would be advised.

Cannabinoids for Tourette's syndrome

Tourette's syndrome (TS) is a neurological disorder characterized by repetitive involuntary movements called tics. A French neurologist named Dr. George Gilles de la Tourette first described the condition in 1885 found in an 86-year-old female. TS is a chronic condition that may have its beginning in childhood and later develops into the shoulder jerking, eye movements, and facial grimacing that is characteristic of the disorder. These movements can be worse during times of excitement or anxiety. To date, no one medication has been helpful to all TS patients, and the most common side effects of neuroleptic medications (drugs used to treat psychotic disorders) are sedation, weight gain, and reduced cognition.

Cannabis treatment of Tourette's syndrome tics and compulsive behaviors was first mentioned in 1988 when three patients smoking marijuana cigarettes had improvement in symptoms [44], and another patient reported being symptom-free for a year while smoking marijuana daily [45].

Cannabis sativa THC was identified as beneficial in reducing tics and behavioral issues seen in Tourette's syndrome by Muller-Vahl [46,47]. Both human and animal studies suggest that CB1 is involved in regulating attention, memory, and cognition, so THC provided over a six-week period in gradually increased doses was beneficial in controlling tics with no significant negative influence on cognition or memory, resulting in Muller-Vahl recommending THC for TS in adults when other treatments have failed to improve patient management [48].

Over 100,000 Americans have Tourette's syndrome with some of them manifesting attention deficit hyperactivity disorder (ADHD). These individuals have problems paying attention to tasks at hand, sitting still, and finishing a project they started. Some may be diagnosed with dyslexia or obsessive-compulsive behaviors since no blood, laboratory, or imaging tests can diagnose TS, according to the National Institute of Neurological Disorders and Stroke. Many patients can be self-diagnosed after years of experiencing symptoms; therefore, treatment with THC could be an option for improved quality of life for Tourette's syndrome sufferers.

Cannabinoids for dystonia

Dystonia is a neurological condition associated with abnormal muscle twitching and turning. Dystonia can affect one muscle, a muscle group, or the entire body, with more women than men being prone to the disorder. Symptoms can include a dragging leg, involuntary neck twitch, uncontrollable blinking, speech difficulties, or cramping in a foot. Causes of dystonia are nonspecific, but research indicates the problem is in the basal ganglia of the brain.

In 1981, Marsden reported improvement in a patient with cervical dystonia who improved by smoking cannabis [49] followed by several other reported uses of cannabis in dystonia [50,51]. CBD showed improvement in some patients reported by Uribe Roca et al. [51], but high doses resulted in tremor or hypokinesis. Nabilone, a synthetic oral form of delta-9-THC, was not found to be effective, and dronabinol, another synthetic form of delta-9-THC, did not improve symptoms in dystonia. Zadikoff concluded that cannabinoid use in dystonia may be dependent on dose and form of administration for dystonia patients [52].

Cannabinoids for Huntington's disease

Huntington's disease (HD) is a slow, progressive neurodegenerative disease that is an inherited disorder on chromosome 4 with physical, emotional, behavioral, and cognitive effects. This genetic defect is dominant, meaning anyone who inherits it from a parent with HD will eventually develop the disease. HD was named for George Huntington, the physician who described it in the 1800s. The defective gene causes development of excessive huntingtin proteins, which lead to brain changes and the development of symptoms. The onset of symptoms usually starts between ages 30 and 50, but individuals have been found as young as 2 years old or as late as 80 [53].

The three main categories of HD symptoms are memory (cognitive), mood (emotional), and movement (physical motor issues called chorea). As the disease progresses, movement disorders such as involuntary writing or jerking (chorea) or muscle rigidity (dystonia) increase. Cognitive inability to organize and focus on tasks declines, and speech slowness, or searching for words, can result. Patients with HD gradually lose their functional ability and live out their lives confined to bed, unable to speak.

Scientists identified the defective gene that causes HD in 1993, and a diagnostic test is now available. The huntingtin gene defect results in extra repeats of one chemical code on chromosome 4. The normal huntingtin gene codes for 17–20 repetitions, while the defective gene codes for 40 or more repeats. Genetic testing can measure the number of repeats to confirm a diagnosis. Research is ongoing to understand the normal function of the huntingtin protein and how extra repeats lead to the devastating symptoms of Huntington's disease [54].

Treatment currently focuses on symptom management since there is no cure. Some patients are treated with neuroleptics, but anecdotal reports indicate young HD patients have used cannabinoids to help control symptoms. A 1991 study of CBD use in the treatment of HD with 15 patients failed to produce significant symptom benefit [55], but by 2007, tremendous progress in understanding the pathogenic mechanisms in HD significantly expanded treatment potential, according to Stack and Ferrante [56].

In 2011, Sagredo et al. [57] reported Sativex as a neuroprotective agent capable of delaying neuron loss in HD. The 1:1 combination of delta-9-THC and CBD had positive effects in a rat study. The oral mucosa spray Sativex has also been proposed as useful in other neurological disorders due to cannabis-based medications providing analgesic, antitumoral, and anti-inflammatory properties [58].

According to Valdeolivas et al. [59], cannabinoids with antioxidant properties protected striated neurons against toxicity caused by mitochondrial complex II inhibitor 3-nitroprropionic (3NP) that leads to oxidative injury. Study data suggest that cannabinoids used as disease-modifying agents should use broad-spectrum cannabinoid combinations for the greatest potential, especially in light of the HD model success.

Cannabinoids for ALS

Amyotrophic lateral sclerosis (ALS) is the most common degenerative disease of the motor neuron system with characteristics of weakness in the extremities (arms and legs) that can eventually lead to dysfunction in chewing, swallowing, and breathing. Symptoms include difficulty walking, leg cramps, twitching, and paralysis in hands, arms and legs. Most ALS patients maintain full cognitive function throughout the progression of their disease. Since there is no cure for ALS, compassionate care using cannabinoid-based medicines has been studied in animal models to access symptom progression delay and prolong survival [60].

The cannabinoid system has been identified in the pathogenesis of ALS. Yiangou et al. [61] described spinal cord motor neuron damage in ALS with CB2 positive microglia/macrophages signaling neuro-inflammation and oxidative cell damage. The possibility that cannabinoids could delay onset and slow progression of the disease through anti-inflammatory and antioxidative actions via CB1 and CB2 were reviewed by Shoemaker et al. [62], Carter et al. [63], and Raman et al. [64] using a combination of THC and/or CBD. Weydt et al. [65] showed that nonpsychotropic cannabinoid cannabinol (CBN) influenced disease progression and survival in a SOD1 mouse model. Consideration needs to be given to nonpsychotropic cannabinoids as beneficial in ameliorating symptoms for ALS patients not wanting the mind-altering effects of THC [66].

Given the severity of their illness and the lack of current effective symptom management agents, many ALS patients consider complementary and alternative medicine (CAM) therapies such as nutrition supplements, acupuncture, energy healing, and cannabis [67]. Since ALS disables and shortens the lifespan of the patient, and the endocannabinoid system has been implicated in the progression of the disease, phytocannabinoids may hold therapeutic promise. The terpenoids, especially limonene and myrcene, along with the phytocannabinoids found in whole plant preparations need to be considered [68].

References

1. Ben-Shabat S, Fride E, Sheskin T et al. An entourage effect: Inactive endogenous fatty acid glycerol esters enhance 2-arachiddonoylglycerol cannabinoid activity. *Eur J Pharm.* 1998;353:23–31.
2. Mechoulam R, Ben-Shabet S. From gan-zi-gun-nu to anandamide and 2-arachidonoylglycerol: The ongoing story of cannabis. *Nat Prod Rep.* 1999;16:131–143.
3. Sanchez-Ramos J. The entourage effect of the phytocannabinoids. *Amer Neurological Assn.* 2015;77(6):1083. doi:10.1002/ana.24402.
4. Elfawal MA, Towler MJ, Reich NG et al. Dried whole-plant Artemesia annua slows evolution of malaria drug resistance and overcomes resistance to artemisinin. *Proc Acad Sci USA.* 2015;112:821–826.
5. Russo EB. History of cannabis and its preparations in saga, science, and sobriquet. *Chem Biodivers.* 2007;4(8):1614–1648.
6. Russo EB. Taming THC: Potential cannabis synergy and phytocannabinoid-terpenoid entourage effects. *Br J Pharmacol.* 2011;163(7):1344–1364.
7. Mechoulam R et al. Early phytocannabinoid chemistry to endocannabinoids and beyond. *Nat Rev Neurosci.* 2014;15(11):757–764.
8. Pertwee RG. The central neuropharmacology of psychotropic cannabinoids. *Pharmacol Ther.* 1988;36(2–3):189–261.

9. Mechoulam R et al. Early phytocannabinoid chemistry to endocannabinoids and beyond. *Nat Rev Neurosci.* 2014;15(11):757–764.

10. Egertova M, Elphick MR. Localisation of cannabinoid receptors in the rat brain using antibodies to the intracellular C-terminal tail of CB. *J Comp Neurol.* 2000;422(2):159–171.

11. Van Laere K et al. Gender-dependent increases with healthy aging of the human cerebral cannabinoid-type 1 receptor binding using [(18)F]MK-9470 PET. *Neuroimage.* 2008;39(4):1533–1541.

12. Fernández-Ruiz J et al. Prospects for cannabinoid therapies in basal ganglia disorders. *Br J Pharmacol.* 2011;163(7):1365–1378.

13. Lanciego JL, Borroso-Chinea P et al. Expression of the mRNA coding the cannabinoid receptor 2 in the pallidel complex of Macaca fascicularis. *J Psychopharmacol.* 2011;25(1):97–104.

14. Fernández-Ruiz J et al. Cannabinoid CB2 receptor: A new target for controlling neural cell survival? *Trends Pharmacol Sci.* 2007;28(1):39–45.

15. Szabo B, Schlicker E. Effects of cannabinoids on neurotransmission. *Handb Exp Pharmacol.* 2005;168:327–365.

16. Sanudo-Pena MC, Tsou K, Walker JM. Motor actions of cannabinoids in the basal ganglia output nuclei. *Life Sci.* 1999;65(6–7):703–713.

17. Freiman I, Szabo B. Cannabinoids depress excitatory neurotransmission between the subthalemic nucleus and the globus pallaidus. *Neuroscience.* 2005;133(1):305–313.

18. Martínez-Orgado J et al. The seek of neuroprotection:introducing cannabinoids. *Recent Pat CNS Drug Discov.* 2007;2:131–139.

19. Beitz JM. Parkinson's disease: A review. *Front Bioscience (Schol Ed).* 2014;6:65–74.

20. Chao J, Leung Y et al. Nutraceuticals and their preventative or potential therapeutic value in Parkinson's disease. *Nut Rev.* 2012;70(7):373–386.

21. Wang Y, Xie CL, Wang WW et al. Epidemiology of complementary and alternative medicine use in patients with Parkinson's disease. *J Clin Neurosci.* 2013;20(8):1062–1067.

22. Lotan I, Treves TA et al. Cannabis (medical marijuana) treatment for motor and non-motor symptoms of Parkinson's disease: An open-label observational study. *Clin Neuropharmacol.* 2014;37(2):41–44.

23. Venderová K et al. Survey on cannabis use in Parkinson's disease: Subjective improvement of motor symptoms. *Mov Discord.* 2004;19(9):1102–1106.

24. Catlow B, Sanchez-Ramos J. Cannabinoids for the treatment of movement disorders. *Current Treatment Options in Neurology.* 2015;17:39.

25. Xu J, Kochanek KD, Murphy SL. National vital statistics reports death:final data for 2007. *Statistics.* 2010;58(3):135.

26. Dorsey ER, Constantinescu R et al. Projected number of people with Parkinson's disease in the most populous nations, 2005–2030. *Neurology.* 2007;68(5):384–386.

27. Tan LCS. Epidemiology of Parkinson's disease. *Neurology Asia.* 2013;18(3):231–238.

28. Zuardi AW, Crippa JAS, Hallak JE et al. Cannabidiol for the treatment of psychosis in Parkinson's disease. *Journal of Psychopharmacology.* 2009;23(8):979–983.

29. Chagas MHN, Zuardi AW, Tumas V et al. Effects of cannabidiol in the treatment of patients with Parkinson's disease: An exploratory double-blind trial. *Journal of Psychopharmacology.* 2014;28(11):1088–1092.

30. Chagas MHN, Eckeli AL, Zuardi AW et al. Cannabidiol can improve ccomplex sleep-related behaviors associated with rapid eye movement sleep disorder in Parkinson's disease patients:a case series. *Journal of Clinical Pharmacy and Therapeutics.* 2014;39(5):564–566.
31. García C, Palomo-Garo C et al. Symptom-relieving and neuroprotective effects of the phytocannabinoid Δ 9-THCV in animal models of Parkinson's disease. *British Journal of Pharmacology.* 2011;163(7):1495–1506.
32. Lastres-Becker I, Molina-Holgado F, Ramos JA et al. Cannabinoids provide neuroprotection against 6-hydroxydopamine toxicity in vivo and in vitro: Relevance to Parkinson's disease. *Neurobiology of Disease.* 2005;19(1–2):96–107.
33. García-Arencibia M, Gonzalez S et al. Evaluation of the neuroprotective effect of cannabinoids in a rat model of Parkinson's disease: Importance of antioxidant and cannabinoid receptor-independent properties. *Brain Research.* 2007;1134(1):162–170.
34. Pan H, Mukhopadhyay P et al. Cannabidiol attenuates cisplatin-induced nephrotoxicity by decreasing oxidative/nitrosative stress, inflammation, and cell death. *Journal of Pharmacology and Experimental Therapeutics.* 2009;328(3):708–714.
35. Watzl B, Scuderi P, Watson RR. Influence of marijuana components (THC and CBD) on human mononuclear cell cytokine secretion in vitro. *Advances in Experimental Medicine and Biology.* 1991;288:63–70.
36. Srivastava MD, Srivastave BIS, Brouhard B. Δ 9 tetrahydrocannabinol and cannabidiol alter cytokine production by human immune cells. *Immunopharmacology.* 1998;40(3):179–185.
37. Mechoulam R, Parker LA, Gallily R. Cannabidiol: An overview of some pharmacological aspects. *Journal of Clinical Phartmacology.* 2002;42(11):11s–19s.
38. Mechoulam R, Peters M et al. Cannabidiol-recent advances. *Chemistry and Biodiversity.* 2007;4(8):1678–1692.
39. Hoogendijk WJG, Sommer IEC et al. Depression in Parkinson's disease: The impact of symptom overlap on prevalence. *Psychosomatics.* 1998;39(5): 416–421.
40. Yamamoto M. Depression in Parkinson's disease: Its prevalence, diagnosis and neurochemical background. *Journal of Neurology.* 2001;248(3):III 5–11.
41. Reijnders JSAM, Ehrt U et al. A systematic review of prevalence studies of depression in Parkinson's disease. *Movement Disorders.* 2008;23(2):183–189.
42. Densson TF, Earleywine M. Decreased depression in marijuana users. *Addictive Behaviors.* 2006;31(4):738–742.
43. Degenhardt L, Hall W, Lynskey M. Exploring the association between cannabis use and depression. *Addiction.* 2003;98(11):1493–1504.
44. Sandyk R, Awerbuch G. Marijuana and Tourette's syndrome. *J Clin Psychopharmacol.* 1988;8:444–445.
45. Hemming M, Yellowlees PM. Effective treatment of Tourette's syndrome with marijuana. *J Psychopharmacol.* 1993;7:389–391.
46. Müller-Vahl KR et al. Delta 9-tetrahydrocannabinol (THC) is effective in the treatment of tics in Tourette's syndome: A 6-week randomized trial. *J Clin Psychiatry.* 2003;64(4):459–465.
47. Müller-Vahl KR. Cannabinoids reduce symptoms of Tourette's syndrome. *Expert Opin Pharmacother.* 2003;4(10):1717–1725.
48. Müller-Vahl KR. Treatment of Tourette's syndrome with cannabinoids. *Behav Neurol.* 2013;27(1):119–124.

49. Marsden CD. Treatment of torsion dystonia. In: Barbeau A, ed. *Disorders of Movement, Current Status of Modern Therapy*. Philadelphia, PA. Lippincott. 1981. 81–104.
50. Chatterjee A, Almahrezi A et al. A dramatic response to inhaled cannabis in a woman with central thalamic pain and dystonia. *J Pain Symptom Manage*. 2002;24:4–6.
51. Uribe Roca MC, Micheli F, Viotti R. Cannabis sativa and dystonia secondary to Wilson's disease. *Mov Disord*. 2005;20:113–115.
52. Zadikoff C et al. Cannabinoid, CB1 agonists in cervical dystonia. Failure in a phase IIa randomized controlled trial. *Basal Ganglia*. 2011;1(2):91–95.
53. Mayo Clinic. Huntington's Disease. www.mayoclinic.org/diseases-conditions/huntingtons-disease
54. Huntington's Disease Society of America. hdsa.org
55. Consroe P et al. Controlled clinical trial of cannabidiol in Huntington's disease. *Pharmacol Biochem Behav*. 1991;40(3):701–708.
56. Stack EC, Ferrante RJ. Huntington's disease: Progress and potential in the field. *Expert Opin Investig Drugs*. 2007;16(12):1933–1953.
57. Sagredo O, Pazos MR, Satta V et al. Neuroprotective effects of phytocannabinoid-based medicines in experimental models of Huntington's disease. *J Neurosci Res*. 2011;89(9):1509–1518.
58. Sagredo O, Pazos MR, Valdeolivas S et al. Cannabinoids: Novel medicines for the treatment of Huntington's disease. *Recent Pat CNS Drug Discov*. 2012;7(1):41–48.
59. Valdeolivas S, Satta V, Pertwee RG et al. Sativex-like combination of phytocannabinoids is neuroprotective in malonate-lesioned rats, an inflammatory model of Huntington's disease: Role of CB1 and CB2 receptors. *ACS Chem Neurosci*. 2012;3(5):400–406.
60. Giacoppo S, Mazzon E. Can cannabinoids be a potential therapeutic tool in amyotropic lateral sclerosis? *Neural Regen Res*. 2016;11(12):1896–1899.
61. Yiangou Y, Facer P, Durrenberger P et al. COX-2, CB2 and P2X7-immunoreactivities are increased in activated microglial cells/macrophages of multiple sclerosis and amyotropic lateral sclerosis spinal cord. *BMC Neurol*. 2006;6:12.
62. Shoemaker JL, Seely KA et al. The CB2 cannabinoid agonist AM-1241 prolongs survival in a transgenic mouse model of amyotropic lateral scherosis when initiated at symptom onset. *J Neurochem*. 2007;101(1):87.
63. Carter GT, Abood ME et al. Cannabis and amyotropic lateral sclerosis: Hypothetical and practical applications, and a call for clinical trials. *Am J Hosp Palliat Care*. 2010;27(5):347–356.
64. Raman C, McAllister SD et al. Amyotropic lateral sclerosis: Delayed disease progression in mice by treatment with cannabinoid. *Amyotroph Lateral Scel Other Motor Neuron Disord*. 2004;5(1):33–39.
65. Weydt P, Hong S et al. Cannabinol delays symptom onset in SOD1(G93A) transgenic mice without affecting survival. *Amyotroph Lateral Scler Other Motor Neuron Disord*. 2005;6(3):182–184.
66. Iuvone T, Esposito G et al. Cannabidiol: a promising drug for neurodegenerative disorders? *CNS Neurosci Ther*. 2009;Winter 15(1):65–75.
67. Bedlack RS, Joyce N, Carter G et al. Complementary and alternative therapies in ALS. *Neurol Clin*. 2015;33(4):909–936.
68. Russo EB. Taming THC: Potential synergy and phytocannabinoid-terpenoid entourage effects. *Br J Pharmacol*. 2011;163(7):1344–1364.

chapter five

Cannabinoids and the entourage effect

Betty Wedman-St. Louis

Contents

Tetrahydrocannabinol (THC) and cannabidiol (CBD) have been the primary focus of cannabis research since 1964 when Raphael Mechoulam isolated and synthesized THC, which later led to synthetic pharmaceutical products available as prescriptions. But less attention has been paid to the entourage effect, which is a term used to describe the enhancement of efficacy and improvement in therapeutic effectiveness of other phytocannabinoids [1]. Besides CBD, phytocannabinoids exerting clinically useful effects without psychoactivity are tetrahydrocannabivarin, cannabigerol, and cannabichromene [2]. Cannabis-derived terpenes, including limonene, myrcene, α-pinene, linalool, β-caryophyllene, caryophyllene oxide, nerolidol, and phytol, add flavor and fragrance along with therapeutic effects [3].

The phytocannabinoid-terpene synergy increases the likelihood of new therapeutic benefits to treat pain and inflammation. Phytocannabinoids and terpenes are produced in the cannabis plant by secretory cells in the glandular trichomes with the highest concentration noted in unfertilized female flowers [4]. Acid forms of phytocannabinoids have important biochemical properties and are important in their own right.

Ben-Shabat et al. [5] first described the function of active and inactive synergistic compounds in cannabis, and a short time later, Mechoulam and Ben-Shabat refined their analogy as "this type of synergism may play a role in the widely held (but not experimentally based) view that in some cases plants are better drugs than the natural products isolated from them" [6].

Dr. Dustin Sulak, director of Integr8 Health, cofounder of Healer.com, and a practicing osteopath, discussed cannabis and the potential health benefits of THC and psychoactivity as "more isn't always better." He went on to say "a lot of us think more equals more in our lives but that's not the case with cannabis, based on what I've observed in my patients." The dose response curve should be carefully considered, including the role that raw cannabinoids such as THCA and CBDA play. "I've been extremely impressed with the acidic cannabinoids … they're effective at reducing symptoms, sometimes at a tenth or even a hundredth of the dose that would be required if they were using the neutral or decarboxylated cannabinoids THC and CBD" [7].

Phytocannabinoids beyond THC and CBD

Over 60 phytocannabinoids have been identified in various cultivars of the cannabis plant [8]. Of great interest for clinical application are delta-9-tetrahydrocannabivan (THCV), cannabichromene (CBC), and cannabigerol (CBG). Innovative plant breeding has yielded cannabis chemotypes that contain high amounts of these components that can have beneficial therapeutic effects.

Delta-9-tetrahydrocannabivan (THCV) has been shown to work with CBD to modulate the effects of THC via a direct blockade of cannabinoid CB1 receptors. THCV also has a high affinity for CB2 receptors, which differs from CBD activity [9]. Bolognini et al. [10] reported that THCV can behave as a CB2 receptor agonist in vitro and established that THCV can reduce signs of inflammatory pain and inflammation. The important recent findings that THCV can induce both CB1 receptor antagonism in vivo and in vitro, with signs of CB2 receptor activation in vitro at low concentrations, has a potential for management of disorders such as chronic liver disease and inflammation-associated obesity [11].

Cannabichromene (CBC) and cannabidiol (CBD) are known to modulate in vitro activity of proteins involved in nociceptive pain mechanisms [12]. Nociceptive pain is the most common form of pain caused by harmful stimuli by nociceptors around the body. (Neuropathic pain is associated with damage to the neurons following an infection or injury to the area, resulting in pain messages sent to the central nervous system and brain.)

Cannabichromene is a nonpsychotropic plant cannabinoid with anti-inflammatory and analgesic properties, described in the 1980s [13,14]. Both cannabichromene and cannabigerol have been shown to have antifungal and antidepressant activity [15]. CBG has demonstrated modest antifungal properties and recently has been shown to be an effective cytotoxin on human epithelial carcinoma [16] and an effective phytocannabinoid against breast cancer along with CBD [17]. Russo further describes antidepressant, antihypertensive, and MRSA antagonist activities of cannabigerol [18].

Cannabinol (CBN) has a low affinity for CB1 and CB2 but produced a sedative effect as well as anticonvulsant with anti-inflammation properties [19–21].

Tetrahydrocannabinolic acid (THCA), cannabidiolic acid (CBCA), and cannabigerolic acid (CBGA) produce necrosis in plant cells [22] and have proven to be insecticidal [23].

Phytocannabinoid activity summary

CBC cannabichromene	Antifungal, antidepressant
CBG cannabigerol	GABA uptake inhibitor, antifungal, antidepressant, effective against MRSA
THCV tetrahydrocannabivain	Treatment of metabolic syndrome, anticonvulsant
CBV cannabidivarin	Anticonvulsant
CBN cannabinol	Sedative, effective against MRSA, TRPV2 agonist for burns

Terpenoids

Terpenoids form the largest group of plant chemicals numbering between 15 and 20,000 [24], with over 200 reported in cannabis, but only a few have been studied [25]. Terpenoids, also known as isoprenoids, are essential for the viability of plants and have a variety of functions. As flavors or scents, terpenoids also act as a growth regulator, a defense secretor, and a pollinator attractant [26]. Large terpenoid molecules are essential components of human metabolism, including the lipid soluble vitamins A, E, and K. Terpenes are classified based on their chemical structure.

Monoterpenes are volatile, aromatic, colorless, and oily substances that are not soluble in water. This group includes limonene, linalool, α-pinene, β-myrcene, and humulene.

- Limonene has expectorant and sedative activity and demonstrated antineoplastic activity in pancreatic and breast cancer, in addition to a solvent of gallstones [27–29].
- Pinene is an irritant that is used in insecticides and as a bronchodilator in humans.
- Linalool is antiseptic and fungistatic with sedative properties [30].

- Myrcene occurs in highly fragrant plants and herbs (mango, hops, bay leaves) and provides a sedative, anti-inflammatory, analgesic, and antimutagenic benefit [31].
- Humulene is the essential oil in hops with antibacterial, anti-inflammatory, and antitumor properties.

Sesquiterpenes total in the thousands of compounds found in plants and are responsible for producing fungal pheromones along with playing a defensive role in plant–insect interactions [32]. This group includes β-caryophyllene. Beta-caryophyllene is found in several commonly available herbs and spices such as black pepper, cinnamon, cloves, and others. It binds to CB2 receptors for a strong anti-inflammatory and analgesic effect [33]. Other studies show that β-caryophyllene is effective in reducing neuropathic pain and promotes a Th1 immune response to control neuroinflammation [34].

The yield of terpenoids in a cannabis assay is small, less than 1%, but can be as high as 10% of trichome content [35]. Monoterpenes predominate and are lost at a rate of 5% before processing [36] and diminish substantially with drying and storage [37], resulting in a higher proportion of sesquiterpenoids (especially β-caryophyllene). Terpenoid production increases with light exposure but decreases with soil fertility [38]. They have GRAS (Generally Recognized As Safe) status by the U.S. Food and Drug Administration for use as food additives and food extracts.

Cannabis terpenoid components above a 0.05% concentration are considered for pharmacological interest [39,40]. Mice exposed to terpenoid odors inhaled from ambient air for one hour demonstrated effects on activity level, even at low concentrations. Ingestion and percutaneous absorption have been documented in humans.

Flavonoids

Like cannabinoids and terpenes, flavonoids contribute to the therapeutic effects of cannabis. Flavonoids are a group of phytonutrients that contribute to the entourage effect through color, smell, and taste to provide a highly bioactive role in plant cultivation and consumption.

Over 6000 flavonoids have been identified with many of them found in foods eaten daily such as vegetables, fruits, and herbs. Many flavonoids have high antioxidant benefits that support detoxification to reduce chronic diseases and certain cancers.

Flavonoids are polyphenolic molecules containing 15 carbon atoms soluble in water. They are divided into six subtypes: chalones, flavones, isoflavonoids, flavonoids, anthoxanthins, and anthocyanins—which vary in color from yellow to purple–red. In a plant, flavonoids attract pollinating insects and support nitrogen fixation for growth. Some flavonoids inhibit fungal spores to protect against disease. Examples of foods high in flavonoids consumed by humans include onions, parsley, blueberries, bananas, and green tea.

Daily human consumption of flavonoids is emphasized for the antioxidant properties of fruits, vegetables, and herbs that provide benefits of

- Antiviral
- Anticancer
- Anti-inflammatory

Regular consumption of flavanols has shown increased activity of erythrocyte superoxide dismutase (an antioxidant enzyme found in red blood cells), a decrease in lymphocyte DNA damage, a decrease in urinary 8-hydroxy-2-deoxyguanosine (a marker of oxidative damage), and an increase in plasma antioxidant capacity (the ability to scavenge free radicals) [41]. The number of flavonoids in foods is affected by plant type, growth, season, light, degree of ripeness, food preparation, and processing [42].

Flavonoid glycosides in cannabis

Standards for most flavonoid glycosides are not readily available so they are seldom tested in cannabis products, but Flores-Sanchez and Verpoorte reported no flavonoids detected in cannabis roots with variations from plant to plant [43]. Flowers and leaves did not differ significantly between genders and varieties. As plants grew, the cannabinoid levels increased, but the flavonoid content declined.

Twenty-one flavonoids have been reported in cannabis plants, according to Ross and ElSohly [44]. They are grouped as

- Aglycones
- Conjugated O-glycosides: apigenin, luteolin, quercetin, kaempferol
- C-glycosides: orientin, vitexin, isovitexin

Flavonoid glycosides are considered beneficial in treatment of conditions with capillary bleeding and as powerful antioxidants [45]. They also have inhibitory activities against HIV [46].

Research is underway to distinguish cannaflavins from flavonoids in common foods. The cannabis flavonoids cannaflavin A and cannaflavin B were included in the pharmaceutical composition and method of manufacturing patent US 9044390 B1 for extraction and administration of a pharmaceutical dosage form [47]. Future study will reveal how the presence of cannabis flavonoids such as β-sitosterol, vitexin, isovitexin, apigenin, kaempferol, quercetin, luteolin, and orientin work with cannabinoids and terpenes.

Cannabis constituents

Cannabis is one of the oldest plants known in medicine, and its phytochemistry has been well studied [48]. A total of 483 constituents have been identified of which only 66 are cannabinoids, 21 flavonoids, and 120 terpenes. A brief listing of cannabis constituents follows:

• Cannabinoids	66
• Nitrogenous compounds	27
• Carbohydrates	34
• Fatty acids	22
• Terpenes	120
• Flavonoids	21

Final thought about entourage effect

David Wright, President and CEO of AltMed of Sarasota, FL, explained in an interview with Cannabis Insider, "We believe in the entourage effect of the plant. Typically, in a pharmaceutical biotech company, you need a single isomer, a single chemical. For example, the drug Marinol, which is on the market, is a high THC product, but it's only THC. The physicians I've talked to who have prescribed this say patients come back and say it doesn't work. Actually, smoking of the product or taking it in an edible or an oil does work. One of the things we're looking at from a genetic perspective is to separate out different levels of THC and CBD, different CBD, CBN, what's the relationship between CBD and CBN and THC, and the effects it has on specific conditions" [49].

Mr. Wright further explains that cannabis "is a very complex plant and produces a very complex medicine. There are over 86 cannabinoid receptors in the human body and we have no concept today of what parts of the plant and what is the relationship between these cannabinoids on the body. It's very unlikely that any drug product made from the plant will soon be as effective as the whole plant."

References

1. Fine PG, Rosenfeld MJ. The endocannabinoid system, cannabinoids, and pain. *Rambam Maimonides Med J*. 2013;4(4):e0022.
2. Russo EB. Taming THC: Potential cannabis synergy and phytocannabinoid-terpenoid entourage effects. *Br J Pharmacol*. 2011;163:1344–1364.
3. Gertsch J, Pertwee RG, Di Marzo V. Phytocannabinoids beyond the cannabis plant—do they exist. *Br J Pharmacol*. 2010;160:523–529.
4. Potter D. Growth and morphology of medicinal cannabis. In: Guy GW, Whittle BA, Robson R (eds). *Medicinal Uses of Cannabis and Cannabinoids*. Pharmaceutical Press, London. 2004. p 17–54.

5. Ben-Shabat S, Fride E, Sheskin T et al. An entourage effect: Inactive endogenous fatty acid glycerol esters enhance 2-arachidonoyl-glycerol cannabinoid activity. *Eur J Pharmacol.* 1998;353:23–31.

6. Mechoulam R, Ben-Shabat S. From gan-zi-gun-nu to anadamide and 2-arachidonoylglycerol: the ongoing story of cannabis. *Nat Prod Rep.* 1999;16:131–143.

7. Sulak D. Project CBD: Dr. Dustin Sulak: Cannabis Dosing. http://www. projectcbd.org

8. Hanus L. Pharmacological and therapeutic secrets of plant and brain (endo) cannabinoids. *Med Res Rev.* 2008;29:213–271.

9. McPartland JM, Duncan M, Di Marzo V et al. Are cannabidiol and Δ-9-tetrahydrocannabivarin negative modulators of the endocannabinoid system? A systematic review. *Br J Pharmacol.* 2015;172(3):737–753.

10. Bolognini D, Costa B, Maione S et al. The plant cannabinoid Δ-9-tetrahydrocannabivarin can decrease signs of inflammation and inflammatory pain in mice. *Br J Pharmacol.* 2010;160(3):677–687.

11. Pertwee RG. The diverse CB1 and CB2 receptor pharmacology of three plant cannabinoids: Δ-9-tetrahydrocannabinol, cannabidiol and Δ-9-tetrahydrocannabivarin. *Br J Pharmacol.* 2008;153(2):199–215.

12. Malone S, Piscitelli F, Gatta L et al. Non-psychoactive cannabinoids modulate the descending pathway of antinociception in anaesthetized rats through several mechanisms of action. *Br J Pharmacol.* 2011;162(3):584–596.

13. Wirth PW, Watson ES, ElSohly M et al. Anti-inflammatory properties of cannabichromene. *Life Sci.* 1980;26:1991–1995.

14. Davis WM, Hatoum NS. Neurobehavioral actions of cannabichromene and inter-actions with delta-9-tetrahydrocannabinoid. *Gen Pharmacol.* 1983;14:247–252.

15. ElSohly HN, Turner CE, Clark AM et al. Synthesis and antimicrobial activities of certain cannabichromene and cannabigerol related compounds. *J Pharm Sci.* 1982;71:1319–1323.

16. Baek SH, Kim YO, Kwag JS et al. Boron trifluoride etherate on silica-A modified Lewis acid reagent (VII). Antitumor activity of cannabigerol against human oral epitheloid carcinoma cells. *Arch Pharm Res.* 1998;21:353–356.

17. Ligresti A, Moriello AS, Starowicz K et al. Antitumor activity of plant cannabinoids with emphasis on the effect of cannabidiol on human breast carcinoma. *J Pharmacol Exp Ther.* 2006;318:1375–1387.

18. Russo EB. Taming THC: Potential cannabis synergy and phytocannabinoid-terpenoid entourage effects. *Br J Pharmacol.* 2011;163:1344–1364.

19. Musty RE, Karniol IG, Shirikawa I et al. Interactions of delta-9-tetrahydrocannabinol and cannabinol in man. In: Braude MC, Szara S (eds). *The Pharmacology of Marihuana,* vol 2. Raven Press, NY. 1976. p 559–563.

20. Turner CE, ElSohly MA, Boeren EG. Constituents of Cannabis sativa L. XVII. A review of the natural constituents. *J Nat Prod.* 1980;43:169–234.

21. Evans FJ. Cannabinoids: The separation of central from peripheral effects on structural basis. *Planta Med.* 1991;57:S60–S67.

22. Shoyama Y, Sugawa C, Tanaka H et al. Cannabinoids act as necrosis-inducing factors in Cannabis sativa. *Plant Signal Behav.* 2008;3:1111–1112.

23. Sirikantaramas S, Taura F, Tanaka Y et al. Tetrahydrocannabinolic acid synthase, the enzyme controlling marijuana psychoactivity, is selected into the storage cavity of the grandular trichomes. *Plant Cell Physiol.* 2005;46:1578–1582.

24. Langenheim JH. Higher plant terpenoids: A phytocentric overview of their ecological roles. *J Chem Ecol.* 1994;20:1223–1279.
25. Russo EB. Taming THC: Potential cannabis synergy and phytocannabinoid-terpenoid entourage effects. *Br J Pharmacol.* 2011;163:1344–1364.
26. Hoffmann D. *Medical Herbalism- The Science and Practice of Herbal Medicine.* Healing Arts Press, Rochester, VT. 2003.
27. Crowell PL, Gould MN. Chemoprevention and therapy of cancer by d-limonene. *Critical Reviews in Oncogenesis.* 1994;5(1):1–22.
28. Crowell PL, Siar Ayoubi A, Burke YD. Antitumorigenic effects of limonene and perillyl alcohol against pancreatic and breast cancer. *Advances in Experimental Medicine and Biology.* 1996;401:131–136.
29. Igimi H, Tamura R, Toraishi K et al. Medical dissolution of gallstones. Clinical experience of d-limonene as a simple, safe and effective solvent. *Digestive Diseases and Sciences.* 1991;36(2):200–208.
30. Harbone JB, Baxter H. *Photochemical Dictionary: A Handbook of Bioactive Compounds from PLants.* Taylor & Francis, London. 1993.
31. Russo EB. Taming THC: potential cannabis synergy and phytocannabinoid-terpenoid entourage effects. *Br J Pharmacol.* 2011;163:1344–1364.
32. Harbone JB, Baxter H. *Photochemical Dictionary: A Handbook of Bioactive Compounds from Plants.* Taylor & Francis, London. 1993.
33. Gertsch J, Leonti M, Raduner S et al. Beta-Caryophyllene is a dietary cannabinoid. *Proc Natl Acad Sci USA.* 2008;105:9099–9114.
34. Dinarello CA. Immunological and inflammatory functions of the interleukin-1 family. *Annu Rev Immunol.* 2009;27:519–550.
35. Potter DJ. The propagation, characterisation and optimisation of Cannabis sativa L. as a phytopharmaceutical. *PhD, King's College,* London. 2009.
36. Gershenson J. Metabolic costs of terpenoid accumulation in higher plants. *J Chem Ecol.* 1994;20:1281–1328.
37. Ross SA, ElSohly MA. The volatile oil composition of fresh and air-dried buds of cannabis sativa. *J Nat Prod.* 1996;59:49–51.
38. Langenheim JH. Higher plant terpenoids: A phytocentric overview of their ecological roles. *J Chem Ecol.* 1994;20:1223–1279.
39. Buchbauer G. Biological activities of essential oils. In: Baser KHC, Buchbauer (eds). *Handbook of Essential Oils: Science, Technology, and Application.* CRC Press, Boca Raton, FL. 2010. p 235–280.
40. Adams TB, Taylor SV. Safety evaluation of essential oils: A constituent-based approach. In: Basser KHC, Buchbaucher G (eds). *Handbook of Essential Oils.* CRC Press, Boca Raton, FL. 2010. p 185–208.
41. Williamson G, Manach C. Bioavailability and bioefficacy of polyphenols in humans. Review of 93 intervention studies. *Amer J Clin Nutr.* 2005;81:243S–255S.
42. Heneman K, Zidenberg-Cherr S. Nutrition and Health Info-Sheet-Some Facts About Flavonols. *UC Cooperative Extension Center for Health and Nutrition Research, Dept of Nutr U of California Davis.* Oct 2008.
43. Flores-Sanchez IJ, Verpoorte R. PKS activities and biosynthesis of cannabinoids and flavonoids in Cannabis sativa L. Plants. *Plant Cell Physiol.* 2008;49(12):1767–1782.
44. Ross S, ElSohly MA. Constituents of Cannabis sativa L. XXVIII. A Review of the natural constituents: 1980–1994. *Zagazig Journal of Pharmaceutical Sciences.* 1995;4(2):1–10.

45. Dewick PM. *Medicinal Natural Products: A Biosynthetic Approach.* Wiley & Sons Hoboken, NJ, 2012. p 149–152.

46. Tewtrakul S, Nakamura N, Hattori M et al. Flavaanone and flavonol glycosides from the leaves of thevetia peruviana and their HIV-1 reverse transcriptase and HIV-1 integrase inhibitory activities. *Chem Pharm Bull.* 2002;50:630–635.

47. Speier GT, Eden Prairie MN. Pharmaceutical composition and methods of manufacturing U.S. Patent No. US 9044390 B1, Washington, D.C. 2015.

48. Turner CE, ElSohly MA, Boeren EG. Constituents of Cannabis sativa L. XVII. A review of the natural constituents. *J Nat Prod.* 1980;43:169–234.

49. Kind M. Interviews with the leading voices of the Cannabis Industry- David Wright, CEO of AltMed of Sarasota, FL. http://www.cannainsider.com/altmed.

chapter six

Terpenes

Betty Wedman-St. Louis

Contents

While there are over 100 known phytocannabinoids in cannabis, more than 200 terpenes have been identified as the source of flavor and fragrance in the cannabis plant [1]. Terpenes are thought to work synergistically with the cannabinoids to produce therapeutic responses ranging from lowering inflammation and regulating blood glucose to protection of neurons and gastric cells [2]. Terpenoid properties even include cancer chemoprotective effects [3].

Terpenes are fragrant oils that are secreted in the flower's sticky resin glands—the same ones that produce THC, CBD, and other cannabinoids. Terpenes are not unique to cannabis and can be found in many other herbs, fruits, and plants. Cannabis is unique in that each strain has a unique profile of terpenes, which exhibit medicinal properties independent from cannabinoids [4].

Terpene profile differences can be used to distinguish between cannabis strains, according to Casano et al. [5]. Biotype "mostly indica" strains have high levels of β-myrcene, while "mostly sativa" strains have more complex terpene profiles, which include α-pinene as the dominant terpenoid. Further research is needed to assess the potential medical value of these terpenoid biotypes and analyze their biological activity.

Horticulturalists believe that plants developed terpenes to repel predators and lure pollinators. Many factors influence a plant's terpene production such as climate, weather, age, fertilizers used in production, and even soil content. Terpenes are volatile aromatic molecules that evaporate easily and make up the odorous oily substance that repels insects and prevents fungal growth.

Importance in health

Terpenes are healthy for humans as well as plants, according to Ethan Russo, MD, of GW Pharmaceuticals, Salisbury, Wiltshire UK [6]. Monoterpenes usually predominate (limonene, β-myrcene, α-pinene) but can be diminished with drying, irradiation, and storage of cannabis [7]. Lower leaves of Cannabis sativa have higher concentrations of bitter sesquiterpenoids that repel grazing animals, according to Potter [8], and give terpenoid balance to the mixture.

The European Pharmacopeia Sixth Edition in 2007 [9] listed 28 essential oils that are lipophilic with activity in cell membranes, neuronal and muscle ion channels, neurotransmitter receptors, and messenger systems, which included cannabis terpenoids. Animal studies by Buchbauer [10] show support for cannabis terpenes having a pharmacological effect on the brain. Russo [11] and Huestis [12] yield insight into human pain therapeutic effects provided by terpenes.

Most common cannabis terpenes

Limonene [13]
   Aroma: Lemon, citrus
   Effects: Elevated mood, stress relief
   Medical value: Antifungal, antibacterial, gastrointestinal issues, apoptosis of breast cancer cells, antidepressant

β-Myrcene [13]
   Aroma: Cloves, musky, earthy
   Effects: Sedating, relaxing
   Medical value; Antioxidant, anticarcinogenic, muscle relaxant, sedative, pain, inflammation

α-Pinene [13]
   Aroma: Pine
   Effects: Alertness, memory
   Medical value: Antibiotic, bronchodilator, insect repellant, anti-inflammatory, acetylcholinesterase inhibitor

β-Caryophyllene [13]
   Aroma: Black pepper, spicy, cloves, cinnamon leaves
   Effects: Binds to CB2 receptor as agonist
   Medical value: Gastroprotective, anti-inflammatory, dermatitis, chronic pain

D-Linalool [13]
   Aroma: Floral, lavender

Effects: Anxiety relief, sedation
Medical value: Anticonvulsant, antidepressant, antiglutamatergic, seizure reduction

Humulene [14]
Aroma: Hops (beer)
Effects: Used in Chinese medicine for thousands of years
Medical value: Antitumor, antibacterial, anti-inflammatory, anorectic/suppresses appetite

Terpenes and cannabinoids

Terpenes, like cannabinoids, can increase blood flow, enhance cortical activity, and kill respiratory pathogens along with modulating pain and inflammation [15]. Terpenoid profiles of cannabis plants vary from strain to strain, but studies have shown that the cannabinoid–terpenoid interactions improve the beneficial effects of cannabis. A validated method for analysis of both terpenes and cannabinoids in cannabis is critical to ensure quality of active compounds. Since the requirements for an acceptable cannabis assay have changed over the years, Giese, Lewis et al. in the Journal of AOAC International [16] provide guidance in this analysis so that patients can be assured of the benefits in their product.

Terpene odor and law enforcement

The distinct odor of cannabis terpenes has allowed law enforcement agencies to incarcerate millions of people, according to Small [17]. Drug enforcement personnel recognize the odor with the help of devices and sniffer dogs to detect the volatile terpene odor. As more patients are approved for medical cannabis use, regulatory restrictions need to be modified to avoid unreasonable search and seizure.

References

1. Hendriks H et al. Mono-terpene and sesqui-terpene hydrocarbons of the essential oil of Cannabis sativa. *Phytochem* 1975; 14, 814–815.
2. Schug KA. Into the Cannabinome. *The Analytical Scientist* Feb 2017. www.theanalyticalscientist.com
3. Paduch R, Kanderfer-Szerszen M et al. Terpenes: Substances useful in human healthcare. *Archivum Immunologiae et Therapiae Experimentalis* 2007; 55, 315–327.
4. Cannabinoid and Terpenoid Reference Guide. n.d. www.Steephilllab.com/science/terpenes
5. Casano S, Grassi G et al. Variations in terpene profiles of different strains of cannabis sativa L. Acta Hortic. *Acta Horticulturae* 2011; 925, 115–121.

6. Russo EB. Taming THC: Potential cannabis synergy and phytocannabinoid-terpenoid entourage effects. *British Journal of Pharmacology* 2001; 163(7), 1344–1364.

7. Ross SA, El Sohly MA. The volatile oil composition of fresh and air-dried buds of Cannabis sativa. *J Nat Prod* 1996; 59, 49–51.

8. Potter DJ. The propagation, characturisation and optimisation of Cannabis sativia L. as a phytopharmaceutical. PhD, King's College, London, 2009.

9. Pauli A, Schilcher H. In vitro antimicrobial activities of essential oils monographed in the European Pharmacopoeia, 6th ed. In Baser KHC, Buchbauer G ed. *Handbook of Essential Oils: Science, Technology and Applications.* CRC Press, Boca Raton, FL, 2010, 353–548.

10. Buchbauer G, Jirovetz L et al. Fragrance compounds and essential oils with sedative effects on inhalation. *J Pharm Sci* 1993; 82, 660–664.

11. Russo EB. The solution to the medicinal cannabis problem. In: Schatman EM ed. *Ethical Issues in Chronic Pain Management.* Taylor Francis, Boca Raton, FL, 2006, 165–194.

12. Huestis MA. Human cannabinoid pharmacokinetics. *Chem Biodivers* 2007; 4, 1770–1804.

13. Russo EB. Taming THC: Potential cannabis synergy and phytocannabinoid-terpenoid entourage effects. *British Journal of Pharmacology* 2001; 163(7), 1344–1364.

14. Casano S, Grassi G et al. Variations in terpene profiles of different strains of cannabis sativa L. Acta Hortic. *Acta Horticulturae* 2011; 925, 115–121.

15. McPartland JM, Russo EB. Cannabis and cannabis extracts: Greater than the sum od their parts? *Journal of Cannabis Therapeutics* 2002; 1, 103–132.

16. Geise MW, Lewis MA et al. Development and validation of a relaible and robust method for the analysis of cannabinoids and terpenes in cannabis. *J of AOAC International* 2015; 98(6), 1503–1522.

17. Small E. *Cannabis—A Complete Guide.* 2017. CRC Press, Boca Raton, FL, 179–189.

Other references

Bonamin F, Moraes TM et al. The effect of a minor constituent of essential oil from Citrus aurantium: The role of β-myrcene in preventing peptic ulcer disease. *Chemico-Biological Interactions* 2014; 212, 11–19.

Chen W, Liu Y et al. Anti-tumor effect of α-pinene on human hepatoma cell lines through inducing G2/M cell cycle arrest. *Journal of Pharmacological Sciences* 2015; 127(3), 332–338.

Horvath B, Mukhopadhyay P et al. β-Caryophyllene ameliorates cisplatin-induced nephrotoxicity in a cannabinoid 2 receptor-dependent manner. *Free Radical Biology and Medicine* 2012; 52(8), 1325–1333.

Ma J, Xu H, Wu J et al. Linalool inhibits cigarette smoke-induced lung inflammation by inhibiting NF-χB activation. *International Immunopharmacology* 2015; 29(2), 708–713.

Rohr AC, Wilkins CK et al. Upper airway and pulmonary effects of oxidation products of (+) alpha-pinene, d-limonene, and isoprene in BALB/c mice. *Inhalation Toxicology* 2002; 14(7), 663–684.

Sabogal-Guaqueta AM, Osorio E, Cardona-Gomez GP. Linalool reverses neuropathological and behavioral impairments in old triple transgenic Alzheimer's mice. *Neuropharmacology* 2016; 102, 111–120.

chapter seven

Cannabis and pain

Michelle Simon and Betty Wedman-St. Louis

Contents

Pain is the symptom that signals the brain that an injury has occurred whether it is due to an accident or illness. Over 1.5 billion people throughout the world are affected by chronic pain according to the American Academy of Pain Medicine, and more than 100 million Americans have pain-related long-term disability.

Pain signals travel to the brain through three main pathways that produce different pain sensations [1]:

- *Somatic pain* is sent by receptors located throughout the body via peripheral nerves to the brain, resulting in a constant, dull ache in the injured area.
- *Visceral pain* occurs when tissues/organs in the abdominal cavity are inflamed due to disease or injury, resulting in feelings of pressure deep within the abdomen.
- *Neuropathic pain* occurs when nerves are injured, which results in a burning sensation when touched.

Cannabinoids have been shown to help block pain in experimental animals, but few human studies have been conducted due to legal and ethical constraints. Chronic pain is the most common disorder that patients reported medical cannabis was used to reduce [2]. Boehnke et al. reported that pain patients in a Michigan medical cannabis dispensary were using marijuana to reduce their opioid use [3]. A meta-analysis by Whiting et al. [4] provided a comprehensive review of cannabinoids and their effect on chronic pain, which was identified as neuropathy, although cancer pain, multiple sclerosis, arthritis, and musculoskeletal issues were also included. Improvement noted from inhaled cannabis in the Whiting meta-analysis was noted as approximately 40%.

Most of the studies compared in the Whiting analysis used nabiximols and were done outside the United States. Cannabis studies for pain in the United States are limited and evaluated cannabis in a flower form provided by the National Institute for Drug Abuse (NIDA) for smoking and vaping [5]. The dose and strain of products used in the U.S. studies are not comparable to what is available for sale in state medical cannabis clinics. Chronic pain patients also use topical forms of cannabis in the form of creams and patches, which have not been evaluated for efficacy or dose.

In many diseases such as multiple sclerosis and cancer, prolonged pain begins to deteriorate the quality of life for individuals with the disease. Inflammation is the cause of injury to the peripheral tissue or nerves in the central nervous system. Current treatments are only partially effective but are accompanied with side effects [6,7].

Alternative approaches for chronic pain

A new option of treatment using cannabinoids is being considered for pain featuring the therapeutic activity of cannabidiol (CBD) to control inflammation in animal models reported by Costa et al. [8] and Maione et al. [9]. The complete mode of action and analgesic effects of CBD have not elucidated in animal models nor how this will translate into human therapeutic benefit. Medical literature reviews indicate that cannabinoids and medical cannabis can provide some analgesic benefit despite inadequate data on concentration, dose frequency, and delivery route [10].

The recent trend in the use of cannabinoids for pain is associated with the decreased incidence of opioid mortality [11]. Healthcare professionals are becoming emboldened to favor prescribing/ recommending cannabis as a means to promote less harm in pain management [12]. Prescriptions for opioids in the United States are estimated at over 200 million a year, with the cost of developing new drugs a disincentive to research new therapeutics [13]. Research supports the use of cannabis, specifically cannabidiol (CBD), for treatment of pain to avoid the addiction potential [14].

Yasmin Hurd blames the reluctance to acknowledge CBD's effectiveness on the scientific community's exclusion from policymaking discourse. "Legalization has outpaced the science … this is one of the first times in U.S. history that the question of whether a plant (or any drug) is an effective medicine has been decided at the ballot box" [15].

Greg Miller in the special section Pain Research in Science 2016 quoted Sir John Reynolds, house physician to Queen Victoria and late president of the Royal College of Physicians in London, who praised the use of cannabis in The Lancet in 1890: "In almost all painful maladies I have found Indian hemp by far the most useful of drugs" and went on to say "the bane of many opiates and sedatives is this, that the relief of the moment, the hour, or the day, is purchased at the expense of tomorrow's misery. In no one case to which I have administered Indian hemp have I witnessed any such results" [16]. But the misery caused from prescription opioids still survives today 125 years later.

Cannabinoids and safety

Research and prolonged exposure to cannabinoids in animals and humans have shown they have a high therapeutic index without any toxicity of any cannabinoid, even at very high doses [17]. But numerous studies report the cognitive, psychotomimetic and substance abuse effects associated with delta-9-tetrahydrocannabidiol (THC) [18–23]. These adverse effects can be avoided by eliminating the THC component of cannabis and using only the nonpsychoactive cannabinoid—cannabidiol (CBD) [24].

Value of cannabinoids for pain

Since the discovery of a cannabinoid receptor in the brain, medical research has focused on the CB1 (central nervous system) and CB2 (peripheral tissues) receptors and the G-protein coupled receptor group that comprises the binding sites for many pain mediating drugs [25]. Gertsch's description of the cannabinoid system and how it relates to inflammation reveals "an ancient lipid signaling network which in mammals modulates neuronal functions, inflammatory processes, and is involved in the etiology of certain human lifestyle diseases, such as Crohn's disease, atherosclerosis and osteoarthritis." The system is able to downregulate stress-related signals that lead to chronic inflammation and certain types of pain, but it is also involved in causing inflammation-associated symptoms, depending on the psychological context [26].

The CB1 receptors are predominately found in the brain and appear to be responsible for mood-enhancing effects of cannabis and the dysphoria experienced by some individuals [27].

The CB2 receptors are viewed as important to immune function and inflammation [28]. Evidence has shown that CB2 receptor activation has reduced harmful stimuli in the nervous system and thereby modulates neuropathic pain. Evidence continues to increase about the impact of cannabinoids having an inhibitory effect on stimuli that cause pain and inflammation, but it remains unclear if different cannabinoids have different effects on the components of pain [29].

The psychoactive cannabinoid—THC—has preferred binding to CB1 receptors [30]. Synthetic compounds such as dronabinol and nabilone are available by prescription for anorexia treatment in AIDS and reduction of nausea and vomiting during chemotherapy. Nabilone has been used in fibromyalgia with modest results [31]. Cannabidiol (CBD) agonist activity at the CB2 receptors account for the anti-inflammatory benefits experienced in CBD products [32].

Taking a closer look at pain

As the Washington Post reported in 2015, chronic pain affects more people than cancer, diabetes, heart attack, and stroke combined [33]. The Institute of Medicine estimates there are more than 100 million chronic pain sufferers in the United States costing in the range of $635 billion a year in medical treatment and lost productivity [34].

Richard W. Rosenquist, chairman of the Cleveland Clinic Department of Pain Management, indicates that pain-causing factors can be genetic, social status related, or exercise related [35]. Chronic pain can be so debilitating that it destroys the patient's quality of life and is subjective and hard to define. If the resulting tissue damage causing the pain is ignored, it can be fatal.

Pain is a universal experience with occurrence, severity, duration, response to treatment, and disabling consequences varying with each individual [36]. Pain is the warning sign of injury or infection that healthcare professionals have a moral and ethical responsibility to treat. All people are at risk of chronic pain, which can be a disorder in its own right. Pain can be caused by age (e.g., arthritis), from genetic predisposition (e.g., migraine), as a component of another chronic disease (e.g., cancer, heart disease), as a result of surgery (e.g., severed nerves), or post injury (e.g., low back pain, neck pain) [36].

Psychological and cognitive effects need to be considered when determining approaches for treatment of pain because anxiety, depression, anger, and cost all can be factors in resolution and response to treatment. Those with chronic pain need to be acknowledged as having a serious condition. Large numbers of Americans receive inadequate pain prevention and treatment because clinicians and patients seldom realize pain care needs to be personalized.

Both patients and healthcare professionals need educational programs on pain management to transform expectations, beliefs, and physiological implications that can affect treatment. Pain is a syndrome that is poorly understood, and research on pain is poorly funded [37]. Further research is needed into whether inflammatory and neuropathic pain are similar or distinct [38,39], how chronic pain arises in peripheral tissues, and what genetic factors influence pain symptoms [40,41].

As Fine and Rosenfeld [42] reviewed, pain is an unpleasant human experience. It frequently leads to avoidance behaviors, decreased mobility, altered functional status, diminished self-efficacy, and social limitations. The experience of pain can impart tremendous financial, psychological, emotional, social, and occupational impact related to

- Loss of income
- Decreased productivity
- Low self-esteem
- Inability to concentrate
- Fatigue/irritability
- Increased health costs
- Impaired relationships
- Increased suicide risk
- Sexual dysfunction
- Insomnia
- Depression/anxiety/frustration

We all deal with pain in different ways. Thoughts and emotions affect path pathways. Older people tend to have a lower pain threshold due to brain degeneration with age. Women have a higher sensitivity to pain than men. Fatigue and stress can make dealing with pain more of a challenge. Millions of people are living with debilitating pain, whether from accidents or illness, and need safe and effective forms of relief to carry on their activities of daily living. A pain assessment tool can be useful in evaluating the need for medication and its effectiveness. Numeric pain ratings are one way of measuring pain intensity on a scale of 0–10.

Pain scale

0	Pain-free	Feeling normal
1–3	Minor pain	Nagging, annoying pain but no interference with ADLs No meds needed
4–6	Moderate pain	Interferes significantly with ADLs Patient remains independent but unable to adapt to pain
7–10	Severe pain	Disabled and unable to perform ADLs Unable to function independently

Lack of research

In the United States, there are 29 states and the District of Columbia that have legalized medical marijuana, but there is no state-wide collection of data on how patients are using cannabis or whether they have benefited from its use because marijuana is still declared illegal by federal law [43]. As Greg Miller reported in 2016, Ryan Vandrey, a behavioral pharmacologist at Johns Hopkins University, Baltimore, MD, declared, "It's mind-boggling that we have millions of people in the U.S. using cannabis for medicine and we not only don't have the proper data to help them take it appropriately, we're not doing a good job collecting it."

The University of Colorado Anschutz Medical Campus in Aurora, CO, will be the first study to compare cannabis and opioid painkillers in patients with back and neck pain under the direction of Emily Lindley, neurobiologist. The research grant from the state of Colorado was funded by tax collected on marijuana sales, but the research faces many regulatory obstacles, and it has taken years from the time she received her grant to get the approval to start the research project because of the Schedule I restrictions on marijuana research [43].

Mindfulness and cannabis

Mindfulness is making its way into medical care as a possible way to reduce the stress of pain symptoms. Mindfulness activities such as breathing exercises and visualizing thoughts and feelings can reduce stress by focusing on the present moment [44]. The Mindfulness-Based Stress Reduction (MBSR) programs developed in 1979 by Jon Kabat-Zinn, an MIT scientist, have been taught in most U.S. states and in over 30 countries. Healthcare professionals have been recommending it to help patients cope with anxiety, depression, stress, and pain.

The techniques taught in mindfulness may help chronic pain patients deal with the 24/7 aspects of their symptoms. According to Ellen Langer, mindfulness generates a more positive result no matter whether you are eating a sandwich, writing a report, or planning activities for the day. Mindful management can lead to finding alternatives and better balance in life experiences which reduce stress and inflammation [45].

References

1. Marijuana and Pain. *Marijuana As Medicine? The Science Beyond the Controversy.* The National Academies Press, Washington, DC, 2000.
2. Light MK, Oreno A, Lewandowski B et al. Market size and demand for marijuana in Colorado. http://gov/pacific/sites/default/files/market.pdf.
3. Boehnke KF, Litinas E, Clauw DJ. Medical cannabis use is associated with decreasing opiate medication use in a retrospective cross-sectional survey of patients with chronic pain. *Journal of Pain* 2016;17(6):739–744.
4. Whiting PF, Wolff RF, Deshpande S et al. Cannabinoids for medical use: A systematic review and meta-analysis. *Journal of the American Medical Assoc* 2015;313(24):2456–2473.

5. Therapeutic Effects of Cannabis and Cannabinoids. *The Health Effects of Cannabis and Cannabinoids: The Current State of Evidence and Recommendations for Research.* National Academy of Sciences. Washington, DC, 2017.

6. Benyamin R, Trescot AM, Datta S et al. Opioid complications and side effects. *Pain Physician* 2008;11(2Supple):S105–S120.

7. Sindrup SH, Jensen TS. Efficacy of pharmacological treatments of neuropathic pain: An update and effect related to mechanism of drug action. *Pain* 1999;83:389–400.

8. Costa A, Trovato AE, Comelli F et al. The non-psychactive cannabis constituent cannabidiol is an orally effective agent in rat chronic inflammatory and neuropathic pain. *Eur J Pharmacol* 2007;556:75–83.

9. Maione S, Piscitelli F, Gatta L et al. Non-psychoactive cannabinoids modulate the descending pathway of antinociception in anesthetized eats through several mechanisms of action. *Br J Pharmacol* 2011;162:584–596.

10. Deshpaande A, Mailis-Gagnon A, Zoheiry N et al. Efficacy and adverse effects of medical marijuana from chronic noncancer pain: Systematic review of randomized controlled trials. *Can Fam Physician* 2015;61(8):e372–81.

11. Bachhuber MA, Saloner B, Cunningham CO et al. Medical cannabis laws and opioid analgesic overdose mortality in the United States, 1999–2010. *JAMA Intern Med* 2014;174(10):1668–73.

12. Hurd YL. Cannabidiol: Swinging the marijuana pendulum from "weed" to medication to treat the opioid epidemic. *Trends Neurosci* 2017;40(3):124–127.

13. Skolnick P, Volkow ND. Re-energizing the development of pain therapeutics in light of the opioid epidemic. *Neuron* 2016;92:294–297.

14. Hurd YL et al. Early phase in the development of cannabidiol as a treatment for addiction: Opioid relapse takes initial center stage. *Neurotherapeutics* 2015;12:807–815.

15. Hurd YL. Cannabidiol: Swinging the marijuana pendulum from "weed" to medication to treat the opioid epidemic. *Trends Neurosci* 2017;40(3):124–127.

16. Miller G. Pot and pain—Hints are emerging that cannabis could be an alternative to opioid painkillers. *Science* 2016;354(6312):566–568.

17. Fine PG, Rosenfeld MJ. The endocannabinoid system, cannabinoids, and pain. *Rambam Maimonidesa Med J* 2013;4(4):e0022.

18. Malone DT, Hill Mn, Rubino T. Adolescent cannabis use and psychosis: Epidemiology and neurodevelopmental models. *Br J Pharmacol* 2010;160:511–522.

19. Ashtari M, Avants B, Cyckowski L et al. Medical temporal structures and memory functions in adolescents with heavy cannabis use. *J Psychiatric Res* 2011;45:1055–1066.

20. Cohen M, Rasser PE, Oeck G et al. Cereebellar gray-matter deficits, cannabis use and first-episode schizophrenia in adolescents and young adults. *Int J Neuropsychopharmacol* 2012;15:297–307.

21. Fergusson DM. Is there a causal linkage between cannabis use and increased risks of psychotic symptoms? *Addiction* 2010;105:1336–1337.

22. Solowij N, Battisti R. The chronic effects of cannabis on memory in humans: A review. *Curr Drug Abuse Rev* 2008;1:81–98.

23. Yucel M, Solowij N, Respondek C et al. Regional brain abnormalities associated with long-term heavy cannabis use. *Arch Gen Psychiatry* 2008;65:694–701.

24. Cuhha JM, Carlini EA, Pereira AE. Chronic administration of cannabidiol to healthy volunteers and epileptic patients. *Pharmacology* 1980;21:175–185.

25. Overington JP, Al-Lazikani B, Hopkins AL. How many drug targets are there? *Nat Rev Drug Discov* 2006;5:993–996.
26. Gertsch J. Anti-inflammatory cannabinoids in the diet: Towards a better understanding of CB(2) receptor action? *Commun Integ Biol* 2008;1:526–528.
27. Glass M, Faull RLM, Dragunow M. Cannabinoid receptors in the human brain: A detailed anatominical and quantitative autoradiographic study on the fetal, neonatal and adult brain. *Neuroscience* 1997;77:299–318.
28. Hulsebosch CE. Special issue on microglia and chronic pain. *Exp Neurol* 2012;234:253–254.
29. Iverson L, Chapman V. Cannabinoids: A real prospect for pain relief? *Curr Opin Pharmacol* 2002;2:50–55.
30. Gaoni Y, Mechoulam R. Isolation, structure and partial synthesis of an active constituent of hashish. *J Amer Chem Society* 1964;86:1646–1647.
31. Skrabek RQ, Galimova L, Ethans K et al. Nabilone for treatment of pain in fibromyalgia. *J Pain* 2008;9:164–173.
32. Thomas A, Baillie GL, Phillips AM et al. Cannabidiol displays unexpectedly high potency as an antagonist of CB1 and CB2 receptor agonists in vitro. *Br J Pharmacol* 2007;150:613–623.
33. http://www.washingtonpost.com/national/health/scsience/chronic-pain-notonly-hurts-italso-causes-isolation-anddepression-but-theres-hope/2015/01/12.
34. Institute of Medicine (US) Committee on Advancing Pain, Research, Care, and Education. *Relieving Pain in America: A Blueprint for Transforming Prevention, Care, Education, and Research*. National Academies Press, Washington, DC, 2011.
35. Health.ClevelandClinic.org/2015/12women-likely-suffer-chronicpain.
36. Institute of Medicine (US) Committee on Advancing Pain, Research, Care, and Education. *Relieving Pain in America: A Blueprint for Transforming Prevention, Care, Education, and Research*. Wash DC, National Academies Press, 2011.
37. Grosser T, Woolf CJ, Fitzgerald GA. Time for nonaddictive relief of pain-greater insight into the biology of pain will likely identify potential drug targets. *Science* 2017;355(6329):1026–1027.
38. Chiu IM, Heester BA, Ghasemlow N et al. Bacteria activate sensory neurons that modulate pain and inflammation. *Nature* 2013;501(7465):52–57.
39. Smith-Edwards KM, DeBerry JJ, Saloman JL et al. Profound alterations in cutaneous primary afferent activity produced by inflammatory mediators. *eLife* 2016;5:e20527.
40. Volkow ND, McLellan AT, Koob GF. Neurobiologic advances from the brain disease model of addiction. *N Engl J Med* 2016;374:1253.
41. Trost Z, Strachan E, Sullivan M et al. Heritability of pain catastrophizing and associations with experimental pain outcomes: A twin study. *Pain* 2015;156(3):514–520.
42. Fine PG, Rosenfeld MJ. The endocannabinoid system, cannabinoids, and pain. *Rambam Maimonidesa Med J* 2013;4(4):e0022.
43. Miller G. Pot and pain—hints are emerging that cannabis could be an alternative to opioid painkillers. *Science* 2016;354(6312):566–568.
44. Pickert K. The Mindful Revolution. *Time* January 23, 2014.
45. Beard A. Mindfulness in the age of complexity. *Harvard Business Review* March 2014.

chapter eight

Cannabis and mindfulness
A method of harm reduction

Amanda Reiman

Contents

The use of mindfulness practice in addressing substance dependence is rooted in the ability of the individual to make a mind–body connection. This connection then facilitates control over their substance use. Cannabis has long been used as a conduit to this mind–body connection. The use of cannabis in spiritual practice is thousands of years old. The modern framing of cannabis as an illicit substance with no medical value has driven it away from this traditional therapeutic use.

The issue of substance abuse and dependence is complex. A large part of that complexity exists in the arena of treatment programs. Debates over treatment philosophies, along with the moral sanctions imposed by society for using illicit substances, stifles innovation and often demonizes treatment programs that do not adhere to abstinence-only models. Additionally, those engaged in treatment as patients are often left out of the conversation. Their desires regarding their substance use and its trajectory are not considered. Rather, top-down, authoritarian-style programs impose treatment upon patients, who can be released from the program for nonadherence.

One treatment philosophy that has diverged from this model is harm reduction. In a harm reduction framework, the patient drives the treatment program, making decisions about the trajectory of their substance use. Rather than focusing on the use itself, harms associated with use are the focus of the treatment. Patients may continue using substances while reducing likelihood of other harms. For example, using a clean syringe every time one injects heroin reduces the likelihood of contracting HIV or hepatitis C, even if the patient continues to use heroin. Similarly, setting use parameters around such things as days and times of use, geographic locations of use, and using peers can assist the patient in reducing overall use and the harms associated with using at particular days and times, places, or with certain people [1].

Some patients practice harm reduction by substituting a less harmful substance for a more harmful one. For many patients, cannabis is a substance that poses little risk and leads to fewer harms than most other substances. Medical cannabis patients have been known to substitute cannabis for alcohol, prescription, and illicit drugs [2–4].

Another innovative treatment venue that diverges from the traditional model is mindfulness practice. Mindfulness practice refers to an awareness of the relationship between thoughts and bodily sensations. The goal of mindfulness practice is to quiet outside noise and focus on enhancing that connection, often through breathing exercises and other meditations. In treating substance use disorders (SUDs), mindfulness practices such as meditation are used to control cravings, help participants focus on the relationship between their addictive voice and their physical self, and aid in relapse prevention [5,6]. Furthermore, it is posited that the act of stress reduction associated with mindfulness practice can reduce the likelihood of straying outside one's self-imposed drug use boundaries [7].

As previously mentioned, many medical cannabis patients are using cannabis as a substitute for a more harmful substance. Reasons most often cited include less negative side effects from cannabis and less chance of dependence and withdrawal from cannabis [2,3]. Indeed, cannabinoids such as tetrahydrocannabinol (THC) and cannabidiol (CBD) have been shown to block craving receptors in animal models for substances such as nicotine and opiates [8–10]. The endocannabinoid system has been shown to play a role here as well through modulation of the brain's reward center [11]. It can then be hypothesized that the use of mindfulness practice in conjunction with cannabis use might facilitate a greater chance of abstaining from or reducing the use of other substances.

However, the area of mindfulness and cannabis is not only in reference to the hazardous use of other substances. Indeed, mindfulness around cannabis use can help reduce the chance of having a negative cannabis experience. While the risks of dependence with cannabis are significantly lower than the risks of dependence on other substances, mindfulness can help ensure that one's cannabis use results not only in harm reduction but benefit maximization [12]. The mindless use of a substance increases the chance of harmful use while decreasing the chance of beneficial use. Food is a perfect example. Sitting down with a bag of potato chips and mindlessly eating the whole bag is a very different experience for the mind and body than selecting a chip, looking at it, savoring it, and thinking about what it is doing for you in that moment. In a society where consumption is a national pastime and people are constantly barraged with marketing and consumer pressures, the ability to gain mindfulness is becoming increasingly important. Along with mindfulness, cannabis can be powerful tool for centering the individual and slowing down impulses that may not be healthy.

Several years ago, I conducted a study on cannabis and mindfulness as a method for reducing methamphetamine use. During the prestudy interviews, I asked each participant how cannabis helped them reduce their use of methamphetamine. Even though none of the participants heard the others' answers, they were uniformly the same. "When I have been up for a few days, and I am tired, and I know I should go to sleep. But this little voice in my head keeps telling me to call my guy and get more meth. I know I shouldn't, but that voice is loud and strong. So, if I smoke a joint right then, the voice gets softer, and I can think better. Then I make the better decision, and I just go to sleep. Then, when I wake up, I feel good about myself, like I did something good for my health."

References

1. Principles of Harm Reduction. 2017. Harm Reduction Network. Viewed August 1, 2017, from www.harmreduction.org.
2. Reiman A. Cannabis as a substitute for alcohol and other drugs. *Harm Reduction Journal*, 2009; 6: 35.
3. Lucas P, Reiman A, and Earleywine M. Cannabis as a substitute for alcohol and other drugs: A dispensary-based survey of substitution effect in Canadian medical cannabis patients. *Journal of Addiction Theory and Research*, 2013; 435–442. doi: 10.3109/16066359.2012.733465. Published Online November 20, 2012.
4. Reiman A, Welty M, and Solomon P. Cannabis as a substitute for opioid-based pain medication: Patient self report. *Cannabis and Cannabinoid Research*, 2017; 2(1): 160–166. doi: 10.1089/can.2017.0012.
5. Appel J and Kim-Appel D. Mindfulness: Implications for substance abuse and addiction. *International Journal of Mental Health Addiction*, 2009; 7: 506–512.
6. Witkiewitz K, Marlatt G, and Walker D. Mindfulness-based relapse prevention for alcohol and substance use disorders. *Journal of Cognitive Psychotherapy: An International Quarterly*, 2005; 19: 212–228.
7. Marcus M and Zgierska A. Mindfulness-based therapies for substance use disorders: Part 1. *Substance Abuse*, 2009; 30: 263–265.
8. Muldoon P, Lichtman A, and Damaj I. The role of 2-AG endocannabinoid neurotransmission in nicotine reward and withdrawal. *21st Annual Symposium on the Cannabinoids*, 2011; 24. Research Triangle Park, NC: International Cannabinoid Research Society.
9. Blume L, Bass C, Childers S, Dalton G, Richardson J, Selley D, Xiao R, and Howlett A. Cannabinoid receptor interacting protein 1A (CRIP1A) modulates striatal neuropharmacology and signal transduction in cannabinoid, dopamine and opioid receptor systems. *21st Annual Symposium on the Cannabinoids*, 2011; 21. Research Triangle Park, NC: International Cannabinoid Research Society.
10. Ramesh D, Owens R, Kinsey S, Cravatt B, Sim-Selley L, and Lichtman A. Effects of chronic manipulation of the endocannabinoid system on precipitated opioid

withdrawal. *21st Annual Symposium on the Cannabinoids*, 2011; 22. Research Triangle Park, NC: International Cannabinoid Research Society.

11. Parsons L and Hurd Y. Endocannabinoid signaling in reward and addiction. *National Revue of Neuroscience*, 2015; 16(10): 579–594.

12. Gable RS. The toxicity of recreational drugs. *American Scientist*, 2006; 94(3): 208. Research Triangle Park, NC: Sigma Xi, The Scientific Research Society, May–June 2006.

chapter nine

Cannabis and addiction

Betty Wedman-St. Louis

Contents

For thousands of years, cannabis has been used medically and spiritually throughout Asia. Current awareness of cannabinoids and their increasing importance as medicinal agents has led to use as a treatment for pain and spasticity [1]. A more widespread use of cannabis is for pleasure, but that hardly ever gets a mention [2]. More emphasis is given to adverse problems caused by cannabis such as addiction, cognitive impairment, and possible psychotic issues [3].

Cannabis is a plant known by numerous descriptions—Purple Haze, grass, marijuana, weed—and most research has been focused on two of over 100 cannabinoids produced in its growing. These two compounds, Δ-9-THC and CBD (Δ-9-tetrahydrocannabinol and cannabidiol, respectively), have opposite effects on the human brain and behavior [4]. THC impairs learning, produces psychosis-like effects, and increases anxiety [5]. CBD enhances learning and has antipsychotic and antianxiety properties in humans [6,7].

Endocannabinoid signaling

Innate brain endocannabinoid signaling is critical for human survival because it produces signals for eating, exercise, and sexual activity [8]. The G protein-coupled receptors in the endocannabinoid system (ECS) make up the CB1 and CB2 receptors that are abundant in the adult brain and immune system. Glass et al. [9] outlines the dense CB1 receptors known for reward, addiction, and cognition function as amygdala, cingulate cortex, prefrontal cortex, ventral pallidum, caudate putamen, nucleus accumbens, ventral tegmental area, and lateral hypothalamus. The CB2 receptors are mainly expressed in immune cells of neurons, glia, and endothelial cells in the brain [10].

Cannabis is one of the most widely used illicit substances in the world, and animal models have shown that Δ-9-THC and synthetic CB1 receptor agonists enhance brain reward function [11]. Evidence in mice indicates CB2 receptors have an inhibitory influence on cocaine and alcohol reward [12], but it is possible that disparate observations in rats may be caused from species differences [13].

Animal studies have collectively indicated that alcohol, nicotine, and opiates alter brain endocannabinoid content and influence behavioral effects [14]. Ducci and Goldman [15] implicate genetic influences in the development of substance use disorders and pathological forms of eating, sexual behavior, and gambling. Initial drug use may be influenced by pleasure, while prolonged drug exposure progressively blunts the reward system and leads to escalated frequency and increased quantity of cannabis consumption. Morgan et al. [16] suggests that CBD protects against cannabis addiction.

Gateway theory

It is widely believed that cannabis is a gateway to harder drugs such as cocaine and heroin. This theory is based on a sequential progression from one drug to another [17]. According to Ferguson et al. [18], the progression of use from cannabis to other drugs is supported especially when cannabis use is during adolescence. A twin study described by Lynskey et al. [19] casts doubt on genetic or environmental factors causing the progression. Rat studies have shown that adolescent exposure to Δ-9-tetrahydrocannabinol results in increased opiate consumption [20].

As Curran et al. [21] point out, causality is difficult and challenging. It encompasses everything from availability to regulations controlling sale of cannabis and other drugs. MacCoun and Reuter [22] point out that in the Netherlands where the sale of cannabis is regulated, the rate of cocaine use among people who have used cannabis is lower (22%) than in the United States (33%).

Only a minor number of cannabis users become addicted, according to Freeman and Winstock [23]; therefore, other factors need to be considered in vulnerability to cannabis dependence. Tobacco use in adolescence has been identified in several studies [24–26] with males at a faster and greater risk of addiction.

Early exposure to cannabinoids in adolescent rats decreases the reactivity of brain dopamine reward centers late in adulthood [27]. However, most people who use cannabis do not go on to use other drugs, since alcohol and nicotine also prime the brain for a heightened response [28].

The March 17, 1999, report from the Institute of Medicine found no evidence that the medical use of cannabis would increase use in the general population, nor was it a "gateway drug" leading to cocaine or heroin use [29]. Bioethicist William Stempsey, MD, indicates that the government's view that street drug availability is related to prescription drug availability is false [30]. He states that morphine, like other narcotics, is available only by prescription to limit availability, and this has not led to increased use of morphine.

JC van Ours of Tilburg University analyzed a dataset in Amsterdam that identifies cannabis users starting at ages 18–20, while cocaine use started at 20–25. The study found there was little difference in the probability that cocaine users had ever used cannabis. The use of drugs was linked to personality characteristics and a predilection to experimentation [31].

Legalizing medical marijuana

Some people will review the legalizing of medical marijuana as condoning and encouraging the use of cannabis as a recreational drug, but the intent of the legalization is to relieve pain and suffering that cannot be relieved by currently approved medications. As Clark et al. [32] discusses, the misinterpretation of the legalization of medical marijuana could be corrected through public education.

The specific value of legalizing medical marijuana is relieving pain and suffering associated with life-threatening disorders. The downside of achieving that goal is the possibility that some will view this as condoning and encouraging illegal drug use. Ethicist Richard McCormick's criteria of proportionate reason [33] is cited as rationale why legalizing medical marijuana should be every patient's right in medical care

> to allow physicians to prescribe marijuana. First, the most comprehensive scientific analysis to date by the Institute of Medicine cautioned that the benefits of smoking marijuana were limited because smoke itself is toxic, but recommended that it be given, on a short-term basis under close supervision, to patients who do not respond to other therapies. The possible damage to an individual's lungs is a legitimate health concern; however, the patients who would benefit from smoking marijuana are suffering from cancer, AIDS, MS, etc. Many of these conditions are terminal and the treatments they are undergoing

also have toxic effects- chemotherapy, radiation, the
AIDS cocktail, etc. The point is that the benefit of the
treatments outweighs the burden [34].

Research funded by the National Institute on Drug Abuse (NIDA)
and the National Institute on Alcohol Abuse and Alcoholism (NIAAA),
both part of the National Institutes of Health, indicates that legalizing
medical marijuana use has increased illicit cannabis use and cannabis
use disorders among adults [35]. State-specific policy changes may be a
contributing factor, investigators noted. These findings underscore the
importance of considering the negative effects of cannabis as regulations
throughout the United States continue to change.

Risks and consequences of cannabis abuse

According to Levine, "despite the perceived low risk of cannabis use by
the general public, there is growing clinical awareness about the spectrum
of behavioral and neurobiological disturbances associated with cannabis
exposure such as anxiety, depression, psychosis, cognitive deficits, social
impairments, and addiction" [36].

The psychoactive cannabinoid THC targets the endocannabinoid
system and plays a key role in brain development. Studies have assessed
the long-term effect of cannabis on neurodevelopment, behavior, and
immunological and reproductive processes in subsequent generations of
offspring whose parents were exposed to cannabis before mating [37–40].
Knowledge of how gene expression is regulated by the cellular network of
DNA elements, epigenetic modifiers, and transcription factors is evolving
along with contributing to the understanding of how these processes are
coordinated throughout the lifespan of the individual [41].

Sparse research is available on epigenetic processes and behavioral
consequences of cannabis exposure. Most neurobiological studies have
targeted the adult brain and memory. Since marijuana use is cited by the
NIDA as widespread among adolescents and young adults, more research
and education is needed in this age group [42]. According to the NIDA,
teens' perceptions of the risks of marijuana use has steadily decreased over
the past decade, although a decline in marijuana use has been seen since
the 1990s. The report states that in 2016 9.4% of eighth graders reported
marijuana use in the past year and 5.4% in the past month. Tenth graders
were reported as 23.9% having used marijuana in the past year and 14.0% in
the past month. Rates among the twelfth graders were the highest at 35.6%
using within the past year and 22.5% using in the past month. Johnson
reports 6% of twelfth graders used marijuana daily or near-daily [43].

Adolescence and early adulthood are periods when many begin to
experiment with substances of abuse such as cannabis, but it is during

this time period that neural substances that underlie the development of cognition and behavior are most active [44]. Cannabis and other drugs used during this period may interfere in social and academic functioning.

Since cannabis use is on the rise globally, in addition to the increase in potency of cannabis sold in legal markets and the black market, it is crucial that innovative ways are needed to reduce harm [45]. Cannabidiol, the nonpsychoactive cannabinoid (CBD), has been found to reduce the negative effects of cannabis use, but it needs to be better understood. The positive effects of CBD and its safety profile have been reported by Iffland and Grotenhermen [46]. Chronic use and high doses of CBD up to 1500 mg per day were well tolerated by humans with no psychological or psychomotor functions adversely affected.

Medical cannabis and opioid overdoses

Opioid overdose mortality continues to rise in the United States because of more prescriptions for chronic pain [47]. Bachhuber reports that three states—California, Oregon, and Washington—had medical cannabis laws prior to 1999, with 10 additional states—Alaska, Colorado, Hawaii, Maine, Michigan, Montana, Nevada, New Mexico, Rhode Island, and Vermont—enacting medical cannabis laws from 1999 to 2010. The states with medical cannabis laws had a 24.8% lower mean annual opioid overdose mortality rate compared to states without medical cannabis laws.

The availability of alternative nonopioid treatments needs to be considered to reduce opioid overdose rates, since chronic noncancer pain prescriptions for opioids have almost doubled over the last decade. Daubresse et al. noted that if medical cannabis laws lead to a decrease in polypharmacy, particularly with benzodiazepines, in people taking opioid analgesics, overdose risk would be decreased [48].

An accumulation of pain, distress, and social dysfunction in the lives of Americans in the blue collar economic sector took hold in the 1970s and continued through the 2008 financial crisis with slow recovery today [49]. Case and Deaton describe this trend as a contributor to "deaths of despair"—death by drugs, alcohol, and suicide. These deaths are rising in men and women throughout the country and at every level of urbanization. Further research is needed to address the needs of this population and reduce drug use.

Mindfulness and addiction

Researchers at the University of Washington showed that a program based on mindfulness was more effective in preventing drug-addiction relapse than 12-step programs [50]. Smith reported that mindfulness training was twice as effective as a behavioral antismoking program. Mindfulness trains people to acknowledge cravings but not react to them so they can overcome the urge to indulge whether it is food, drugs, sex, or exercise.

Psychoactive drugs to "enhance" daily life

The use of psychoactive drugs is as old as recorded history, but there is an emerging trend to increase their use in healthy individuals. Lifestyle use of novel psychoactive substances (NPS) indicates the desire for enhanced cognitive function, creativity, pleasure, and motivation [51]. In Europe, synthetic cannabinoids are the popular NPS, and they have accounted for almost 70% of the seizures reported in 2014. Synthetic cannabinoids (also known as "spice") are used as replacements for cannabis so they cannot be detected on a drug screen.

Soussan and Kjellgren conducted a survey of NPS users to understand motivation for use [52]. Synthetic cannabinoid use in the United States was the least appreciated NPS drug studied by Palamar and Acosta and the least likely to be used again, probably due to severe side effects [53]. Their study identified synthetic cannabinoid use was motivated by price, legal status, and availability, in addition to nondetectability in screening tests.

Synthetic cannabinoids contain compounds that are more potent than THC found in traditional cannabis, with the likelihood of abuse and addiction a major concern [54]. The long-term effects on health and the high numbers of emergency department visits should make these compounds subject to immediate review [55]. One study reported emergency medical treatment to be 30 times greater following the use of synthetic cannabinoids than traditional cannabis [56]. Johnson acknowledged that among adolescents in the United States, synthetic cannabinoids were the most popular choice after cannabis [57].

No studies have reported cognitive deficits from synthetic cannabinoid use, but a 2016 study about long-term (more than five times a week for at least a year) synthetic cannabinoid use was associated with white matter abnormalities in adolescents and young adults [58]. Papanti reported psychosis associated with synthetic cannabinoids [59].

The use of novel psychoactive substances such as synthetic cannabinoids, especially by adolescents and young adults, has changed the drug scene in the past decade. With increased availability, legal status, and lower cost, their popularity will only grow. The use of drugs by healthy people to enhance cognition, creativity, motivation, and pleasure is also changing society.

Kratom

Like cannabis, kratom is a psychoactive botanical that healthcare professionals may need to consider when evaluating pain treatment options. It has a long history of use with its own abuse and addiction potential. It is included here because cannabis and kratom have many similarities and can be used intermittently.

Kratom (Mitragyna speciosa) is an indigenous tree in Southeast Asia that has been used for hundreds of years to relieve pain and is increasingly used for self-management of opioid withdrawal in the United States [60]. The leaves can be eaten raw or crushed for brewing into a tea as well as made into capsules, tablets, and liquids. In low doses, kratom can be a stimulant to increase energy and sexual desire, but high doses have a sedative effect.

Mitragyna speciosa/kratom is metabolized in humans similar to cannabis [61]. It is very bitter, so sweeteners are used to make it palatable. Some states have made it illegal, but anecdotal reports suggest kratom is less addictive than opioids and can be used for opioid withdrawal and pain [62]. Kratom has been touted by many as a safe and legal psychoactive product to improve mood along with pain relief, but hospital visits and deaths in several countries have caused more current attention [63].

Mitragyna speciosa has been used medically throughout Asia, Africa, and Oceania in formulations of topical balms or tinctures [64]. The tree and leaves are currently illegal in four countries, but it is legal and widely available in the United States [65]. Vardi et al. [66] showed that kratom-based drugs had analgesic effects but fewer side effects, slower development of tolerance, and lower potential for dependence than morphine in a mouse model. The therapeutic benefits of kratom can be noted in several United States patents issued from 1964 to 2009 [67–69].

As more people turn to kratom to avoid street opioids [70], the Drug Enforcement Agency (DEA) announced in August 2016 that kratom and mitragynine would be added to Schedule I status, drugs that have no valid medical use and high potential for abuse. Opposition was so great that the DEA had to withdraw its intent to ban kratom [71].

How serious is the abuse and addictive potential of kratom and are kratom products safe? Prozialeck describes the pharmacologically active compounds and potential toxicities but states that "moderate doses of less than 10–15 grams pure leaf kratom appears to be relatively benign in the vast majority of uses" [72].

Healthcare professionals need to be aware of any botanical products their patients may be using for analgesic properties including those that may be promoted to reduce opioid dependence.

References

1. Whiting PF, Wolf RF, Deshpande S et al. Cannabinoids for medical use: a systematic review and meta-analysis. *JAMA*. 2015;313(24):2456–2473.
2. Curran HV, Morgan CJA. Desired and undesired effects of cannabis on the human mind and psychological well-being. In *Handbook of Cannabis* (ed. Pertwee RG). Oxford University Press, Oxford, England, 2014.

3. Hall W. What has research over the past two decades revealed about the adverse health effects of recreational cannabis use? *Addiction*. 2015;110:19–35.

4. Curran HV, Freeman TP, Mokrysz C et al. Keep off the grass? Cannabis, cognition and addiction. *Nature Reviews/Neuroscience*. 2016;17(5):293–306. www.nature.com/nrn

5. D'Souza DC, Perry E, Mc Dougall L et al. The psychtomimetic effects of intravenous Δ-9-tetrahydrocannabidol in healthy individuals: implications for psychosis. *Neuropsychopharmacology*. 2004;29(8):1558–1572.

6. Leweke F, Piomelli D, Pahlisch F et al. Cannabidiol enhances anandamide signaling and alleviates psychotic symptoms of schizophrenia. *Trans Psychiatry*. 2012;2:e94.

7. Bergamaschi MM, Queiroz RH, Chagas MH et al. Cannabidiol reduces the anxiety induced by stimulated public speaking in treatment-naive social phobia patients. *Neuropsychopharmacology*. 2011;36(6):1219–1226.

8. Parsons LH, Hurd YL. Endocannabinoid signaling in reward and addiction. *Nat Rev Neurosci*. 2015;16(10):579–594.

9. Glass M, Dragunow M, Faull RL. Cannabinoid receptors in the human brain: a detailed anatomical and quantitative autoradiographic study in fetal, neonatal, and adult brain. *Neuroscience*. 1997;77:299–318.

10. Atwood BK, Macki K. CB2: A cannabinoid receptor with an identity crisis. *Br J Pharmacol*. 2010;160:467–479.

11. Vlachou S, Panagis G. Regulation of brain reward by the endocannabinoid system: a critical review of behavioral studies in animals. *Curr Pharm Des*. 2014;20:2072–2088.

12. Xi ZX, Peng X-Q, Li X, Song R et al. Brain cannabinoid CB(2) receptors modulate cocaine's actions in mice. *Nat Neurosci*. 2011;14:1160–1166.

13. Zhang HY, Bi GH, Li J et al. Species differences in cannabinoid receptor 2 and receptor responses to cocaine self-administration in mice and rats. *Neuropsychopharmacology*. 2015;40(4):1037–1051.

14. Parsons LH, Hurd YL. Endocannabinoid signaling in reward and addiction. *Nat Rev Neurosci*. 2015;16(10):579–594.

15. Ducci F, Goldman D. The genetic basis of addictive disorders. *Psychiatr Clin North Am*. 2012;35:495–519.

16. Morgan CJ, Freeman TP, Schafer GL et al. Cannabidiol attenuates the appetitive effects of Δ-9-tetrahydrocannabinol in humans smoking their chosen cannabis. *Neuropsychopharmacology*. 2010;35:1879–1885.

17. Kandel DB. *Stages and Pathways of Drug Involvement: Examining the Gateway Hypothesis*. Cambridge University Press, Cambridge, England, 2002.

18. Ferguson DM, Boden JM, Horwood LJ. Cannabis use and other illicit drug use: testing the cannabis gateway hypothesis. *Addiction* 2006;101:556–559.

19. Lynsky MT, Heath AC, Bucholz KK et al. Escalation of drug use in early-onset cannabis users versus co-twin controls. *JAMA*. 2003;289:427–433.

20. Cadoni C, Simola N, Espa E et al. Strain dependence of adolescent cannabis influence on heroin reward and mesolimbic dopamine transmission in adult Lewis and Fisher 344 rats. *Addict Biol*. 2015;20:132–142.

21. Curran HV, Freeman TP, Mokrysz C et al. Keep off the grass? Cannabis, cognition and addiction. *Nature Reviews/Neuroscience*. 2016; 17(5):293–306. www.nature.com/nrn

22. Mac Coun R, Reuter P. Evaluating alternative cannabis regimes. *Br J Psychiatry*. 2001;178:123–128.

23. Freeman T, Winstock A. Examining the profile of high-potency cannabis and its association with severity of cannabis dependence. *Psychol Med* 2015;45:3181–3189.

24. Coffey C, Carlin JB, Lynsky M et al. Adolescent precursors of cannabis dependence: Findings from the Victorian Adolescent Health Cohort Study. *Br J Psychiatry*. 2003;182:330–336.

25. Hines LA, Morley KI, Strang J et al. Onset of opportunity to use cannabis and progression from opportunity to dependence: Are influences consistent across transitions? *Drug Alcohol Depend*. 2016;160:57–64.

26. Hindocha C, Shaban ND, Freeman TP et al. Associations between cigarette smoking and cannabis dependence: a longitudinal study of young cannabis users in the United Kingdom. *Drug Alcohol Depend*. 2015;148:165–171.

27. Pistis M, Perra S, Pillolla G et al. Adolescent exposure to cannabinoids induces long-lasting changes in the response to drugs of abuse of rat midbrain dopamine neurons. *Biol Psychiatry* 2004;56(2):86–94.

28. Levinbe A, Huang Y, Drisaldi B et al. Molecular mechanism for a gateway drug: Epigenetic changes initiated by nicotine prime gene expression by cocaine. *Sci Transl Med*. 2011;3:107–109.

29. Joy JE, Watson SJ, Benson JA. *Marijuana and Medicine: Assessing the Science Base*. Institute of Medicine, Wash D.C., 1999 March.

30. Stempsey WE. The battle for medical Marijuana in the war on drugs. *America*. *NY*. 1998;178(12):14–16.

31. Van Ours JC. Is cannabis a stepping stone for cocaine? *J Health Econ*. 2003;22(4):539–554.

32. Clark PA, Capuzzi K, Fick C. Medical marijuana: medical necessity versus political agenda. *Med Sci Monit*. 2011;17(12):RA249–RA261.

33. McCormick R, Ramsey P, (ed). *Doing Evil to Achieve Good*. Loyola Univ Press, Chicago, 1978.

34. Clark PA, Capuzzi K, Fick C. Medical marijuana: medical necessity versus political agenda. *Med Sci Monit*. 2011;17(12):RA249–RA261.

35. Hasin DS, Sarvet AL, Cerda M et al. US adult illicit cannabis use, cannabis use disorder, and medical marijuana laws 1991–1992 to 2012–2013. *JAMA Psychiatry*. 2017;74(6):579–588.

36. Levine A, Clemenza K, Rynn M et al. Evidence of the risks and consequences of adolescent cannabis exposure. *J Am Acad Child Adilesc Psychiatry*. 2017;56(3):214–225.

37. Morris CV, DiNieri JA, Szutorisz H et al. Molecular mechanisms of maternal cannabis and cigarette use in human neurodevelopment. *The European J Neuroscience*. 2011;34:1574–1583.

38. Owen KP, Sutter ME, Albertson TE. Marijuana: respiratory tract effects. *Clin Rev Allergy Immunol*. 2014;46:65–81.

39. Chadwick B, Miller ML, Hurd YL. Cannabis use during adolescent development: susceptibility to psychiatric illness. *Front Psychiatry*. 2013;4:129.

40. Bari M, Battista N, Pirazzi V et al. The manifold actions of endocannabinoids on female and male reproductive events. *Frontiers in Bioscience*. 2011;16:498–516.

41. Dambacher S, deAlmeida GP, Schotta G. Dynamic changes of the epigenetic landscape during cellular differentiation. *Epigenomics*. 2013;5:701–713.

42. What is the scope of marijuana use in the United States? National Institute on Drug Abuse. www.drugabuse.gov/publ;ications/research-reports/marijuana/what-scope-marijuana-use-in-united-states

43. Johnson L, O'Malley P, Miech R et al. Monitoring the future national survey results on drug use: 1975–2016. Overview: Key Findings on Adolescent Drug Use. Institute of Social Research, University of Michigan, Ann Arbor, MI 2016.

44. Giedd JN. The amazing teen brain. *Scientific American*. 2015;312(6):32–37.

45. England A, Freeman TP, Murray RM et al. Can we make cannabis safe? *Lancet Psychiatry*. 2017;4(8):643–648.

46. Iffland K, Grotenherman F. European Industrial Hemp Association (EIHA) review on: Safety and Side Effects of Cannabidiol—A review of clinical data and relevant animal studies. 2017;2(1):139–154.

47. Bachhuber MA, Saloner B, Cunningham CO et al. Medical cannabis laws and opioid analgesic overdose mortality in the United States, 1999–2010. *JAMA Intern Med*. 2014;174(10):1668–1673.

48. Daubresse M, Chang HY, Yu Y et al. Ambulatory diagnosis and treatment of nonmalignant pain in the United States, 2000–2010. *Med Care*. 2013;51(10):870–878.

49. Case A, Deaton SA. Mortality and morbidity in the 21st Century. https://www.brooklings.edu/bpea-articles/mortality-and-morbidity-in-the-21st-century

50. Smith F. The addicted brain. *National Geographic*. 2017;34–51.

51. Camilla d'Angelo L-S, Savulich G, Sahakian BJ. Lifestyle use of drugs by healthy people for enhancing cognition, creativity, motivation and pleasure. *Br J Pharmacology*. 2017; 3251–3267.

52. Soussan C, Kjellgren A. The users of novel psychoactive substances: online survey about their characteristics, attitudes, and motivations. *Int J Drug Pol*. 2016;32:77–84.

53. Palamar JJ, Acousta P. Synthetic cannabinoid use in nationally representative sample of US high school seniors. *Drug Alcohol Depend*. 2015;149:194–202.

54. Le Boisselier R, Alexandre J, Lelong-Boulouard V et al. Focus on cannabinoids and synthetic cannabinoids. *Clin Pharmacol Ther*. 2016; 001:10.1002/cpt.563.

55. Castaneto MS, Gorelick DA, Desrosier NA et al. Synthetic cannabinoids: Epidemiology, pharmacodynamics, and clinical implications. *Drug Alcohol Depend*. 2014;144:12–41.

56. Winstock A, Lynsskey M, Borchmann R et al. Risk of emerging medical treatment following consumption of cannabis or synthetic cannabinoids in a large global sample. *J Psychopharmacol*. 2015;29:698–703.

57. Johnson L, O'Malley P, Miech R et al. Monitoring the future national survey results on drug use: 1975–2016. Overview: Key Findings on Adolescent Drug Use. Institute of Social Research, University of Michigan, Ann Arbor, MI, 2016.

58. Zorlu N, Di Biase MA, Kalayci CC et al. Abnormal white matter integrity in synthetic cannabinoid users. *Eur Neuropsychopharmacol*. 2016;26:1818–1825.

59. Papanti D, Schifano F, Botteon G et al. 'Spiceophrenia': A systematic overview of 'spice'-related psychopathological issues and a case report. *Hum Psychopharmacol*. 2013;28:379–389.

60. Prozialeck WC. Update on the pharmacology and legal status of kratom. *J Amer Osteopathic Assn*. 2016;116:802–809.

61. Warner ML, Kaufman NC, Grundmann O. The pharmacology and toxicity of kratom: from traditional herb to drug of abuse. *Int J Legal Med (Review)*. 2016;130(1):127–138.

62. Prozialeck WC, Jivan JK, Andurkar SV. Pharmacology of kratom: an emerging botanical agent with stimulant, analgesic and opioid-like effects. *J Am Osteopath Assn.* 2012;111(12):792–799.
63. Warner ML, Kaufman NC, Grundmann O. The pharmacology and toxicity of kratom: From traditional herb to drug of abuse. *Int J Legal Med (Review).* 2016;130(1):127–138.
64. Browwn PN, Lund JA, Murch SJ. A botanical, phytochemical and ethnomedicinal review of the genus Mitragyna korth: implications for products sold as kratom. *J Ethnopharmacol.* 2017;202:302–325.
65. Adkins JE, Boyer EW, McCurdy CR. Mitragyna speciosa, a psychoactive tree in Southeast Asia with opioid activity. *Curr Top Med Chem.* 2011;11(9):1165–1175.
66. Varadi A, Marrone GF, Palmer TC et al. Mitragynine/corynantheidine pseudoindoxyls as opioid analgesics with mu arrestin-2. *J Med Chem.* 2016;59(18):8381–8397.
67. Boyer EW, McCurdy CR, Adkins JE. Inventors: University of Mass Medical School. Assignees: University of Mississippi. Methods for treating withdrawal from addictive compounds. US Patent 20100209542, 2016.
68. Takayama H, Kitajima M, Matsumoto K, Horie S. Inventors: National University Corporation Chiba University; Josai University Corporation, assignees. Indole alkaloid derivatives having opioid receptor agonist effect, and therapeutic composition and methods relating to same. US Patent 8247428B2. November 7, 2018.
69. Heyworth BA, inventor; Smith Kline French Lab, assignee. Speciofoline, an alkaloid from Mitragyna speciosa. US Patent 3324111A. August 10, 1964.
70. Swogger MT, Hart E, Erowid F et al. Experiences of kratom users: a qualitative analysis. *J Psychoactive Drugs.* 2015;47(5):360–367.
71. DEA. Withdrawal of notice of intent to temporarily place mitragynine and 7-hydroxymitragynine into Schedule I. *Fed Register.* 2016:59929–59934. 21CFR Part 1308.
72. Prozialeck WC. Update on the pharmacology and legal status of kratom. *J Amer Osteopathic Assn.* 2016;116:802–809.

section two

Clinical Practice

chapter ten

What should we tell our patients about marijuana?

Joseph Pizzorno

Contents

Long-time readers *Integrative Medicine—A Clinician's Journal* are well aware of the many editorials I have written on how a growing body of research is showing that toxins have become a major cause of chronic disease. As I study toxicity, my understanding has broadened to include not only environmental metals and chemicals but also endogenously produced toxins such as those from homocysteine, gut bacteria, and nonoptimally detoxified hormones. To this list I now add what I call "toxins of choice." Few of our patients are intentionally exposing themselves to neurotoxic organophosphate pesticides, endocrine-disrupting polychlorinated biphenyls (PCBs), insulin receptor site-blocking phthalates, or lung-damaging mold from damp buildings. However, many of our patients are intentionally consuming known toxins such as alcohol and marijuana and are unlikely to realize that at modest dosages salt, high-fructose corn syrup, phosphates, and nonsteroidal anti-inflammatory drugs (NSAIDs) are toxic as well. Added to this that by also considering genetic susceptibility, even sources of gluten can be toxic. The huge load of environmental, endogenous, and choice toxins adds up to deplete stores of protective glutathione and cause physiological and structural damage in many ways.

The following is my current list of many toxins that stress physiology and cause disease in our patients.

Exogenous toxins

- OTC and prescription drugs
- Chemicals: inorganic, organic, fluoride, persistent organic pollutants, solvents
- Metals: arsenic, cadmium, lead, mercury
- Microbial
- Mold (damp buildings)
- Particulate matter
- Radiation: light at night, medical, cell phone

Endogenous

- Catecholamines (if COMT SNP)
- Gut-derived toxins
- Homocysteine
- Non-end product metabolites
- Poorly detoxified hormones

Toxins of choice

- Alcohol
- Marijuana
- Food constituents
- High-fructose corn syrup
- Phosphates
- Salt
- Smoking
- Wheat (if zonulin is produced)

Cannabis (marijuana)

Although the federal government has classified cannabis as a controlled substance illegal for use, many states have now decriminalized its use. Twenty-four states and the District of Columbia have passed laws allowing medicinal use of marijuana, and 14 states have decriminalized its use. The percentage of Americans who say they have tried marijuana has steadily increased from 4% to 43% in 2016 [1].

Cannabis production has become a multibillion dollar industry in the United States, and legal markets for cannabis are projected to reach $11 billion by 2019 [2]. The federal illegality of cannabis has resulted in not only limited clinical research but also a production environment with few standards and very little regulation. As most is currently grown indoors, heavy use of agricultural chemicals is common. Toxicity may be due to not only constituents of marijuana itself but also contaminants such as solvents, pesticides, and heavy metals, with most extracts adding solvent residues. This likely helps explain some of the discrepancies in the research.

Toxicity in unadulterated cannabis

Almost 500 compounds have been extracted from cannabis, of which 65 are classified as cannabinoids. The most abundant cannabinoids include delta-9-tetrahydrocannabinoic acid (THCA), cannabidiolic acid (CBDA), cannabigerolic acid (CBGA), and their decarboxylated derivatives delta-9-tetrahydrocannabinol (THC), cannabidiol (CBD), and cannabigerol (CBG) [3]. These compounds are converted into their more active decarboxylated counterparts by heat (smoking, evaporation, baking), light, or natural degradation. THC is the most psychoactive component of cannabis and alters cognition primarily through the activation of CB1 receptors on presynaptic axons, though several other mechanisms have been identified [4,5]. The content of THC in marijuana has increased from 3.1% in 1992 to 5.1% in 2002 [6,7].

THC itself has low toxicity, and modest use has shown minimal long-term physical or psychological effects when not used to excess [8,9]. Acute high-dose intoxication occurs quickly but is short term. Typical symptoms include nausea, anxiety, paranoia, short-term memory loss, confusion, and disorientation [10]. THC impairs gonadal function by blocking gonadotropin-releasing hormone (GnRH) release. This results in lower levels of luteinizing hormone (LH) and follicle-stimulating hormone (FSH), which causes reduced testosterone production by the testicular Leydig cells [11].

The research on the toxicity of whole plant marijuana is inconsistent, probably due to lack of control for contaminants, poor assessment of dosage, small sample size, limited number of heavy users, mode of use, and not adjusting for other factors such as alcohol, tobacco, and other recreational drugs [12].

The method of use significantly affects the toxicity of marijuana. The most common use is inhalation of the smoke of the dried plant. This results in higher risk for adverse effects [13]. The whole-plant smoke contains many hazardous compounds such as ammonia, cyanide, heavy metals, carbon monoxide, mutagens, carcinogens, and polycyclic aromatic hydrocarbons [14]. Surprisingly, the tar from a cannabis cigarette contains higher concentrations of carcinogens such as benzanthracenes and benzopyrenes than does tobacco smoke [15].

Contaminants

Pesticides

For most of the twentieth century, most of the marijuana produced in the United States was grown outdoors. With more aggressive law enforcement, marijuana agriculture moved indoors. Although this provided the benefit of year-round cultivation, it also required the use of agricultural chemicals, typically synthetic fertilizers and pesticides.

Because cannabis cultivation is illegal, there are no pesticides registered for use on cannabis in the United States, meaning there is little research on their use for this purpose [16]. The limited research suggests that this results in higher chemical residue levels [17]. There are apparently no direct studies on how pesticides in cannabis affects consumers of the product. A list of the toxic contaminants that have been found in both medical and recreational marijuana follows. Research has shown that cannabis extracts contain considerable amounts of pesticides [18]. Toxic agricultural chemicals found in cultivated marijuana [19–22] includes

Pesticides: Bifenthrin, chlorpyrifos, diazinon, methamidophos, teflubenzuron
Fungicides: Tebuconazole
Growth Regulator: Ethephon
Mosquito repellant: DEET (N,N-diethyl-meta-toluamide), malathion

Solvents

Many methods are used to concentrate the active constituents in cannabis. The organic solvents benzene, hexane, naphtha, petroleum ether, and butane pose a significant risk of toxic chemical concentration [23]. Hexane and benzene are neurotoxic, and naphtha and petroleum ether are potential carcinogens. Research has shown significant residues in these products [24]. A process called *dabbing* uses butane to produce higher THC content [25].

Safer alternative methods of concentration use ethanol and olive oil. Perhaps best is the use of supercritical CO_2 to extract volatile oils from cannabis, as this leaves no residue. Although there is limited research of the efficacy of these methods, nontoxic solvents are clearly preferable.

Heavy metals

Cannabis has been shown to be especially effective in absorbing metals such as cadmium and copper from contaminated soils [26]. Making matters worse, cannabis is also intentionally contaminated with metals to increase the market weight. In 2008, 150 people in Germany developed lead poisoning as the result of using adulterated cannabis [27].

Microbial

Indoor growth results in increased susceptibility of cannabis to contamination by microbes such as fungi, bacteria, and plant viruses. Growing and drying also increase the risk of microbial contamination [28]. Penicillium species are the predominant microbe contamination in marijuana grown indoors [29]. Cannabis has even been shown to be contaminated with human pathogens such as hepatitis A [30], hepatitis B [31], and salmonella [32]. Chronic pulmonary aspergillosis has been found in immunocompromised individuals using medicinal marijuana [33].

Synthetic cannabinoids

There is limited research on synthetic cannabinoids (SCBs) such as "spice," "K2," "herbal incense," and others. Toxicity reports include tachycardia, hypertension, tachypnea, chest pain, heart palpitations, hallucinations, racing thoughts, and seizures [34]. The most common clinical signs of toxicity are neurologic including agitation, central nervous system depression/coma, and delirium/toxic psychosis [35]. There have been reports of acute renal failure associated with the use of these synthetic analogs [36]. These compounds appear significantly more toxic than cannabis and should be avoided [37].

Detoxification

The liver metabolizes THC through hydroxylation and oxidation reactions catalyzed by cytochrome P450 enzymes, especially CYP2C9 and CYP3A4 [38–40]. Approximately 65% is excreted in the feces and 20% in urine [41]. THC is excreted in the urine primarily as the glucuronic acid conjugate THCCOOH, which has a half-life between 30 and 44 hours [42].

Clinical indications of toxicity

Long-term smoking of marijuana leaf has been shown to cause airway obstruction [43]; squamous metaplasia [44]; impaired psychomotor performance; increased incidence of schizophrenia [45]; cancer of the mouth, jaw, tongue, and lung; and leukemia in children of marijuana-smoking mothers [46]. Although marijuana smoke has been shown to contain carcinogenic compounds, research is unclear about whether a link with lung cancer exists [47].

Population studies in adults show that heavy cannabis use increases the risk of accidents, can produce dependence, and has been associated with poor social outcomes and mental health [48]. Long term daily use has been associated with decreased motivation, impaired ability to learn, and reduced sexual desire [49,50]. Daily heavy inhalation can produce bronchial irritation and may lead to long-term pulmonary damage secondary to the associated hydrocarbon residues [51].

Intervention

As noted previously, marijuana can be considered a "toxin of choice." This means dose and toxicity are under the control of the user. Abstinence is, of course, the most effective way to decrease cannabis toxicity. However, for most patients, management to prevent excessive use and education to choose the least toxic forms is more likely. Research has shown little benefit treating cannabis dependence with prescription drugs such a selective serotonin reuptake inhibitor (SSRI) antidepressants, mixed-action antidepressants, atypical antidepressants (bupropion), anxiolytics (buspirone), and norepinephrine reuptake inhibitors [52].

N-acetyl-cysteine (NAC) at 1200 mg b.i.d. has shown benefits because its induction of glutathione synthesis helps mitigate many of the toxic effects and improve the odds of abstinence [53,54].

Vaporization ("vaping") of extracts appears the preferred method of use as it reduces respiratory exposure to toxic particulates and carcinogens [55]. For those smoking the dried plant (buds, leaf, flowers, etc.), the type of filtration significantly affects toxic chemical residue. Hand-held glass pipes allow the most toxins, unfiltered water pipes are intermediate, and the lowest quantity is found with filtered water pipes [56]. Heating may make many of the contaminants more toxic [57].

Conclusion

Many of our patients are using, and in some cases abusing, cannabis. Our key clinical responsibility is to help those who chose to use marijuana—for whatever reason—to do so responsibly and as safely as possible. The most common ways of obtaining and using marijuana clearly result in clinical toxicity. Interestingly, most of this toxicity appears to be determined by contaminants and the consumption method.

We need to advise our patients to carefully avoid marijuana that is contaminated with agricultural chemicals, metals, microbes, solvents, etc. In addition, damage can be decreased by recommending the least toxic ways of consuming marijuana. Because the primary psychoactive constituent of marijuana, THC, appears to have little toxicity (though it likely plays a major role in the psychological issues), our guidance should focus on ways to limit exposure to everything else. This suggests recommending organically grown product, CO_2 extraction, and vaporization rather than smoking agricultural chemical-laden dried plant.

References

1. Gallop. One in eight U.S. adults say they smoke marijuana. Retrieved from http://www.gallop.com/poll/194195.
2. ArcView Market Research. *The State of Legal Marijuana Markets*. 3rd ed. San Francisco, CA: ArcView Market Research; 2016.
3. Happyana N, Agnolet S, Muntendam R et al. Analysis of cannabinoids in laser-microdissected trichomes of medicinal Cannabis sativa using LCMS and cryogenic NMR. *Phytochemistry. March* 2013;87:51–59.
4. Wilson R, Nicoll R. Endocannabinoid signaling in the brain. *Science.* 2002;296(5568):678–682.
5. Hejazi N, Zhou C, Oz M et al. Delta-9-tetrahydrocannabinol and endogenous cannabinoid anandamide directly potentiate the function of glycine receptors. *Mol Pharmacol.* 2006;69(3):991–997.
6. ElSohly MA, Ross SA, Mehmedic Z et al. Potency trends of delta-9-THC and other cannabinoids in confiscated marijuana from 1980–1997. *J Forensic Sci.* 2000;45:24–30.
7. National Center for the Development of Natural Products. *Quarterly Report, Potency Monitoring Project/NIDA Marijuana Project.* Oxford, MS: University of Mississippi, Research Institute of Pharmaceutical Sciences, School of Pharmacy; 2003.
8. Smith DE, Mehl C. An analysis of marijuana toxicity. *Clin Toxicol.* 1970;3(1):101–105.
9. Smith DE. The acute and chronic toxicity of drugs. *J Psych drugs.* 1968;2(1):37–47.
10. Weil A. Adverse reactions to marijuana: Classification and suggested treatment. *N Engl J Med.* 1970;282:997–1000.
11. Harclerode J. Endocrine efects of marijuana in the male: Preclinical studies. *NIDA Res Monograph.* 1984;44:46–64.
12. Hashibe M, Straif K, Tashkin DP et al. Epidemiologic review of marijuana use and cancer risk. *Alcohol.* 2005;35(3):265–275.
13. Cohn A, Johnson A, Ehlke S et al. Characterizing substance use and mental health profiles of cigar, blunt, and non-blunt marijuana users from the National Survey of Drug Use and Health. *Drug Alcohol Depend. March* 2016;160:105–111.
14. Moir D, Rickert W, Levasseur G et al. A comparison of mainstream and sidestream marijuana and tobacco cigarette smoke produced under two machine smoking conditions. *Chem Res Toxicol.* 2008;21(2):494–502.
15. Wu TC, Scott R, Burnett S et al. Pulmonary hazards of smoking marijuana as compared with tobacco. *N Engl J Med.* 1998;318:347–351.
16. Thomson J. *Medical Marijuana Cultivation and Policy Gaps.* Sacramento, CA: California Research Bureau; 2012.
17. Stone D. Cannabis, pesticides and conflicting laws: The dilemma for legalized states and implications for public health. *Reg Toxicol Pharmacol.* 2014;69(3):284–288.
18. Raber JC, Elzinga S, Kaplan C. Understanding dabs: Contamination concerns of cannabis concentrates and cannabinoid transfer during the act of dabbing. *J Toxicol Sci.* 2015;40(6):797–803.
19. Thompson C, Sweitzer R, Gabriel M et al. Impacts of rodenticide and insecticide toxicants from marijuana cultivation sites of fisher survival rates in the Sietta National Forest, CA. *Conserv Letter.* 2014;7:91–102.

20. Perez-Parada A, Alonso B, Rodriguez C et al. Evaluation of three multiresidue methods for the determination of pesticides in marijuana (Cannabis sativa L.) with liquid chromatography-tandem mass spectrometry. *Chromatographia.* 2016;79(17):1069–1083.

21. United Chemical Technologies. Potency and pesticide content in medical vs. recreational marijuana. Amchro Web site. http://www.armchro.com/uct/Potency_Pesticide_Content_in_Medical_vs_Recreational_Marijuana_0_6101-02-01.pdf. Published 2015.

22. Skeet N. City attorney explains medical marijuana issue on NBC. LA City Attorney Web site. http://lacityorgatty.blogspot.com/2009/10/city-attorney-explains-medical.html. Published October 10, 2009.

23. Rosehthal E, Downs D. *Beyond Buds: Marijuana Extracts- Hash, Vaping, Dabbing, Edibles, and Medicines.* San Francisco, CA: Quick American Archives; 2014.

24. Romano I, Hazekamp A. Cannabis oil: Chemical evaluation of an upcoming cannabis based medicine. *Cannabinoids.* 2013;1(1):1–11.

25. Miller BI, Stogner JM, Miller JM. Exploring butane hash oil use: a research note. *J Psychoactive Drug.* 2016;48(1):44–49.

26. Kozlowski R. Interview with Professor R. Kozlowski, director of the Institute of Natural Fibers. *J Int Hemp Assoc.* 1995;2(2):86–87.

27. Busse F, Omidi L, Timper K et al. Lead poisoning due to adulterated marijuana. *N Engl J Med.* 2008;358(15):1641–1642.

28. Miller JD, Jognson I. Consequences of large-scale production of marijuana in residential buildings. *Indoor Built Environ.* 2012;21:595–600.

29. Martynt JW, Serano K, Schaeffer J et al. Potential exposures associated with indoor marijuana growing operations. *J Occup Environ Hygiene.* 2013;10(11):622–639.

30. Alexander T. Hepatitis outbreak linked to imported pot. *Sinsemilla Tips.* 1987;7(3):22.

31. Cates W, Warren JW. Hepatitis B in Nuremburg, Germany. *JAMA.* 1975;234:930–934.

32. Taylor DN, Washsmuth IK, Shangkuan YH et al. Salmonellosis asscoiated with marijuana. *N Engl J Med.* 1981;306:1249–1253.

33. Gargani Y, Bishop P, Denning DW. Too many moldy joints: Marijuana and chronic pulmonary aspergillosis. *Mediterr J Hematol Infect Dis.* 2011;3(1):e2011005.

34. Wells DL, Ott CA. The 'new' marijuana. *Ann Pharmacother.* 2011;45(3):414–417.

35. Riederer AM, Campleman SL, Carlson RG et al. Acute poisoning from synthetic cannabinoids: 50 US toxicology investigators consortium registry sites, 2010-2015. *MMWR Morb Mortal Wkly Rep.* 2016;65(27):692–695.

36. Gudsoorkar VS, Perez JA Jr. A new differential diagnosis: Synthetic cannabinoid-associated acute renal failure. *Methodist Debakey Cardiovasc J.* 2015;11(3):189–191.

37. Bonnet U, Mayler H. Synthetic cannabinoids: Spread, addiction biology, and current perspective of personal health hazard. *Fortschr Neurol Psychiatr.* 2015;83(4):221–231.

38. Sharma P, Murthy P, Bharath MM. Chemistry, metabolism, and toxicology of cannabis: Clinical implications. *Iran J Psychiatr,* 2012;7(4):149–156.

39. Watanabe K, Yamaori S, Funahashi T et al. Cytochrome P450 enzymes involved in the metabolism of tetrahydrocannabinols and cannabinol by human hepatic microsomes. *Life Sci.* 2007;80(15):1415–1419.

40. Stout SM, Cimino NM. Exogenous cannabinoids as substrates, inhibitors, and inducers of human drug metabolizing enzymes: A systematic review. *Drug Metab Rev.* 2014;46(1):86–95.
41. Lemberger L, Axelrod J, Kopin IJ. Metabolism and disposition of delta-9-tetrahydrocannbinol in man. *Pharmacol Rev.* 1971;23:371–380.
42. Goulle JP, Saussereau E, Lacroix C. Delta-9-tetrahydrocannabinol pharmokinetics. *Am Pharm Fr.* 2008;66(4):232–244.
43. Tshkin DP, Baldwin GC, Sarafiaan T et al. Respiratory and immunologic consequences of marijuana smoking. *J Clin Pharmacol.* 2002;42(11 Suppl):71S–81S.
44. Zhang ZF, Morgenstern H, Spitz MR et al. Marijuana use and increased risk of squamous cell carcinoma of the head and neck. *Cancer Epidiol Biomarkers Prev.* 199;8(12):1071–1078.
45. Kelly M, Wan C, Broussard B et al. Marijuana use in the immediate 5-year premorbid period is associated with increased risk of onset of schizophrenia and related psychotic disorders. *Schizophrenia Res.* 2016;171(1):62–67.
46. Robison LL, Buckley JD, Daigle AE et al. Maternal drug use and risk of childhood nonlymphoblastic leukemia among offspring. *Cancer.* 1989;63(10):1904–1911.
47. Hashibe M, Morgenstern C, Cui Y et al. Marijuana use and the risk of lung and upper aerodigestive tract cancers: Results of a population-based case-control study. *Cancer Epidemiol Prev.* 2006;15(10):1829–1834.
48. Hall W. What has research over the past two decades revealed about the adverse health effects of recreational cannabis use? *Addiction.* 2015;110(1):19–35.
49. Pope HG, Gruber AJ, Hudson JI et al. Cognitive measures in long-term cannabis users. *J Clin Pharmacol.* 2002;42(1 Suppl):41s–47s.
50. Bolla KI, Brown K, Eldreth D et al. Dose-related neurocognitive effects of marijuana use. *Neurology.* 2002;59(9):1337–1343.
51. Bloom JW, Kaltenborn W, Paoletti P et al. Respiratory effects of non-tobacco cigarettes. *Br Med J.* 1987;295(6612):1516–1518.
52. Marshall K, Gowing L, Ali R et al. Pharmacotherapeuties for cannabis dependence. *Cochrane Database Syst Rev.* 2014;12:CD008940.
53. Deepmala, Slattery J, Kumar N et al. Clinical trials of N-acetylcysteine in psychiatry and neurology: A systematic review. *Neurosci Biobehav Rev.* 2015;55:294–321.
54. Asevedo E, Mendes AC, Berk M et al. systematic review of N-acetylcysteine in the treatment of addictions. *Rev Bras Psiquiatr.* 2014;36(2):168–175.
55. Tashkin DP. How beneficial is vaping cannabis to respiratory health compared to smoking? *Addiction.* 2015;110(11):1706–1707.
56. Sullivan N, Elzinga S, Raber J. Determination of pesticide residues in cannabis smoke. *J Toxicol.* 2013;2013:378168.
57. Lorenz W, Bahadir M, Korte F. Thermolysis of pesticide residues during tobacco smoking. *Chemosphere.* 1987;16(2–3):521–522.

chapter eleven

What is a medical marijuana program?

Betty Wedman-St. Louis

Contents

Medical cannabis, or commonly called "medical marijuana," refers to the use of cannabis compounds in the treatment of specific medical conditions. Medical marijuana programs define the medical use, cultivation specifics, and dispensing of cannabis through a physician who certifies that a patient meets the criteria to obtain and use cannabis.

Many doctors today have patients asking about medical cannabis, and they need to get past the obstacles for recommending a Schedule I controlled substance [1]:

- Cannabis was not taught in medical school.
- Cannabis is not covered by insurance.
- How will this affect my medical license?
- What about dosing?
- How much extra paperwork will be required?
- Is training to certify patients required?
- How safe is cannabis?

Safety is usually a critical concern for patients and medical staff because associations with "getting high" from recreational cannabis use predominates awareness. Smoke-free forms of cannabis medication—tinctures, vaporization, capsules, and nasal sprays—are available in both CBD (nonpsychoactive) and low THC (psychoactive) or zero THC forms at local dispensaries. Physicians write a recommendation for a patient who qualifies based on state guidelines, but they cannot dispense it. The patient must secure cannabis at a licensed dispensary.

Guidelines for recommending cannabis for medical purposes

The Medical Board of California developed guidelines for those physicians who choose to recommend cannabis for medical purposes as part of their regular practice of medicine, so they would not be subject to investigation or disciplinary action [2]. Similar state medical boards with medical marijuana programs have compiled rules governing the approved use of cannabis under their jurisdiction. A consent form or medical cannabis agreement form is usually included in the state regulations. An example can be found on pages 105–107.

Physician-patient relationship

The patient and physician relationship is based on a collaborative effort and mutual understanding of shared responsibility for the patient's care [3]. The physician documents and attests to an appropriate relationship prior to recommendation and authorization of cannabis for only the patient but not other family members.

Patient evaluation

A documented medical examination and medical history must be obtained before an authorization of cannabis for medical purposes is given. The history should include past medical and surgical events, alcohol and substance use, family history of addiction, and psychotic or mental health disorders. A periodic review documented at least annually is recommended unless more frequent monitoring is warranted. Consideration needs to be made concerning drug–cannabis interactions that may interfere with drug dosing and effectiveness.

Informed and shared decision making

The recommendation to use cannabis should be a shared decision between the physician and the patient who discuss the risks and benefits of using cannabis. Patients need to be advised about cognitive changes that could affect driving, operation of heavy machinery, or any other hazardous activity. If the patient is a minor, the patient's parent or guardian needs to be informed of the risks and benefits along with full involvement in the treatment program.

Treatment agreement

A treatment plan with clear objectives needs to guide the therapy program. Measurable goals and objectives can be used to evaluate treatment progress such as relief of pain and improved physical or psychosocial function. Patients need to be advised of various cannabis preparations and dosing guidelines.

Physicians need to regularly access the patient's response to cannabis use and overall health. A review of cannabis quality and concentration of the dose is needed to ensure purchase from a licensed dispensary and should be included in the evaluation of treatment.

An "exit strategy" for discontinuing cannabis use should be included in the treatment plan in the event that termination of the cannabis becomes necessary.

Consultation and referrals

A patient with a history of substance use disorder or a mental health disorder may require specialized referral or consultation for pain management, addictive behavior monitoring, or mood disorder counseling.

Medical cannabis consent form

A medical cannabis consent form has been recommended to document the treatment plan discussed between the physician and patient. An example of a form follows [4].

Medical Cannabis Agreement

Date _____

I understand that _____ (clinician name) is helping me with the treatment of my medical illness.

In considering the possibility of using medical cannabis, it is important to recognize that the risks of medical cannabis may be impacted by specific medical conditions and patterns of use. I understand what has been explained to me, and I agree to the following conditions of treatment:

1. I understand that the course of treatment will be re-evaluated regularly after I begin treatment with medical cannabis.
2. I may be asked to reduce my intake of sedative-hypnotic medications to avoid excessive sedation due to the combined effects of cannabis and such drugs.
3. If I am beginning cannabis treatment for pain relief and have been taking opioids for pain, I will follow my doctor's advice on how to reduce the opioid dose so as to avoid experiencing opioid withdrawal symptoms.

4. I must prevent children and adolescents from gaining access to cannabis because of the potential harm to their well-being. I will store cannabis in locked cabinets to prevent anyone else from using it.

5. I recognize that some people cannot control their use of cannabis. One example is using cannabis for reasons other than for the indication for which it was prescribed; another is taking higher doses and doing so more frequently than my doctor recommended. I agree to discuss this with my healthcare provider if this happens to me.

6. Since the effects of cannabis on a fetus are uncertain, women may wish to abstain from cannabis if they become pregnant or are planning to become pregnant.

7. Because cannabis use has been associated with changes in heart rate and blood pressure, and there have been case reports linking heart attacks to cannabis use, I will review my heart health with my doctor to determine if taking cannabis is right for me.

8. Cannabis may not be right for me if I have had a serious mental illness (e.g., schizophrenia, mania, or history of hallucinations or delusions). I will discuss my mental health symptoms with my doctor prior to starting cannabis and report any of these symptoms to my doctor if they occur.

9. Because combining smoking tobacco with smoking cannabis may increase the risk of lung disease, I should avoid tobacco smoking if I take cannabis in smoked form.

10. I will not drive a car or operate heavy machinery while under the influence of cannabis. The issue of when it is safe to drive after cannabis ingestion is an area of uncertainty and can be affected by my experience with cannabis, the type of product that I am using, whether I am inhaling it or ingesting it, the dose and strength of the cannabis, among other things. After taking cannabis, I will wait until any impairing effects have subsided before driving or find alternatives to driving.

11. As the strength and potency of cannabis varies widely, I will use the minimum amount of cannabis needed to obtain relief from symptoms. I will follow my provider's guidance, which will likely include starting with a low dose and increasing it gradually to avoid unwanted side effects.

12. I might notice a withdrawal syndrome for two weeks if I stop cannabis abruptly. Trouble getting to sleep and angry outbursts might be a sign that I should lower the dose of cannabis gradually before stopping it completely. I should consult with my doctor if I experience such symptoms.

13. I will be mindful that use of medical cannabis in public places may place me in jeopardy with the law.

14. Despite the fact that I may be using medical cannabis under a doctor's supervision in a jurisdiction which permits this, my employer may have a different policy about cannabis use and drug testing. It is possible that I may be denied employment or lose my job as a result of an employer's policies if I use cannabis for medical reasons.

Signed: _____

References

1. D'Angelo JB. Cannabis as medicine: Redefining the paradigm of the doctor patient relationship. Available at www.slideshare.net/cannaholdings/cannabis-as-medicine-redefining-the-paradigm-of-the-doctorpatient-relationship.
2. Medical Board of California's Guidelines for the Recommendation of Cannabis for Medical Purposes. Nov 2017. BRD 18-1-9.
3. Fischer B, Jeffries V, Hall W et al. Lower risk cannabis use guidelines for Canada LRCUG: A narrative review of evidence and recommendations. *Can J Public Health*, 2011; 102: 324–327.
4. Wilsey B, Atkinson JH, Marcotte T, and Grant I. The medical cannabis treatment agreement: providing information to chronic pain patients through a written document. *Clinical J of Pain*, 2015; 31(12): 1087–1096.

chapter twelve

The clinical use of cannabinoid therapies in oncology patients

Paul J. Daeninck and Vincent Maida

Contents

Introduction

Patients with malignant diseases represent a cohort within healthcare that have some of the greatest unmet needs despite the availability of a plethora of guideline-driven disease-modulating treatments and pain and symptom management options [1,2]. Cannabinoid therapies are varied and versatile, and they are available as pharmaceuticals (Nabilone [Cesamet™], synthetic delta-9 THC [Marinol™], and THC/CBD extracts [Sativex™]), dried botanical material (marijuana), and edible organic oils infused with cannabis extracts. In some jurisdictions, edibles and topical preparations may also be offered as therapeutic modalities. Cannabinoid therapy regimens for specific patients may be personalized and involve combinations of all the aforementioned modalities. Patients with malignant disease, at all points of their disease trajectory, may be candidates for cannabinoids as supportive monotherapy or as adjuvants to other mainstream treatments. The most studied and established roles for cannabinoid therapies include pain, chemotherapy-induced nausea and vomiting (CINV), and anorexia. Moreover, given their breadth of activity, they may be used to concurrently optimize the management of multiple symptoms, thereby reducing overall polypharmacy. Cannabinoid therapy can also be effective in improving quality of life and malignancy control by direct effects as well as through improving compliance/adherence with disease modulating treatments such as chemotherapy and radiation therapy.

Access to medical cannabis in Canada

Canada is among a growing number of jurisdictions that have legalized access to cannabis for medical purposes [3]. Originally enacted in 2001, the Canadian regulations have undergone a number of revisions and updates that have been shaped by several key Supreme Court rulings [4]. The Access to Cannabis for Medical Purposes Regulations (ACMPR) from August 2016 contains a definition of medical cannabis that includes the dried product (marijuana), fresh buds and flowers, as well as extracts and derivatives such as cannabis infused oils, but as yet excludes edible products [5]. Furthermore, the ACMPR also permits qualifying patients to obtain live plant material or seeds for cultivation for their personal use [5]. The ACMPR further defines how cannabis is produced and marketed for sale to people with medical needs. To access cannabis through this program, patients need to be assessed by a physician or nurse practitioner, and if felt to have an appropriate condition or symptom, would be directed to apply to a licensed producer (LP). This entails applying to the producer in question via their Internet site (LPs are accessible virtually, no storefronts), as well as a medical authorization form completed by the practitioner. The latter includes the patient's name and address, where they were assessed, and how much cannabis product they can use on a daily basis. Patients are free to choose from a variety of strains, over 200 of which are registered by Health Canada and are only available from LPs [5]. The LPs are held to a high standard and are required to regularly submit samples to Health Canada-approved labs for quantifying their cannabinoid profile, as well as testing for heavy metals, microbial contaminants, and pesticide residues. Products that do not meet the standard are removed from the producer and destroyed [5].

Practitioners can approve a reasonable amount of product for daily use, up to the equivalent of 5 g of dried product (marijuana). Amounts beyond this limit are discouraged by both Health Canada and regulatory colleges [5–7], based on opinion as well as evidence [8]. The cannabis product, once ordered and purchased, is then delivered by secure courier to the patient's door or the practitioner's office.

Cannabinoids for pain and symptom management

Despite practice guidelines extolling the virtues of assessment and treatment of pain and other symptoms in those with advanced cancers [1] many patients still have poor symptom control [9]. This situation continues even with a plethora of available pharmaceutical therapies, including opioid analgesics and adjuvant or targeted therapies (e.g., antiepileptic, antidepressant, and N-methyl-D-aspartate receptor agonist therapies). Prior to 2014, patients with cancer-related symptoms made up 6 to 8% of those requesting medical cannabis in Canada [5], but this has increased rapidly with the initiation of the Marihuana for Medical Purposes Regulations (MMPR), enacted in April 2014 and then the transition to the Access to Cannabis for Medical Purposes Regulations (ACMPR). These numbers are expected to increase again, with the impending federal legalization and regulation of marijuana in Canada anticipated for July 2018 [10]. Other centers have also seen an increase in the number of cancer patients requesting or admitting to use of cannabis for medical purposes, given its increasingly widespread availability [11,12]. Many oncology physicians are unaware of the potential medical benefits of cannabis [13] and are unwilling or unable to authorize its use. This results in patients and caregivers seeking out illegal sources ("street marijuana"), which can be fraught with dangerously tainted products and potential social and emotional implications [14–18]. A review of the best supported treatments follows.

Pain

Herbal cannabis and extracts have been used for the treatment of pain for centuries [3]. There is evidence in historical texts and ancient pharmacopeia of treating different pain syndromes, from menstrual cramps to labor pains to headaches [3,19,20]. Indeed, Queen Victoria was thought to regularly use a tincture of cannabis for pain related to menses [19]. In terms of its use in the past 40 years, an emerging preclinical and clinical literature exists, such that systematic reviews are showing benefit in noncancer and cancer-related pain [21–23]. Early studies using pharmaceutical cannabinoids such as dronabinol, nabilone, and levonantradol demonstrated benefit, but methodologies were not as rigorous as more recent trials, so the benefits may have been overcalled [24]. The few trials using cannabinoids in acute pain have shown essentially no benefit and do not support its use in the postoperative setting [25–27].

Cannabinoid therapies for cancer pain have been studied in a few randomized trials, but the evidence has been less than convincing. Studies published earlier than 2000 (reviewed by Campbell et al., 2001 [24]) demonstrated mild benefits, with patients reporting dose-limiting adverse effects. Comparators such as codeine and secobarbital were employed, but these presently are not commonly used in patients with severe cancer pain, so extrapolation of these results is difficult. More recently, cannabis extracts (nabiximols) have been used in two placebo-controlled trials [28,29]. Patients with moderate-to-severe cancer pain were given nabiximols (THC and CBD in combination), THC alone, or placebo in addition to opioids and other adjuvant pain medications. Those receiving the THC/CBD combination demonstrated modest benefits with a minimum of dose-related adverse effects. A second trial using similar methodology but graded dosing demonstrated better pain control and improvement in sleep with the two lower-dosed patient groups (1–4 sprays and 6–10 sprays per day, respectively). Significant adverse events were again seen in the highest dosing group (>10 sprays per day) [29]. Interestingly, a recent report of those study patients continuing long-term nabiximols therapy demonstrated continued benefit without escalation of their cannabinoids or opioids [30]. These results support the use of cannabinoids as adjuvant agents for those with cancer pain proving to be resistant to opioids.

It is chronic neuropathic pain that has received the most research focus, with studies looking at the use of pharmaceutical cannabinoids, cannabis, and extracts in a variety of settings (post-traumatic neuropathies, diabetic neuropathy, AIDS-related neuropathic pain, etc. [23]). These conditions may co-exist in cancer patients or may be caused by the cancer or its treatment (chemotherapy-induced peripheral neuropathy [CIPN]). Indeed, cannabinoids have prevented CIPN when administered to animals subsequently exposed to paclitaxel, vincristine, or cisplatin [31–33]. Several recent systematic analyses have examined the use of cannabinoids in pain, including a wide-ranging review of the use of cannabinoids in several medical conditions [21–23]. The modest quality evidence supported their efficacy, found them to be safe to use in this setting, and were a reasonable option for treating chronic neuropathic pain. This evidence has contributed to the Canadian Pain Society revising their consensus statement to include cannabinoids as a third-line option in the treatment of chronic neuropathic pain [34]. Inhaled or vaporized cannabis has also been examined in patients with chronic neuropathic pain, although again, a paucity of randomized trials exists currently. A recently published meta-analysis postulated 1 in 5 to 6 patients would benefit from the use of inhaled cannabis treatments for neuropathic pain [35].

Nausea and vomiting

Controlling chemotherapy-induced nausea and vomiting (CINV) was one of the first reported studies in the modern literature of medical cannabinoid use. Sallan et al. in 1975 showed that use of oral Δ9-THC could control chemotherapy-induced nausea and almost eliminate emesis [36]. Since then, several larger scale studies, including placebo-controlled randomized trials, have employed dronabinol, nabilone, and cannabis extracts. Systematic reviews examining this topic support the use of pharmaceutical cannabinoids in patients undergoing chemotherapy [37–39]. However, most of these studies were performed prior to the emergence of 5-HT$_3$ antagonists and NK-1 antagonists, which are presently the standard of care [40]. Only one clinical double-blind placebo-controlled trial has compared dronabinol with current standard therapy (ondansetron alone and in combination with dexamethasone) [41]. The authors concluded that dronabinol alone was equally effective as ondansetron alone in treating both nausea and vomiting, but those receiving dronabinol had the lowest nausea scores using a visual analog scale. Interestingly, the dronabinol dose was only 50% of that used in previous trials, resulting in a low incidence of adverse effects [41]. Cannabinoids may be useful in those patients who do not get complete response to current evidence-based therapies and possibly for anticipatory nausea.

When looking at the use of cannabis (smoked or inhaled) or extracts for CINV, the picture is not quite as clear. There is some logic in the use of these products, as their route of administration (inhalation, sublingual, rectal) can bypass the oral route, which is impacted by CINV. In addition, the onset of benefit is faster with inhalation, and patients can self-titrate [37,42]. Most of the published studies to date are observational or uncontrolled, and no large-scale, randomized, controlled trials exist to guide the clinician [43–46]. Despite this, many patients will admit to the acquisition and use of some form of cannabis, either as a prechemotherapy treatment or after experiencing CINV [47,48]. Several share their experiences with others undergoing chemotherapy, resulting in a significant "underground" support system and results in a reduction in anxiety [48]. Given that up to 1 in 5 patients may discontinue their treatments due to poorly controlled nausea [49], cannabinoids may indeed help patients complete their regimens and maximizing their chemotherapy dose.

No study has yet shown benefit for the use of CBD alone in patients undergoing chemotherapy. A phase II study using nabiximols in combination with ondansetron did demonstrate benefit in preventing delayed nausea, but this product contains approximately 1:1 ratio of THC to CBD [50]. Preclinical research has established models for nausea (rats and shrews), and CBD has reduced nausea and vomiting in both of these animal models [42,51]. These models have been particularly useful in studying anticipatory nausea, a conditioned behavioral response to poorly controlled CINV, which can create difficulties for patients undergoing longer-term chemotherapy [42,51]. Cannabidiol, cannabidiolic acid (CBDA), and tetrahydrocannabinolic acid (THCA) have all reduced anticipatory nausea as well as acute nausea [42]. It appears from preclinical studies that CBDA may be as much as 100 to 1000 times more potent than CBD, which may lead to clinical trials of this cannabinoid in the future [42].

Radiotherapy involving specific body areas (abdomen, chest, whole brain) can induce nausea and vomiting (RINV), but very few reports of the use of cannabinoids to treat this condition are found in the literature. Those that are published mainly employ pharmaceutical cannabinoids [52]. A recently published placebo-controlled study demonstrated that global measurement of quality of life for patients undergoing radiotherapy for head and neck cancer is not improved nor worsened using nabilone [53]. Secondary measures of pain, appetite, weight gain, and nausea were also not impacted using nabilone. The authors postulated that nabilone on its own is not potent enough to have impact upon symptoms such as pain and nausea. A second recently published study of patients with previously treated head and neck cancer patients surveyed their use of medical cannabis. Fifteen respondents endorsed the use of cannabis (smoked, vaporized, or eaten) in the treatment of long-term residual effects of radiation, including pain, appetite, and weight maintenance [54].

Appetite stimulation

It is a well-told tale of people expressing a sudden craving for food after using marijuana ("the munchies") [55]. Preclinical research has demonstrated the importance of the endocannabinoid system in feeding, weight gain, and appetite regulation [42]. The data supporting cannabis and cannabinoid use in appetite stimulation in people with malignancy is less conclusive compared with that of pain or nausea. An early phase II study examined the use of dronabinol in cancer patients with anorexia, based on earlier studies of its use in CINV. Thirteen of 19 patients reported improvement in their appetite, but weight gain was not measured [56]. A placebo-controlled study from the North Central Cancer Trial Group compared the use of oral dronabinol to oral megestrol acetate and to a group of patients taking the two drugs together. Final results did not show any statistical improvement in appetite or weight gain with dronabinol, either alone or in combination with the megestrol acetate [57]. A later Swiss-led phase III randomized placebo-controlled trial using cannabis extracts versus dronabinol in cancer patients also did not show benefit in terms of appetite or weight gain and was closed early following a mandated review [58]. A small Canadian study using oral dronabinol in patients with advanced cancer demonstrated improved sense of taste and subsequent increased protein consumption. This did not translate to weight gain, but patients did express improvement in quality of life measurements [59]. Thus far, no good-quality studies regarding the use of smoked or vaporized cannabis for appetite in patients with cancer have been published [39].

More promising but not conclusive results were seen in studies using cannabis and cannabinoids in the noncancer population. A review of trials using cannabinoids to treat HIV wasting syndrome concluded that cannabinoids (smoked cannabis or dronabinol) showed some benefit in terms of weight gain [23]. A study in patients with probable Alzheimer's dementia treated with either dronabinol or placebo documented an increase in appetite, increased weight gain, and modulated aggressive behavior over a 12-week treatment course [76]. These results have not been repeated in subsequent trials [39] and should not be used as the current standard of care.

Cannabinoids as cancer therapy

Although people have been using cannabinoids for symptom management in patients with cancer, these compounds may also have a role in the treatment of malignancies. One of the first published reports of cannabinoids having antitumor effects demonstrated cannabis extracts could inhibit the growth of lung adenocarcinoma cells *in vitro* [61]. An *in vivo* model using cultured mouse cells showed similar findings. Several other types of malignancies demonstrating over expression of CB1 and CB2 receptors (lung, glioma, thyroid, lymphoma, skin, pancreas, endometrial, breast, prostate) [62–64] have been treated with cannabinoids in preclinical studies demonstrating a variety of effects including antiproliferation, prevention of cell transport (antimetastatic effects), antiangiogenesis, and proapoptotic effects (reviewed by Velasco and colleagues [65]).

Cannabis as a whole plant product has not been studied clinically as a treatment for malignancy. Unfortunately, many claims of the "curative" benefits of cannabis (fresh buds, dried cannabis, or oil products) can be found in the lay press, especially the Internet. These reports (mostly anonymously authored), extrapolate the results of preclinical work (employing cell culture or animal models) to humans without any basis in fact. There have been a handful of published case reports [66,67] documenting either prolongation of survival or reduction of cancer burden using cannabinoid products (no objective review of the products used), and curiously, in children. The only peer-reviewed and published clinical study (as of the date of writing) using cannabinoids in human cancer patients enrolled those with glioblastoma multiforme, based on extensive preclinical work done by the same group of investigators [68]. This small study (nine patients) demonstrated the safety of intracranial administration of delta-9 THC, and antiproliferative effects were shown in some of the patients. All patients eventually progressed and died but none due to the effects of the extract. These investigators are actively continuing their clinical and research work, spearheading the focus on CNS tumors [65]. A recently presented poster described the combined use of nabiximols with dose-intense temozolomide in patients with recurrent, previously treated glioblastoma multiforme. Twenty-one patients were enrolled (12 in the active arm, nine in placebo), and an increase in median survival was reported (369 days in the placebo group versus >550 days in the nabiximols treatment group). A significant increase in one-year survival was documented (83% in the CBD:THC group and 56% in placebo group, p = 0.042). Treatment related toxicities reported were dizziness (11/18 patients) and nausea (7/18 patients) [69].

Oncologists are always looking for improved treatments for malignancy. Clinical trials in oncology most often are evaluating and adding newer agents to established protocols to improve patient outcomes. Supportive therapies also must be at least neutral in their effects upon the cancer. Investigators have combined cannabis extracts with a variety of chemotherapy agents *in vitro* and in animal models, demonstrating synergism in reducing cell numbers and no negative impact upon anticancer function. Pancreatic [70], glioma [71], gastric [72], lung [73], and colon cell cultures [74] have been investigated using a range of antineoplastic agents (including gemcitabine, temozolomide, paclitaxel, and 5-fluorouracil). Synergism inducing cancer cell death is a common finding, which bodes well for future human clinical trials [65]. Anecdotal reports of patients who used cannabinoids with chemotherapy resulting in prolonged survival may be a signal of "clinical proof" of this concept [66,67].

Despite this emerging evidence of antineoplastic activity, some older *in vitro* studies demonstrate cancer cell proliferation and loss of immune-mediated cancer suppressor activity when treated with cannabinoid extracts [61,75]. Some studies have demonstrated discordant results with varying dose concentrations of cannabinoids: low doses stimulating cancer proliferation and higher doses demonstrating antineoplastic activity [65]. Thus, conflicting evidence points to the need for sober second thought before outright recommending cannabinoids for any and all cancer patients. To quote Dr. Donald Abrams:

> But again, mice and rats are not people, and what is observed *in vitro* does not necessarily translate into clinical medicine. The preclinical evidence that cannabinoids might have direct anticancer activity is provocative as well, but more research is warranted [13].

As of the date of writing, there are several clinical studies employing cannabinoids in cancer therapy registered at ClinicalTrials.gov. An Israeli group is studying the use of cannabis extracts (cannabidiol) to those patients whose cancers are resistant to the usual chemotherapy protocols (NCT02255292). Two more studies in the preliminary stages include the safety of dexanabinol in patients with advanced cancers (NCT01489826,

NCT02423239) and cannabis (high CBD concentration) for pain and inflammation in lung carcinomas (NCT02675842).

An interesting trial using cannabinoids for adjunctive therapy of graft-versus-host disease (GVHD) has recently been published [76]. Cannabidiol has demonstrated anti-inflammatory and immunosuppressive activity, and isolated extracts of CBD were used in adult patients (n = 48) who were at risk of developing GVHD after allogeneic stem cell transplantation for acute leukemia or myelodysplasia. Those patients given the standard treatment for GVHD prophylaxis as well as CBD 300 mg daily had a lower incidence of grade 2 to grade 4 GVHD compared to those using only the standard therapy. These results again argue for larger randomized controlled trials.

Cannabis and malignant wounds

The integumentary system may manifest both primary skin cancers as well as metastatic deposits from remote primary sites. Worldwide, primary skin cancers (basal cell, squamous cell, and melanoma) are the commonest form of malignancy, with basal cell cancers representing the bulk (79%) of all skin occurrences [77]. However, malignant wounds can be due to primary or metastatic disease, creating significant symptoms for patients, including pain, infection, unpleasant odor, and psychological distress [78]. Approximately 15% of advanced cancer patients referred for palliative care manifest malignant wounds requiring attention from the healthcare team [79].

The growing body of preclinical data demonstrating the anticancer potential of cannabinoids (THC and CBD) and noncannabinoid components of cannabis (especially the terpenes and flavonoids) holds particular promise for a potentiated and synergistic antineoplastic effect when applied upon malignant wounds [80,81]. It has been postulated that both terpenoids and flavonoids exert their antineoplastic actions by acting directly and indirectly upon CB1 and CB2 receptors [81–85].

Several people report benefit from the use of topical cannabis products in the lay press and on the Internet (e.g., use of balms, salves, and Phoenix Tears or Rick Simpson Oil). These reports have, unfortunately, not resulted in peer-reviewed publications but have sparked interest in the preclinical research on peripheral use in animal models [80,82]. A published case report from 2016 demonstrated both pain relief and tumor regression in a patient with advanced squamous cell carcinoma employing the topical application of cannabis extracts in an oil base [86]. The potential of cannabis extracts in oil to successfully manage wound-related pain was further reinforced by a case series of Pyoderma gangrenosum published in 2017 [87].

Topical therapies incorporating cannabis are being touted as a viable option for many conditions [88,89], albeit without objective evidence. There are U.S. patents issued for such preparations [90], and one would hope to see clinical trials in the near future.

Assessment of patients requesting cannabinoid therapy

When a patient is referred to the cancer center for outpatient therapy with a request for medical cannabis or cannabinoids, the medical team should entertain a series of questions:

Is this request for a medical symptom that can be treated using cannabinoids?

Is the patient being led to ask by another person or persons (could be for good intentions—family exploring alternative treatment options—or possibly diversion, sharing of cannabis for recreational purposes)?

Does the patient have any prior knowledge or experience with medical cannabis?

Is the patient appropriate for treatment with cannabinoids? Do they have other medical conditions that may be contraindications to therapy?

Many patients presenting to the clinic have either tried or read about medical cannabis and its role in symptom control. Some want to use it for the reported anti-neoplastic effects. Those who have tried it (recreationally or for medical purposes) can accurately reflect on the benefits or the adverse effects experienced, which makes the discussion somewhat more focused. Those who have little knowledge and less experience require a complete discussion as to the benefits, the possible adverse effects, the process of registering with an LP (Canadian context-see above), and the cost (which is borne by the patient in Canada, as it is not currently covered by provincial medical insurance). Contraindications to authorization are listed in Table 12.1, which are similar to those published by Health Canada

Table 12.1 Contraindications and precautions associated with high THC usage

Contraindications	Precautions
Age under 25	Driving motor vehicles
Pregnancy and lactation	Operating industrial equipment
Schizophrenia	Current use of sedative and hypnotics
Psychosis with recreational cannabis	Hypotension
Compromised cardiac status	Heavy tobacco smokers[a]
History of alcohol/substance abuse	Use of strong CYP 3A4 inhibitors[b]

[a] Risk of cannabis induced arteritis.
[b] Clarithromycin, ketoconazole, indinavir, lopinavir, ritonavir.

[91], the College of Family Physicians [6], and the Canadian Medical Protective Association [7].

It should be noted that no special license or additional certification is necessary in Canada to authorize the use of medical cannabis, but the more extensive the knowledge of the practitioner, the more educated the patient and family. This will always result in greater comfort with use, which will translate in the best clinical results for the individual. Alternatively, if the practitioner is not comfortable or has other reasons not to authorize, consultation with a local expert or a designated medical cannabis clinic (colloquially known as *"pot docs"*) may be necessary.

Once the decision is made to pursue medical cannabis as a complementary therapy, the choice of which product to use may be somewhat difficult. In Canada at the time of writing, there are more than 50 licensed producers listing hundreds of products for sale, which can be confusing and problematic for those who are inexperienced with cannabis or those who are elderly or excessively fatigued due to the malignancy or its treatment. We do not advise patients smoke dried cannabis products due to the potential for pulmonary damage [92] but rather vaporize or ingest, which are likely safer for patients in the long run [93]. At present, the use of cannabis extracts (in oil or capsules) are the desired treatment modality, as these are easy to measure and titrate to benefit, as well as having a longer duration of action. Since there are no published guidelines or dosage studies on the use of medical cannabis, the dictum "start low and go slow" should be employed. Starting doses of no more than 2.5 mg of THC or CBD (regardless of product format) should be used to minimize adverse events. Titration of dose should follow beneficial effects on the symptoms in question (e.g., pain reduction, nausea control). Those patients naïve to cannabis are directed to choose a product that has a balanced THC-to-CBD ratio (e.g., THC 5%: CBD 6% or THC 9%: CBD 9%). Cannabinoid proportions may be guided by available efficacy and research data summarized in Table 12.2. Once patients have started to use the product and document the outcomes, adjustment of the THC-to-CBD ratios and subsequent doses can meet their symptom needs. Follow-up with patients is essential to determine and document benefits, adverse effects, and patient questions about use or strain selection. Inquiring about outcomes can also give the team an idea as to patient benefit. For example, a patient with significant nausea may be able to tolerate increased oral intake or participate in social situations involving eating, which was not possible prior to the use of cannabis. Certainly, if the patient describes adverse effects that are not tolerable, then alternative therapy should be considered. If the desired symptom control is not achieved, then dose modification may be necessary. Discontinuation of cannabis should be considered if an adequate trial does not result in the desired outcome (or dose-limiting adverse effects) as determined by the treating team in discussion with the patient.

Table 12.2 Potential conditions responding to cannabinoid therapies [91–96]

Target Symptom	THC	CBD
Neuropathic pain	+++	+
CIPN[a]	++	?
CINV[b]	+++	Preclinical animal models
Anticipatory nausea	+	Preclinical animal models
Appetite stimulation	++	?
Spasticity/spasms	+++	+
Inflammation	+	++
Seizures	+	+++
Anxiety	+/−	Simulated situations
Depression	+ (adjuvant)	Preclinical models/case reports
Malignancy: Preclinical	++	++
Clinical	Early results in CNS tumors	?

[a] Chemotherapy-induced peripheral neuropathy.
[b] Chemotherapy-induced nausea/vomiting.

The importance of interprofessional collaboration

Interprofessional collaboration is a new paradigm, which has been embraced by modern healthcare systems [94]. Research has demonstrated that interprofessional collaboration is enabled and promoted by interprofessional education (IPE), especially at the undergraduate level [94,95]. Given the emergence of cannabinoids as a novel therapeutic class, cannabinoid education for medical professionals as well as patients and caregivers should be carried out by members of the interprofessional team as per the principles of IPE [95].

In the Canadian model, clinicians (physicians and nurse practitioners) ultimately authorize and prescribe cannabinoid therapies, but valuable insights and inputs about achieving optimal patient outcomes can be derived from other members of the healthcare team. These may include nursing, social workers, counselors, psychologists, rehabilitation therapists, dietitians, and pharmacists. Nurses often have first contact with patients and families expressing interest in medical cannabis. They can play a crucial role in education and advocacy regarding obtaining and using medical cannabis [96]. There are now formal nursing associations dedicated to the area of cannabis nursing, e.g., American Cannabis Nurses Association, which can support those working in oncology settings [96].

Pharmacists can play a central role in this process, as they have the training to assess and corroborate the appropriate and safe use of medical cannabinoids with the patient's present medications. They have access to the patient electronic medical records to facilitate medical reconciliation [97] and can access advanced database tools capable of assessing potential drug–drug interactions and cytochrome P-450 interactions, which may be particularly important for cancer patients undergoing chemotherapy [98,99]. Furthermore, pharmacies (in-hospital and community-based) are designed to ensure proper storage and security of controlled medications. Pharmacists are also well positioned to comprehensively counsel patients and caregivers on the optimal storage and disposal methods for opioids and by extension, cannabis products to limit diversion and unintentional exposure to other family members, including children [100]. Moreover, the development of institutional cannabis use policy will require input from many members of the team, often with pharmacists playing a leading role [101–103].

Cannabinoid therapies as a harm reduction strategy

This topic is addressed in more detail elsewhere in this book. Industrialized countries are experiencing exponential increases in the utilization of opioids [104,105]. This is generating major public health issues, especially related to drug diversion, opioid addiction, and death from opioid overdose [104,105]. Currently, opioids remain the mainstay of cancer pain management, meaning increased cancer survival and painful sequelae from cancer therapies translates into patients using opioids for longer periods of time [106]. High-dose and long-term opioid therapy in cancer patients is becoming a concern given the observed risks such as polyendocrinopathies, osteoporosis, and immunosuppression [107]. Preclinical studies have demonstrated that certain opioids such as codeine, morphine, methadone, and remifentanil may be associated with worsening of malignancies and infections [108]. Opioid-induced hyperalgesia syndrome is also being reported with increased incidence, especially in patients with advanced cancer and escalating pain [106]. Despite the widespread use of opioids, 50 to 80% of advanced cancer patients still die with unmet pain needs [109]. Thus, it behooves physicians to explore options that allow for improved overall pain relief while curbing the use of opioids. Observational studies in advanced cancer cohorts have demonstrated that cannabinoid therapies are associated with opioid sparing and improved analgesia [109,110]. A recent American study demonstrated that the death rate from accidental opioid overdoses has been reduced in those states where medical cannabis is legal [111]. Since medical cannabis generally tends to have a higher ratio of CBD to THC, it would be expected to be associated with a lower predilection to diversion, less addiction potential, and lower overall harm scores than recreational cannabis [112]. A further benefit for cancer patients, who have an element of compromised immunity, is a reliably safe and uncontaminated source of cannabis. There are several reports of fungal and other serious infections in those using cannabis from unsanctioned sources, resulting in serious morbidity and sometimes mortality [14,113–115]. Laboratory testing of cannabis products, produced using Good Agricultural Principles, can reduce the risk of exposure to pesticide and microbial contaminants [113]., and, as shown previously, cannabis products may have multiple uses for cancer patients, thus reducing their need for polypharmacy with its inherent safety benefits [116].

Summary and future directions

The integration of cannabinoid therapies within the domain of oncology, including palliative care, can result in improved healthcare outcomes for patients and economic savings for healthcare programs [116]. One could argue that medical use of cannabinoids could lead to greater safety for society, as better understanding and acceptance would reduce the illicit production and use [111,116]. Patient-reported outcomes of improvement in quality of life, especially for those undergoing intensive chemotherapy or radiation treatment regimens, may be key to patients continuing with life-saving/life-prolonging therapies. Cannabinoids can help cancer patients throughout their disease trajectory, but evidence is still lacking as to the ideal time for their initiation. Development of and enrollment of patients in well-designed clinical trials (such as those for children with seizure disorders) [117,118] will help answer many of these questions, which may increase support from the medical community as the public's acceptance of medical cannabis use broadens. Such research is necessary to guide oncology and palliative care teams in their pursuit of excellence in cancer and symptomatic care.

Acknowledgments

The authors wish to thank Anna Mann (librarian) and Sheena Pang (pharmacy resident) at the William Osler Health System in Toronto for their assistance with literature searches.

References

1. American Society of Medical Oncology (ASCO) Practice and Guidelines. http://www.asco.org/practice-guidelines/quality-guidelines/guidelines/supportive-care-and-treatment-related-issues. Accessed October 10, 2017.
2. National Comprehensive Cancer Network (NCCN) NCCN Guidelines® for Supportive Care. https://www.nccn.org/professionals/physician_gls/f_guidelines.asp#supportive. Accessed October 9, 2017.

3. Pertwee, R.G. *Handbook of Cannabis*. Oxford University Press, 2014. ISBN 978-0-19-966268-5.
4. Rudoi, D. and Priebe, S. The development of medical marihuana law in Canada and its effect on Michigan marihuana statutes. *Michigan State International Law Review*, 2017; 25: 335–373.
5. https://www.canada.ca/en/health-canada/topics/cannabis-for-medical-purposes.html. Accessed October 30, 2017.
6. College of Family Physicians of Canada. *Authorizing Dried Cannabis for Chronic Pain or Anxiety: Preliminary Guidance*. Mississauga, ON: College of Family Physicians of Canada, 2014.
7. Medical marijuana: Considerations for Canadian doctors. Published online: https://www.cmpa-acpm.ca/en/advice-publications/browse-articles/2014/medical-marijuana-new-regulations-new-college-guidance-for-canadian-doctors. Accessed November 9, 2017.
8. Hazekamp, A., Ware, M.A., Muller-Vahl, K.R., Abrams, D., and Grotenhermen, F. The medicinal use of cannabis and cannabinoids—An international cross-sectional survey on administration forms. *J Psychoactive Drugs*, 2013; 45: 199–210. doi: 10.1080/02791072.2013.805976.
9. Smith, T.J., Temin, S., Alesi, E.R. et al. American Society of Clinical Oncology provisional clinical opinion: The integration of palliative care into standard oncology care. *J Clin Oncol*, 2012; 30: 880–887. doi: 10.1200/JCO.2011.38.5161.
10. Bill C-45: Cannabis Act. An Act respecting cannabis and to amend the Controlled Drugs and Substances Act, the Criminal Code and other Acts. Sponsored by: Jody Wilson-Raybould, https://openparliament.ca/bills/42-1/C-45/. Accessed Oct 9, 2017.
11. Swift, W., Gates, P., and Dillon, P. Survey of Australians using cannabis for medical purposes. *Harm Reduction J*, 2005; 2: 18–28. doi: 10.1186/1477-7517-2-18.
12. Pergam, S.A., Woodfield, M.C., Lee, C.M. et al. Cannabis use among patients at a comprehensive cancer center in a state with legalized medicinal and recreational use. *Cancer*, 2017; 123: 4488–4497. doi: 10.1002/cncr.30879.
13. Abrams, D.I. Integrating cannabis into clinical cancer care. *Curr Oncol*, 2016; 23(S2): S8–S14. doi: http://dx.doi.org/10.3747/co.23.3099.
14. McLaren, J., Swift, W., Dillon, P., and Allsop, S. Cannabis potency and contamination: A review of the literature. *Addiction*, 2008; 103: 1100–09. doi: 10.1111/j.1360-0443.2008.02230.x.
15. Cescon, D.W., Page, A.V., Richardson, S. et al. Invasive pulmonary aspergillosis associated with marijuana use in a man with colorectal cancer. *J Clin Onc*, 2008; 26: 2214–2215. doi: 10.1200/JCO.2007.15.2777.
16. Bottorff, J.L., Bissell, L.J.L., Balneaves, L.G. et al. Perceptions of cannabis as a stigmatized medicine: A qualitative descriptive study. *Harm Reduction J*, 2013; 10: 2. doi: 10.1186/1477-7517-10-2.
17. Vandrey, R., Raber, J.C., Raber, M.E. et al. Cannabinoid dose and label accuracy in edible medical cannabis products. *J Amer Med Assn*, 2015; 313: 2491–2493.
18. Perrier, L. Why I chose to use cannabis. *Curr Oncol*, 2016; 23(S2): S7. doi: http://dx.doi.org/10.3747/co.23.3104.
19. Guy, G.W., Whittle, B.A., and Robson, P.J. *The Medicinal Uses of Cannabis and Cannabinoids*. Pharmaceutical Press, 2004. ISBN 0-85369-517-2.
20. Grotenhermen, F. and Russo, E. *Cannabis and Cannabinoids*. The Haworth Therapeutic Press, Binghampton, NY, 2002. ISBN 0-7890-1507-2.

21. Lynch, M. and Campbell, F. Cannabinoids for treatment of chronic, non-cancer pain; a systematic review of randomised trials. *Brit J Clin Pharmacol*, 2011; 72: 735–744.

22. Lynch, M. and Ware, M. Cannabinoids for the treatment of chronic non-cancer pain: An updated systematic review of randomized controlled trials. *J Neuroimmune Pharmcol*, 2015; 10(2): 293–301. doi: 10.1007/s11481-015-9600-6.

23. Whiting, P.F., Wolff, R.F., Deshpande, S. et al. Cannabinoids for medical use: A systematic review and meta-analysis. *JAMA*, 2015; 313: 2456–2473. doi: 10.1001/jama.2015.6358.

24. Campbell, F.A., Tramer, M.R., Carroll, D. et al. Are cannabinoids a safe and effective treatment option in the management of pain? A qualitative systematic review. *Brit Med J*, 2001; 323; 1–6. doi: 10.1136/bmj.323.7303.13.

25. Jain, A.K., Ryan, J.R., McMahon, F.G., and Smith, G. Evaluation of intramuscular levonantradol and placebo in acute postoperative pain. *J Clin Pharmacol*, 1981; 21: S320–S326.

26. Beaulieu, P. Effects of nabilone, a synthetic cannabinoid, on postoperative pain. *Can J Anaesthesiology*, 2006; 53: 769–775. doi: 10.1007/BF03022793.

27. Beaulieu, P., Boulanger, A., Desroches, J., and Clark, A.J. Medical cannabis: Considerations for the anesthesiologist and pain physician. *Can J Anesthesiology*, 2016; 63: 608–624. doi: 10.1007/s12630-016-0598-x.

28. Johnson, J.R., Burnell-Nugent, M., Lossignol, D. et al. Multicenter, double-blind, randomized, placebo-controlled, parallel-group study of the efficacy, safety, and tolerability of THC:CBD extract and THC extract in patients with intractable cancer-related pain. *J Pain Symptom Manage*, 2010; 39: 167–179.

29. Portenoy, R.K., Ganae-Motan, E.D., Allende, S. et al. Nabiximols for opioid-treated cancer patients with poorly-controlled chronic pain: A randomized, placebo-controlled, graded-dose trial. *J Pain*, 2012; 13: 438–449.

30. Johnson, J.R., Lossignol, D., Burnell-Nugent, M. et al. An open-label extension study to investigate the long-term safety and tolerability of THC/CBD oromucosal spray and oromucosal THC spray in patients with terminal cancer-related pain refractory to strong opioid analgesics. *J Pain Symptom Manage*, 2013; 46: 207–218.

31. Ward, S.J., McAllister, S.D., Kawamura, K. et al. Cannabidiol inhibits paclitaxel-induced neuropathic pain through 5-HT1A receptors without diminishing nervous system function or chemotherapy efficacy. *Brit J Pharmacol*, 2014; 171: 636–645.

32. Rahn, E.J., Makriyannis, A., and Hohmann, A.G. Activation of cannabinoid CB1 and CB2 receptors suppresses neuropathic nociception evoked by the chemotherapeutic agent vincristine in rats. *Br J Pharmacol*, 2007; 152: 765–777.

33. Khasabova, I.A., Khasabov, S., Paz, J. et al. Cannabinoid type-1 receptor reduces pain and neurotoxicity produced by chemotherapy. *J Neurosci*, 2012; 32: 7091–7101.

34. Moulin, D.E., Boulanger, A., Clark, A.J. et al. Consensus statement: Pharmacological management of chronic neuropathic pain: Revised consensus statement from the Canadian Pain Society. *Pain Research Manage*, 2014; 19: 328–335.

35. Andreae, M.H., Carter, G.M., Shaparin, N. et al. Inhaled cannabis for chronic neuropathic pain: A meta-analysis of individual patient data. *J Pain*, 2015; 16: 1221–1232.

36. Sallan, S.E., Zinberg, N.E., and Frei, E. Antiemetic effect of delta-9-tetrahydrocannabinol in patients receiving cancer chemotherapy. *New Engl J Med*, 1975; 293: 795–797.

37. Tramer, M.R., Carroll, D., Campbell, F.A. et al. Cannabinoids for control of chemotherapy induced nausea and vomiting: Quantitative systematic review. *Brit Med J*, 2001; 323: 16–21.

38. Machado Rocha, F.C., Stefano, S.C., De Cassia Haiek, R. et al. Therapeutic use of cannabis sativa on chemotherapy-induced nausea and vomiting among cancer patients: Systematic review and meta-analysis. *Eur J Cancer Care*, 2008; 17: 431–443.

39. National Academies of Sciences, Engineering, and Medicine. 2017. *The health effects of cannabis and cannabinoids: The current state of evidence and recommendations for research*. Washington, DC: The National Academies Press. doi: 10.17226/24625.

40. Hesketh, P.J., Kris, M.G., Basch, E. et al. Antiemetics: American Society of Clinical Oncology clinical practice guideline update. *J Clin Oncol*, 2017; 35: 3240–3261. https://doi.org/10.1200/JCO.2017.74.4789.

41. Meiri, E., Jhangiani, H., Vredenburgh, J.J. et al. Efficacy of dronabinol alone and in combination with ondansetron versus ondansetron alone for delayed chemotherapy-induced nausea and vomiting. *Curr Med Res Opin*, 2007; 23; 533–543.

42. Parker, L.A. *Cannabinoids and the Brain*. MIT Press, Boston, 2017. ISBN 978-0-262-03579-8.

43. Chang, A.E., Shiling, D.J., Stillman, R.C. et al. Delta-9-tetrahydrocannabinol as an antiemetic in cancer patients receiving high-dose methotrexate: A prospective, randomized evaluation. *Ann Intern Med*, 1979; 91: 819–824.

44. Musty, R.E. and Rossi, R. Effects of smoked cannabis and oral Δ9-tetrahydrocannabinol on nausea and emesis after cancer chemotherapy: A review of state clinical trials. *J Cannabis Therapeutics*, 2001; 1: 29–56.

45. Vinciguerra, V., Moore, T., and Brennan, E. Inhalation marijuana as an antiemetic for cancer chemotherapy. *N Y State J Med*, 1988; 88: 525–527.

46. Levitt, M., Faiman, C., Hawks, R., and Wilson, A. Randomized double blind comparison of delta-9-tetrahydro-cannabinol (THC) and marijuana as chemotherapy antiemetics. *Proc Amer Soc Clin Onc*, 1984; 3: 81.

47. Todaro, B. Cannabinoids in the treatment of chemotherapy-induced nausea and vomiting. *J Natl Compr Canc Network*, 2012; 10; 487–492.

48. Casarett, D. *Stoned: A Doctor's Case for Medical Marijuana*. Current Press, 2015. ISBN 978-1-59184-767-0.

49. Andrews, P.L. and Horn, C.C. Signals for nausea and emesis: Implications for models of upper gastrointestinal diseases. *Autonomic Neuroscience*, 2006; 125: 100–115.

50. Duran, M., Perez, E., Abanades, S. et al. Preliminary efficacy and safety of an oromucosal standardized cannabis extract in chemotherapy-induced nausea and vomiting. *Brit J Clin Pharmacol*, 2010; 70: 656–63.

51. Parker, L.A., Rock, E.M., and Limebeer, C.L. Regulation of nausea and vomiting by cannabinoids. *Brit J Pharmacol*, 2011; 163: 1411–1422.

52. Priestman, T.J. and Priestman, S.G. An initial evaluation of nabilone in the control of radiotherapy-induced nausea and vomiting. *Clinical Radiology*, 1984; 35: 265–266.

53. Côté, M., Trudel, M., Wang, C., and Fortin, A. Improving quality of life with nabilone during radiotherapy treatments for head and neck cancers: A randomized double-blind placebo-controlled trial. *Ann Otology, Rhinol & Laryngol*, 2016; 125; 317–324.

54. Elliott, D.A., Nabavizadeh, N., Romer, J.L., Chen, Y., and Holland, J.M. Medical marijuana use in head and neck squamous cell carcinoma patients treated with radiotherapy. *Support Care Cancer*, 2016; 24: 3517–3524. doi: 10.1007/s00520-016-3180-8.

55. Stromberg, J. *A scientific explanation of how marijuana causes the munchies.* https://www.smithsonianmag.com/science-nature/scientific-explanation-how-marijuana-causes-munchies-180949660/, Accessed October 15, 2017.

56. Nelson, K., Walsh, D., Deeter, P. et al. A phase II study of delta-9-tetrahydrocannabinol for appetite stimulation in cancer-associated anorexia. *J Palliat Care*, 1994; 10: 14–18.

57. Jatoi, A., Windschitl, H.E., Loprinzi, C.L. et al. Dronabinol versus megestrol acetate versus combination therapy for cancer-associated anorexia: A North Central Cancer Treatment Group study. *J Clin Oncol*, 2002; 20: 567–573.

58. Strasser, F., Luftner, D. et al. Cannabis-In-Cachexia-Study-Group. Comparison of orally administered cannabis extract and delta-9-tetrahydrocannabinol in treating patients with cancer-related anorexia-cachexia syndrome: A multicenter, phase III, randomized, double-blind, placebo-controlled clinical trial from the Cannabis-In-Cachexia-Study group. *J Clin Oncol*, 2006; 24: 3394–3400.

59. Brisbois, T.D., de Kock, I.H., Watanabe, S.M. et al. Delta-9-tetrahydrocannabinol may palliate altered chemosensory perception in cancer patients: Results of a randomized, double-blind, placebo-controlled pilot trial. *Ann Oncol*, 2011; 22: 2086–2093.

60. Volicer, L., Stelly, M., Morris, J., McLaughlin, J., and Volicer, B.J. Effects of dronabinol on anorexia and disturbed behavior in patients with Alzheimer's disease. *Intl J Geriatric Psych*, 1997; 12: 913–919.

61. Munson, A.E., Harris, L.A., Friedman, M.A., Dewey, W.L., and Carchman, R.A. Antineoplastic activity of cannabinoids. *J Natl Cancer Inst*, 1975; 55: 597–602.

62. Carracedo, A., Gironella, M., Lorente, M. et al. Cannabinoids induce apoptosis of pancreatic tumor cells via endoplasmic reticulum stress-related genes. *Cancer Res*, 2006; 66: 6748–6755.

63. Sarfaraz, S., Adhami, V.M., Syed, D.N., Afaq, F., and Mukhtar, H. Cannabinoids for cancer treatment: Progress and promise. *Cancer Res*, 2008; 68: 339–342.

64. Alexander, A., Smith, P.F., and Rosengren, R.J. Cannabinoids in the treatment of cancer. *Cancer Letters*, 2009; 285: 6–12.

65. Velasco, G., Sanchez, C., and Guzman, M. Anticancer mechanisms of cannabinoids. *Curr Oncol*, 2016; 23(S2): S23–S32.

66. Foroughi, M., Hendson, G., Sargent, M.A., and Steinbok, P. Spontaneous regression of septum pellucidum/forniceal pilocytic astrocytomas—Possible role of cannabis inhalation. *Childs Nerv Syst*, 2011; 27: 671–679. doi: 10.1007/s00381-011-1410-4.

67. Singh, Y. and Bali, C. Cannabis extract treatment for terminal acute lymphoblastic leukemia with a Philadelphia chromosome mutation. *Case Rep Oncol*, 2013; 6: 585–592. doi: 10.1159/000356446.

68. Guzman, M., Duarte, M.J., Blazquez, C. et al. A pilot clinical study of delta 9-tetrahydrocannabinol in patients with recurrent glioblastoma multiforme. *Br J Cancer*, 2006; 95: 197–203.
69. Twelves, C., Short, S., and Wright, S. A two-part safety and exploratory efficacy randomized double-blind, placebo-controlled study of a 1:1 ratio of the cannabinoids cannabidiol and delta-9-tetrahydrocannabinol (CBD:THC) plus dose-intense temozolomide in patients with recurrent glioblastoma multiforme (GBM). *J Clin Oncol*, 2017; 35: (suppl; abstr 2046).
70. Donadelli, M., Dando, I., Zaniboni, T. et al. Gemcitabine/cannabinoid combination triggers autophagy in pancreatic cancer cells through a ROS-mediated mechanism. *Cell Death Dis*, 2011; 2: e152.
71. Torres, S., Lorente, M., Rodriguez-Fornes, F. et al. A combined preclinical therapy of cannabinoids and temozolomide against glioma. *Mol Cancer Ther*, 2011; 10: 90–103.
72. Miyato, H., Kitayama, J., Yamashita, H. et al. Pharmacological synergism between cannabinoids and paclitaxel in gastric cancer cell lines. *J Surg Res*, 2009; 155: 40–47.
73. Preet, A., Qamri, Z., Nasser, M.W. et al. Cannabinoid receptors, CB1 and CB2, as novel targets for inhibition of non–small cell lung cancer growth and metastasis. *Cancer Prev Res*, 2010; 4: 65–75. doi: 10.1158/1940-6207.CAPR-10-0181.
74. Gustafsson, S.B., Lindgren, T., Jonsson, M. et al. Cannabinoid receptor-independent cytotoxic effects of cannabinoids in human colorectal carcinoma cells: Synergism with 5-fluorouracil. *Cancer Chemother Pharmacol*, 2009; 63: 691–701.
75. Preet, A., Ganju, R.K., and Groopman, J.E. D(9)-tetrahydrocannabinol inhibits epithelial growth factor-induced lung cancer cell migration in vitro as well as its growth and metastasis in vivo. *Oncogene*, 2008; 27: 339–46.
76. Yeshurun, M., Shpilberg, O., Herscovici, C. et al. Cannabidiol for the prevention of graft-versus-host-disease after allogeneic hematopoietic cell transplantation: Results of a phase II study. *Biol Blood Marrow Transplant*, 2015; 21: 1770–1775. doi: http://dx.doi.org/10.1016/j.bbmt.2015.05.018.
77. Cancer Facts and Figures, 2017. American Cancer Society. http://ww.cancer.org/acs/groups/content/@editorial/documents/document/acspc-048738.pdf. Accessed November 5, 2017.
78. Maida, V., Ennis, M., Kuziemsky, C., and Trozzolo, L. Symptoms associated with malignant wounds: A prospective case series. *J Pain Symptom Manage*, 2009; 37: 206–211. doi: 10.1016/j.jpainsymman.2008.01.009.
79. Maida, V., Corbo, M., Irani, S., Dolzhykov, M., and Tozzolo, L. Wounds in advanced illness: A prevalence and incidence study based on a prospective case series. *Int Wound Journal*, 2008; 5: 305–314.
80. Casanova, M.L., Blazquez, C., Martinez-Palacio, J. et al. Inhibition of skin tumor growth and angiogenesis in vivo by activation of cannabinoid receptors. *J Clin Invest*, 2003; 111: 43–50.
81. Oddi, S. and Maccarrone, M. Endocannabinoids and skin barrier function: Molecular pathways and therapeutic opportunities. In Wondrak, G.T. (ed). *Skin Stress Response Pathways, 301-323.* Springer International, Switzerland, 2016 ISBN 978-3-319-43155-0.
82. Blázquez, C., Carracedo, A., Barrado, L. et al. Cannabinoid receptors as novel targets for the treatment of melanoma. *FASEB J*, 2006; 20: 2633–2635. doi: 10.1096/fj.06-6638fje.

83. Ständer, S., Schmelz, M., Metze, D., Luger, T., and Rukwied, R. Distribution of cannabinoid receptor 1 (CB1) and 2 (CB2) on sensory nerve fibers and adnexal structures in human skin. *J Dermatol Sci*, 2005; 38; 177–188.

84. Huang, M., Lu, J.J., Huang, M.Q., Bao, J.L., Chen, X.P., and Wang, Y.T. Terpenoids: Natural products for cancer therapy. *Expert Opin Invest Drugs*, 2012; 21: 1801–1818.

85. Batra, P. and Sharma, A.K. Anti-cancer potential of flavonoids: Recent trends and future perspectives. *Biotech*, 2013; 3: 439–459.

86. Maida, V. Medical cannabis in the palliation of malignant wounds—A case report. *J Pain Symptom Manage*, 2017; 53: e4–e6. doi: 10.1016/j.jpainsymman.2016.09.003.

87. Maida, V. and Corban, J. Topical medical cannabis: A new treatment for wound pain—Three cases of Pyoderma gangrenosum. *J Pain Symptom Manage*, 2017; 54; 732–736. doi: 10.1016/j.jpainsymman.2017.06.005.

88. http://www.cannabiscure.info/. Accessed November 7, 2017.

89. http://www.cannalifebotanicals.ca/product/cannabis-salve/?age-verified=15508520f6. Accessed November 7, 2017.

90. Composition of cannabinoids, odorous volatile compounds, and emu oil for topical application, and a method for cannabinoid transdermal delivery. US 9526752 B1. https://www.google.com/patents/US9526752. Accessed November 7, 2017.

91. Consumer Information-Cannabis. Published online: http://www.hc-sc.gc.ca/dhp-mps/alt_formats/pdf/marihuana/info/cons-eng.pdf. Accessed November 6, 2017.

92. Ribeiro, L.I.G. and Ind, P.W. Effect of cannabis smoking on lung function and respiratory symptoms: A structured literature review. *Primary Care Resp Med*, 2016: 26: 16071. doi: 10.1038/npjpcrm.2016.71.

93. Solowij, N., Broyd, S.J., van Hell, H.H., and Hazekamp, A. A protocol for the delivery of cannabidiol (CBD) and combined CBD and Δ 9-tetrahydrocannabinol (THC) by vaporisation. *BMC Pharmacology and Toxicology*, 2014, 15: 58. doi: http://www.biomedcentral.com/2050-6511/15/58.

94. Zwarenstein, M., Goldman, J., and Reeves, S. Interprofessional collaboration: Effects of practice-based interventions on professional practice and outcomes. *Cochrane Database Syst Rev*, 2009 Jul; 8(3): CD000072. doi: 10.1002/14651858. CD000072.pub2.

95. Reeves, S., Perrier, L., Goldman, J., Freeth, D., and Zwarenstein, M. Interprofessional education: Effects on professional practice and healthcare outcomes (update). *Cochrane Database Syst Rev*. 2013 Mar; 28(3): CD002213. doi: 10.1002/14651858.CD002213.pub3.

96. Sheldon, L.K. Cannabis guidelines. *Clin J Onc Nurs*, 2017; 21: 409. doi: 10.1188/17.CJON.409.

97. Karnon, J., Campbell, F., and Czoski-Murray, C. Model-based cost-effectiveness analysis of interventions aimed at preventing medication error at hospital admission (medicines reconciliation). *J Eval Clin Practice*, 2009; 15: 299–306.

98. Seamon, M.J. Fass, J.A., Maniscalco-Feichtl, M., and Abu-Shraie, N.A. Medical marijuana and the developing role of the pharmacist. *Am J Health-Syst Pharm*, 2007; 64: 1037–1044.

99. Isaac, S., Saini, B., and Charr, B.B. The role of medicinal cannabis in clinical therapy: Pharmacists perspectives. *PLoS ONE*; 11(5): e0155113. doi: 10.1371/journal.pone.0155113.

100. Sznitman, S.R., Goldberg, V., Sheinman-Yuffe, H., Fletcher, E., and Bar-Sela, G. Storage and disposal of medical cannabis among patients with cancer: Assessing the risk of diversion and unintentional digestion. *Cancer*, 2016; 122: 3363–3370. doi: 10.1002/cncr.30185.

101. Durkin, M. Medical marijuana…in the hospital? *ACP Hospitalist*, January 2017. https://acphospitalist.org/archives/2017/01/marijuana-policies-hospital. htm. Accessed November 9, 2017.

102. Braun, I. and Nibati, L. Developing institutional medical marijuana guidelines: Understanding law and science (abstract). *J Pain Symptom Manage*, 2016; 51: 396–397, SA524.

103. Saskatoon Health Region, Policy 7311-60-032, Medical Marijuana. https://www.saskatoonhealthregion.ca/about/RWPolicies/7311-60-032.pdf. Accessed November 9, 2017.

104. Kuo, Y.F., Raji, M.A., Chen, N.W., Hasan, H., and Goodwin, J.S. Trends in opioid prescriptions among Part D Medicare recipients from 2007 to 2012. *Am J Med*, 2016; 129: 221.e21–221e30. doi: 10.1016/j.amjmed.2015.10.002.

105. Mehendale, A.W., Goldman, M.P., and Mehendale, R.P. Opioid overuse syndrome (OOPS): The story of opioids, Prometheus unbound. *J Opioid Manage*, 2013; 9: 421–438.

106. Carmona-Bayonas, A., Jiminez-Fonseca, P., Castanon, E. et al. Chronic opioid therapy in long-term cancer survivors. *Clin Transl Oncol*, 2017; 19: 236–250, doi: 10.1007/s12094-016-1529-6.

107. Owens, M.R., Simmons, B., Gibson, P.S., and Weeks, D. A longitudinal study of pain in hospice and pre-hospice patients. *Am J Hospice Palliat Care*, 2001; 18: 124–128.

108. Sacerdote, P. Opioids and the immune system. *Pall Med*, 2006 (Suppl 1); 20: s9–s15.

109. Maida, V., Ennis, M., Irani, S., Corbo, M., and Dolzhykov, M. Adjunctive nabilone in cancer pain and symptom management: A prospective observational study using propensity scoring. *J Support Onc*, 2008; 6: 119–124.

110. Cudmore, J. and Daeninck, P.J. Use of medical cannabis to reduce pain and improve quality of life in cancer patients. *J Clin Oncol*, 2015; 33: 29s (suppl; abstr 198).

111. Bachhuber, M.A., Saloner, B., Cunningham, C.O., and Barry, C.L. Medical cannabis laws and opioid analgesic overdose mortality in the United States, 1999–2010. *JAMA*, Oct 2014; 174: 1668–1673.

112. Collen, M. Prescribing cannabis for harm reduction. *Harm Reduction Journal*, 2012; 29: 1. doi: 10.1186/1477-7517-9-1.

113. Thompson, G.R., Tuscano, J.M., Dennis, M. et al. A microbiome assessment of medical marijuana. *Clin Microbiol Infection*, 2017; 23; 269–270. doi: 10.1016/j.cmi.2016.12.001.

114. Ruchlemer, R., Amit-Kohn, M., Raveh, D., and Hanuš, L. Inhaled medicinal cannabis and the immunocompromised patient. *Support Care Cancer*, 2015; 23: 819–822. doi: 10.1007/s00520-014-2429-3.

115. Babu, T.M., Griswold, M.K., Urban, M.A., and Babu, K.M. Aspergillosis presenting as multiple pulmonary nodules in an immunocompetent cannabis user. *J Toxicol Pharmacol*, 2017; 1: 004.

116. Bradford, A.C. and Bradford, W.D. Medical marijuana laws reduce prescription medication use in Medicare Part D. *Health Affairs*, 2016; 35: 1230–1236. doi: 10.1377/hlthaff.2015.1661.

117. Devinsky, O., Marsh, E., Friedman, D. et al. Cannabidiol in patients with treatment-resistant epilepsy: An open-label interventional trial. *Lancet Neurol*, 2016; 15: 270–278. doi: 10.1016/S1474-4422(15)00379-8.
118. Devinsky, O., Cross, J.H., Laux, L. et al. Trial of cannabidiol for drug-resistant seizures in the Dravet syndrome. *New Engl J Med*, 2017; 376: 2011–2020. doi: 10.1056/NEJMoa1611618.

chapter thirteen

Clinical rationale for CBD in cardiovascular, brain, and liver function and optimal aging

Betty Wedman-St. Louis

Contents

On October 7, 2003, the U.S. Patent Office issued Patent No.: US 6,630,507 B1 for cannabinoids as antioxidants and neuroprotectants [1]. Booz elaborates on the use of cannabidiol (CBD) for reducing inflammation due to oxidative stress in pain, diabetic complications, hypertension, ischemia reperfusion injury, depression, neurodegenerative diseases, obesity, and atherosclerosis [2]. Renewed interest in CBD post its discovery as an antioxidant, anti-inflammatory, and neuroprotective compound has resulted in new learning about CB1 and CB2 receptors for treatment of a growing list of diseases.

Cannabidiol has been shown to be more protective than either alpha-tocopherol or vitamin C in an *in vitro* model [3]. According to Booz, the therapeutic antioxidant properties of CBD are not based on its chemistry alone but its ability to modulate cell signaling that underlies the inflammatory process [4].

Oxidative stress

Oxidative stress is an imbalance between the production of free radicals and the human body's ability to detoxify their harmful effects through the use of antioxidants. Without repair of the damage done by the free radicals, injury or stress to cells, mitochondria, and DNA occurs. Every day oxidation occurs when cells use glucose for energy or when the immune system is responding to a bacterial infection, but when the body is physically and/or emotionally stressed, the number of free radicals can exceed the antioxidant level available, resulting in damage to cells, proteins, and genes.

The accumulative damage done by free radicals inadequately neutralized by antioxidants can result in neurological disorders such as anxiety, depression, addiction, and pain. Cannabidiol may have a therapeutic value despite only a small number of clinical studies currently reported [5].

Mode of action

Cannabinoid receptors play a vital role in the body, but cannabidiol (CBD) has little affinity for either of the cannabinoid receptors: CB1 and CB2. The CB1 receptors are primarily located in the brain (hippocampus, cerebellum, and cerebrum), while CB2 receptors are throughout the body (spleen, tonsillar, and immune cells). Instead, CBD activates noncannabinoid receptors and ion channels by delaying the reuptake of endogenous neurotransmitters (anandamide and adenosine) and by enhancing or inhibiting the binding action of certain G-coupled protein receptors. Further research is needed to validate this neuroprotective activity [5].

Thomas et al. [6] further elaborates that cannabidiol has low affinity for both CB1 and CB2 receptors in a mouse model. Its ability in induce CB2 receptor inverse agonism may contribute to the anti-inflammatory properties of CBD.

CBD may also act via serotonin (5-HT) receptors according to Russo et al. [7]. The 5-HT 1A (hydroxytryptamine) receptor is coupled to G-protein where it is implicated in numerous biological and neurological processes such as anxiety, addiction, appetite, sleep, pain, nausea, and vomiting [8–10].

Vanilloid receptors known as TRPV1, which were named for the vanilla bean, respond to CBD as a stimulant or agonist to function in pain perception and inflammation [11]. Capsaicin, the pungent compound in hot chili peppers, also activates the TYP1 receptor.

Peroxisome proliferation activated receptors (PPARs) that are on the cell nucleus surface can be activated by CBD to exert an anticancer effect. This antiproliferation effect and tumor cell regression activity indicate CBD can inhibit tumor cell viability according to Ramer et al. [12]. PPAR-gamma activation degrades amyloid-beta plaque, a key molecule linked to Alzheimer's disease development, so CBD may be a useful therapeutic intervention in controlling the disease [13–15].

Cannabidiol's anti-inflammatory and antianxiety effects are attributed to its inhibition of adenosine reuptake in the cell. CBD competes with endogenous endocannabinoids, which are fatty acids for the transport of anandamide into the cell. Once inside the cell, anandamide is broken down by fatty acid amide hydrolase (FAAH), but CBD slows down this process. Thereby, the endocannabinoid levels in the brain's synapses are raised, which reduces seizure activity and provides other health benefits [16].

Studies have shown that cannabidiol directly activates 5-HT1A and TRPV, while other research indicates CBD functions as an antagonist by blocking/deactivating G-protein receptor GPR 55 found in the brain cerebellum. GPR 55 modulates blood pressure, bone density, and cancer cell proliferation [17,18].

Neuroprotective properties

As a neuroprotectant, CBD helps reduce damage to the brain and nervous system while encouraging new neuron development. Oxidative stress from numerous disorders can lead to neuronal damage, but studies have shown that CBD can protect against damage and improve recovery [19–23] in:

- Ischemia
- Traumatic brain injuries
- Hepatic stellate cell death
- Hepatitis C virus
- Ventricular arrhythmias and infarct
- Diabetes complications
- Elevated blood pressure
- Lipolysis

Potential addiction treatment

Drug rehabilitation is the process of medical and psychological treatment for dependency on psychoactive substances from alcohol, cocaine, heroin, and amphetamines to cigarettes and food. Addiction is considered a brain disorder because of the effect the drug makes on the brain neurons by targeting the brain's reward system with increased dopamine that regulates movement, emotion, cognition, motivation, and feelings of pleasure. Overstimulation with dopamine produces the euphoric effect that leads to repeat behavior.

Cannabinoids derived from the marijuana plant have potential for therapeutic benefits according to Hurd et al. [24]. While delta-9-tetracannabinol is known to hence reward stimulation, CBD appears to inhibit drug-seeking behavior and may assist as a treatment option with drug addiction. Cannabidiol has also been shown to reduce the number of cigarettes smoked during treatment [25].

Safety and use in clinical practice

Cannabidiol is the nonpsychoactive component of Cannabis sativa and constitutes up to 40% of the extracts of the plant [26]. CBD concentrations vary based on growing conditions, species phenotype, and the part of the plant that is analyzed [27]. Human studies reported by Bergamaschi et al. [28] for chronic oral administration of 10 mg CBD for 21 days did not induce any clinical or neurological changes. Epileptic patients tolerated 200–300 mg daily of CBD for 135 days with no signs of toxicity or side effects detected on physical and neurological exams.

Consroe et al. [29] obtained plasma levels of cannabidiol in 14 Huntington's disease patients in a trial of oral CBD (10 mg/kg/day = about 700 mg/day) for six weeks. Mean plasma levels of CBD ranged from 5.9–11.2 ng/mL over the six weeks, with CBD levels averaging 1.5 ng/mL one week after CBD was discontinued. The half-life of CBD was estimated to be two to five days with no difference in genders.

Cannabidiol was tolerated in a multiphase study of healthy volunteers and epileptic patients who received a dose of 3 mg/kg daily for 30 days. No signs of toxicity or serious side effects were noted [30].

Gallily et al. [31] reviewed the dose range for CBD's effectiveness in animal and human studies and concluded that CBD in the presence of other plant constituents improved dose-response, especially for inflammatory conditions.

Side effects of CBD

CBD has a few side effects that need to be reviewed with patients along with consideration of other medications they may be taking. According to Consroe et al. [32], side effects of CBD were mild and included hypotension, dry mouth, psychomotor slowing, lightheadedness, and sedation on an oral dose increasing from 100 to 600 mg/day over a six-week period in a preliminary open pilot study of movement disorder patients.

Induction of human CYP 1A1 expression by CBD has been reported, which could affect hepatic drug metabolism requiring cytochrome P450. High doses of CBD could neutralize the P450 enzymes and alter effectiveness similar to eating/drinking grapefruit [33,34]. The cytochrome P450 enzymes include about a dozen enzymes belonging to the CYP 1, 2, and 3 family that are responsible for biotransformation of 70%–80% of all drugs in clinical use [35]. Genetics, epigenetics, and dose needs to be considered when using CBD with patients on multiple medications that require P450 enzymes.

References

1. Hampson, A.J., Axelrod, J., and Grimaldi, M. Cannabinoids as antioxidants and neuroprotectants. US 6,630,507 B1. October 7, 2003. U.S. Department of Health and Human Services, Washington, DC.
2. Booz, G.W. Cannabidiol as an emergent therapeutic strategy for lessening the impact of inflammation on oxidative stress. *Free Radic Biol Med*, 2011; 51(5): 1054–1061.
3. Hampson, A.J., Grimaldi, M., Lolic, M. et al. Neuroprotective antioxidants from marijuana. *Ann NY Acad Sci*, 2000; 899: 274–282.
4. Booz, G.W. Cannabidiol as an emergent therapeutic strategy for lessening the impact of inflammation on oxidative stress. *Free Radic Biol Med*, 2011; 51(5): 1054–1061.
5. Bih, C.I., Chen, T., Nunn, A.V.M. et al. Molecular targets of cannabidiol in neurological disorders. *Neurotherapeutics*, 2015; 12(4): 699–730.
6. Thomas, A., Baillie, G.L. et al. Cannabidiol displays unexpectedly high potency as an antagonist of CB1 and CB2 receptor agonists *in vitro. Br J Pharmacol* 2007; 150(5): 613–623.
7. Russo, E.B., Burnett, A., Hall, B. et al. Agonistic properties of cannabidiol at 5-HT 1a receptors. *Neurochem Res*, 2005; 30: 1037–1043.
8. Soares, V. deP., Campos, A.C., Bortoli, V.C. de et al. Intra-dorsal periaqueductal gray administration of cannabidiol blocks panic-like response by activating 5-HT 1A receptors. *Behav Brain Res*, 2010; 213: 225–229.
9. Yang, K.-H., Galadari, S. et al. The non-psychoactive cannabinoid cannabidiol inhibits 5-hydroxytryptamine 3 A receptor-mediated currents in Xenopus laevis oocytes. *J Pharm Exp Ther*, 2010; 333: 547–554.
10. Zanelati, T.V., Biojone, E. et al. Antidepressant-like effects of cannabidiol in mice: Possible involvement of 5-HT 1A receptors. *Br J Pharmacol*, 2010; 159: 122–128.
11. Iannotti, F.A., Hill, C.L., Leo, A. et al. Nonpsychotropic plant cannabinoids, cannabidivarin (CBDV) and cannabidiol (CBD), activate and desensitize transient receptor potential vanilloid 1 (TRPV 1) channels *in vitro*: Potential for the treatment of neuronal hyperexcitability. *ACS Chem Neurosci*, 2014; 5: 1131–1141.
12. Ramer, R., Heinemann, K. et al. COX-2 and PPAR-γ confer cannabidiol-induced apoptosis of human lung cancer cells. *Mol Cancer Ther*, 2013; 12: 69–82.
13. Hsieh, H.-L., and Yang, C.-M. Role of redox signaling in neuroinflammation and neurodegenerative diseases. *Biomed Res Int*, 2013; 2013: 484–613.
14. Sosa-Ortiz, L., Acosta-Castillo, I., and Prince, M.J. Epidemiology of dementia and Alzheimer's disease. *Arch Med Res*, 2012; 43: 600–608.
15. Hardy, J.A. and Higgins, G.A. Alzheimer's disease: Amyloid cascade hypothesis. *Science*, 1992; 256: 184–185.
16. Di Marzo, V., Fontane, A., Cadas, H. et al. Formation and inactivation of endogenous cannabinoid anandamide in central neurons. *Nature*, 1994; 372: 686–691.

17. Whyte, L.S., Ryberg, E., Simss, N.A. et al. The putative cannabinoid receptor GPR55 affects osteoclast function *in vitro* and bone mass *in vivo*. *Proc Natl Acad Sci USA*, 2009; 106(38): 16511–16516.

18. Ford, L.A., Roelofs, A.J., Anavi-Goffer, S. et al. A role for L-α-lysophosphatidylinositol and GPR 55 in the modulation of migration, orientation and polarisation of human breast cancer cells. *Brit J Pharmacol*, 2010; 160: 762–771.

19. Pazo, M.R., Mohammed, N., Lafuente, H. et al. Mechanisms of cannabidiol neuroprotection in hypoxic-ischemic newborn pigs: Role of 5-HT 1A and CB2 receptors. *Neuropharmacology*, 2013; 71: 282–291.

20. Liput, D.J., Hammell, D.C. et al. Transdermal delivery of cannabidiol attenuates binge alcohol-induced neurodegeneration in a rodent model of an alcohol use disorder. *Pharmacol Biochem Behav*, 2013; 111: 120–127.

21. Lim, M.P., Devi, L.A., and Rozenfield, R. Cannabidiol causes activated hepatic stellate cell death through a mechanism of endoplasmic reticulum stress-induced apoptosis. *Cell Death Dis*, 2011; e170.

22. Lowe, H.I., Toyang, N.J., and McLaughlin, W. Potential of cannabidiol for the treatment of viral hepatitis. *Pharmcognosy Res*, 2017; 9(1): 116–118.

23. England, T.J., Hind, W.H. et al. Cannabinoids in experimental stroke: a systemic review and meta-analysis. *J Cerb Blood Flow Metab*, 2015; 35(3): 348–358.

24. Hurd, Y.L., Yoon, M., Manini, A.F. et al. Early phase in the development of cannabidiol as a treatment for addiction: Opioid relapse takes initial center stage. *Neurotherapeutics*, 2015; 12(4): 807–815.

25. Morgan, C.J., Das, R.K., Joye, A. et al. Cannabidiol reduces cigarette consumption in tobacco smokers: preliminary findings. *Addict Behav*, 2013; 38(9): 2433–2436.

26. Grlie, A. A comparative study on some chemical and biological characteristics of various samples of cannabis resin. *Bull Narcot*, 1976; 14: 37–46.

27. Mehmedic, Z., Chandra, S., Slade, D. et al. Potency trends of Δ9-THC and other cannabinoids in confiscated cannabis preparations from 1993 to 2008. *J Forsenic Sci*, 2010; 55: 1209–1217.

28. Bergamaschi, M.M., Queiroz, R.H.C., Crippa, J.A.S., and Zuardi, A.W. Safety and side effects of cannabidiol, a cannabis sativa constituent. *Current Drug Safety*, 2011; 6(4): 237–249.

29. Consroe, P., Kennedy, K., and Schram, K. Assay of plasma cannabidiol by capillary gas chromatography/ion trap mass spectroscopy following high-dose repeated daily oral administration in humans. *Pharmacology Biochemistry and Behaviour*, 1991; 40(3): 517–522.

30. Cunha, J.M., Carlini, E.A., Pereira, A.E. et al. Chronic administration of cannabidiol to healthy volunteers and epileptic patients. *Pharmacology*, 1980; 21(3): 175–185.

31. Gallily, R., Yekhtin, Z., and Hanus, L.O. Overcoming the bell-shaped dose-response of cannabidiol by using cannabis extract enriched in cannabidiol. *Pharmacology & Pharmacy*, 2015; 6: 75–85.

32. Consroe, P., Sandyk, R., and Snider, S.R. Open label evaluation of cannabidiol in dystonic movement disorders. *Int J Neurosci*, 1986; 30(4): 277–284.

33. Yamaori, S., Kinugasa, Y., Jiang, R. et al. Cannabidiol induces expression of human cytochrome P450 1A1 that is possibly mediated through aryl hydrocarbon receptor signaling in Hep G2 cells. *Life Sci*, 2015; 136: 87–93.

34. Yamaori, S., Kushihara, M. et al. Characterization of major phytocannabinoids, cannabidiol and cannabinol, as isoform-selective and potent inhibitors of human CYP1 enzymes. *Biochem Pharmacol*, 2010; 79(11): 1691–1698.
35. Zanger, U.M. and Schwab, M. Cytochrome P450 enzymes in drug metabolism: Regulation of gene expression, enzyme activities, and impact of genetic variation. *Pharmacology & Therapeutics*, 2013; 138(1): 103–141.

chapter fourteen

Clinical rationale for CBD use on mood, depression, anxiety, brain function, and optimal aging

Chris D. Meletis and Betty Wedman-St. Louis

Contents

The astronomical growth in cannabis research can be seen in the 22,000 published studies or reviews in the scientific literature referencing the cannabis plant and its cannabinoids, with nearly 50% of them published within the past 10 years according to Pub Med Central, the U.S. government repository for peer-reviewed scientific research [1].

According to the U.S. Hemp Business Journal, hemp industry sales for food, body care, and CBD products grew to $688 million in 2016 and are estimated to top $800 million by 2020. Of the $688 million market was food at 19%, hemp CBD at 19%, supplements at 4%, personal care product at 24%, consumer textiles at 14%, industrial application at 18%, and other consumer products at 2% [2].

The growth of hemp CBD at $130 million in sales contributed significantly to the $688 million market. The CBD sales were in natural and specialty products, smoke shops, and on-line purchases. CBD-based pet care products, estimated at $2,470,000, is considered a definite growth category to watch [2].

Robson [3] details how cannabis has been a known medicine for several thousand years but has become mired in disrepute and legal controls in the early twentieth century within Western medicine. Despite suppression, cannabis has remained available, allowing many thousands of patients to rediscover the power of cannabis to alleviate symptoms of many diseases. Research today is extending beyond symptom management to disease modification with great promise in the treatment of inflammatory and neurodegenerative conditions.

Brain function

The average human brain has about 100 billion neurons (nerve cells) that are supported and protected by neuroglia (glial cells), and it weighs about three pounds (1300–1400 g). By comparison, an elephant brain = 6000 g, chimpanzee brain = 420 g, and a rat brain = 2 g. The 100,000,000,000 neurons = 1000 km or approximately 600 miles [4]. Optimizing neuron function can have profound influences on behavior, visual acuity, auditory function, neurotransmitter response time, and the neuronal membrane system.

In 1990, U.S. President George Bush designated the 1990s as the Decade of the Brain to "enhance public awareness of the benefits to be derived from brain research" [5]. Research evolving since then has shown that each brain neuron may be connected to up to 10,000 other neurons, passing signals to each other via as many as 1000 trillion synaptic connections, equivalent by some estimates to a computer with a 1 trillion bit per second processor. Estimates of the human brain memory capacity vary widely from 1 to 1000 terabytes. For perspective, the U.S. Library of Congress has 10 terabytes of data [6].

Memory disorders

Memory disorders range from mild to severe, but they all result from neurological damage to brain structures and hinder memory storage, retention, and recollection. Memory disorders such as Alzheimer's disease and Huntington's disease result from high levels of oxidative stress and inflammation, while other neurodegenerative diseases such as Parkinson's disease and vascular dementia usually have motor function deficits [7]. Over 24 million people suffer from dementia in today's aging society with Alzheimer's disease (AD) being the most common (50%–60%).

In the increasing aging population, the incidence of Alzheimer's disease, Parkinson's disease, and Huntington's disease is rising, but the etiologies of these disorders differs based on their neurodegenerative components. Current therapies focus on the treatment of symptoms to alter the progression of the disease, but modulation of the endocannabinoid system is an emerging option in the treatment of neurodegeneration whether it is caused from neuroinflammation, excitotoxicity, and/or mitochondrial dysfunction [8].

Over 4000 years ago, the hemp plant was used in China and India for its medicinal effects, but it has only been recently regarded as important to elicit anti-inflammatory action in Western medicine. Because of the broad impact of endocannabinoids on signaling and involvement with inflammation, they need to be considered for treatment regimens despite limited clinical trials because cannabinoids have been used for neurological and psychiatric disorders for centuries [9].

Antioxidant effects have been ascribed to cannabidiol (CBD) due to its influence on anandamide [10]. CBD was shown to protect against A-β induced neurotoxicity in vitro as well as an antioxidant compound in lipid peroxidation [11]. According to Bedse et al. [12], the endocannabinoid system signaling is a major modulator in Alzheimer's disease and needs to be the therapeutic target for disease management. The therapeutic effects of cannabidiol is also emerging as a novel treatment in ophthalmology based on animal studies of inflammatory retinal diseases, including diabetic retinopathy [13].

Gary L. Wenk, PhD, professor of psychology and neuroscience and molecular virology, immunology, and medical genetics at the Ohio State University and Medical Center, has been studying the consequences of chronic brain inflammation in animal models of Alzheimer's disease. He investigated whether components of marijuana (THC) were anti-inflammatory and found that one puff equivalent per day in aged rats was effective in reducing brain inflammation and significantly improving memory but not in young rats who exhibited cognitive impairment [14]. The research was presented at the Society for Neuroscience in Washington, DC.

CBD has been shown in other studies to promote the growth of new brain cells in a process known as neurogenesis. Adult neurogenesis that involved intermediate highly proliferative progenitor cells and the survival and maturation of new neurons was affected by CBD-based compounds [15].

Depression

Littrell [16] describes depression as an inflammatory disorder whose current treatment with antidepressants only increases rather than decreases inflammation. Stress, systemic inflammation, and behavioral symptoms of depression have been identified during the past decade [17,18]. Depressed and anxious patients present with elevations in blood levels of inflammatory cytokines (interleukin-6 or IL-6) and tumor necrosis factor α (TNK-α) plus elevated CRP (C-reactive protein) [19,20]. In addition, depressed individuals exhibit lower levels of anti-inflammatory cytokines [21].

In some studies treatment with pharmaceutical antidepressants have been shown to reduce concentrations of pro-inflammatory cytokines IL-1β, IL-2, and IL-6 while ameliorating depressive symptoms [22].

Proinflammatory cytokines also lower serotonin levels by increasing catabolism of the serotonin precursor tryptophan. Since serotonin plays an important role in regulating mood, motivation, and behavior, cytokine-induced reduction of tryptophan availability may be critical in the etiology of depression [23–25].

Obesity and sleep loss can cause a rise in inflammatory cytokines IL-1β and TNF-α, which have been linked to depression. Metabolic syndrome is also associated with inflammatory markers IL-6 and CRP and is also a risk factor for depression [26].

Deborah Serani, PhD, a clinical psychologist and author of *Living with Depression* and William Marchand, MD, clinical associate professor of psychiatry at the University of Utah School of Medicine and author of *Depression and Bipolar Disorder: Your Guide to Recovery*, both address the cognitive symptoms of depression that interfere with a person's life. They list the cognitive symptoms of depression as:

- Negative or distorted thinking
- Difficulty concentrating
- Distractibility
- Forgetfulness
- Reduced reaction time
- Memory loss
- Indecisiveness

CBD therapeutic considerations

Cannabidiol (CBD) has been described as beneficial for a wide range of psychiatric disorders such as anxiety, psychosis, and depression [27]. The mechanisms responsible for these effects still need further research, but recent findings have shown CBD attenuates the decrease in hippocampal neurogenesis and dendrite spine density caused by chronic stress. Other critical pathways for neuronal survival have also been suggested.

Iseger and Bossong analyzed the ability of CBD to counteract psychotic symptoms and cognitive impairment associated with cannabis use and the pathophysiology of schizophrenia. Cannabidiol treatment with patients for psychotic symptoms has confirmed its safety, but further clinical trials are needed [28]. Campos et al. further summarized the biochemical and molecular mechanisms associated with cannabidiol's effect on synaptic plasticity which facilitates neurogenesis [29].

Cannabidiol inhibits the degradation of the endocannabinoid anandamide and was shown to have significant clinical improvement in schizophrenia [30]. The efficacy of CBD to restore cognition in multiple studies of impairment needs to be further assessed as a treatment for schizophrenia [31].

Cannabis has been suggested as an alternative therapy for refractory epilepsy affecting both children and adults who do not respond to current medications. Since CBD is nonpsychoactive and anticonvulsive, it may offer treatment options in these epilepsy cases [32,33].

CBD has been shown to have anxiolytic effects in humans and animals. Anxiety affects humans in many aspects of life: social life, productivity, and health concerns. It can be defined as a vague and unpleasant feeling to a fear or apprehension caused by a danger or unknown situation. Animal models suggest CBD exhibited antianxiety and antidepressant effects [34,35].

Harnessing the endocannabinoid system (ECS)

The ECS plays a critical role in energy homeostasis in the brain and peripheral tissues of the liver, pancreas, muscle, and adipose tissues. The ECS network of synapse receptors is located in the central nervous system of all vertebrate mammals. An eight-minute video visualization of the ECS sponsored by Phivida is available at http://www.youtube.com/watch?v=jznQfMj9RWM.

References

1. Marijuana. www.ncbi.nlm.nih.gov.
2. Market size: Hemp industry sales grow to $688 million in 2016. www.hempbizjournal.com.
3. Robson P. Human studies of cannabinoids and medicinal cannabis. *Handb Exp Pharmacol* 2005; 168: 719–756.
4. Neuroscience for kids. www.faculty.washington.edu.
5. Presidential Proclamation 6158. July 17, 1990 by the President of the United States of America. www.loc.gov.
6. Hunt M. *Neurons & Synapses. The human memory-what it is, how it works and how it can go wrong. The Universe Within.* Simon & Schuster, New York, 1982.
7. Walther S, Halpern M. Cannabinoids and dementia: a review of clinical and preclinical data. *Pharmaceuticals* 2010; 3(8): 2689–2708.
8. Fagan SG, Campbell VA. The influence of cannabinoids on generic traits of neurodegeneration. *British J Pharmacology* 2014; 171(6): 1347–1360.
9. Pacher P, Batkai S, Kunos G. The endocannabinoid system as an emerging target of pharmacotherapy. *Pharmacol Rev* 2006; 58: 389–462.
10. Iuvone T, Esposito G, De Filippis D et al. Cannabidiol: a promising drug for neurodegenerative disorders? *CNS Neurosci Ther* 2009; 15: 65–75.
11. Iuvone T, Esposito G, Esposito R et al. Neuroprotective effects of cannabidiol a non-psychoactive component of cannabis sativa, on beta-amyloid-induced toxicity in pc12 cells. *J Neurochem* 2004; 89: 134–141.
12. Bedse G, Romano A, Lavecchia AM et al. The role of endocannabinoid signaling in the molecular mechanisms of neurodegeneration in Alzheime's Disease. *J of Alzheimer's Disease* 2015; 43(4): 1115–1136.
13. Liow GI. Diabetic retinopathy: a role of inflammation and potential therapies for anti-inflammation. *World J Diabetes.* 2010; 1(1): 12–18.

14. Scientists are high on idea that marijuana reduces memory impairment. Ohio State University. Press release: 19-Nov-2008.

15. Wolf SA, Bick-Sander A, Fabel K et al. Cannabioid receptor CB1 mediates baseline and activity-induced survival of new neurons in adult hippocampal neurogenesis. *Cell Communication and Signaling* 2010; 8: 12.

16. Littrel JL. Taking the perspective that a depressive state reflects inflammation: implications for the use of antidepressants. *Front Psychol* 2012; 3: 297.

17. Raison CL, Capuron L, Miller AH. Cytokines sing the blues: inflammation and the pathogenesis of depression. *Trends Immunol* 2006; 27: 24–3110.

18. Capuron L, Su S, Miller AH et al. Depressive symptoms and metabolic syndrome: is inflammation the underlying link? *Biol Psychiatry* 2008; 64: 896–90010.

19. Rajagopalan S, Brook R, Rubenfire M et al. Abnormal brachial artery flow-mediated vasodilation in young adults with major depression. *Am J Cardiol* 2001; 88: 196–198.

20. Zorrilla EP, Luborsky L, McKay JR et al. The relationship of depression and stressors to immunological assays: a meta-analytic review. *Brain Behav Immun* 2001; 15: 199–22610.

21. Li Y, Xiao B, Qui W et al. Altered expression of CD4(+) CD25(+) regulatory T cells and its 5-HT(1a) receptor in patients with major depression disorder. *J Affect Disord* 2011; 124: 68–7510.

22. Hernandez ME, Mendieta D et al. Variations in circulating cytokine levels during 52 week course of treatment with SSRI for major depressive disorder. *Eur Neuropsychopharmacol* 2008; 18(12): 917–924.

23. Raison CL, Dantzer R, Kelley KW et al. CSF concentrations of brain tryptophan and kynurenines during immune stimulation with IFN-α: a relationship to CNS immune responses and depression. *Mol Psychiatry* 2010; 15: 393–403.

24. Capuron L, Ravaud A, Neveu P et al. Association between decreased serum tryptophan concentrations and depressive symptoms in cancer patients undergoing cytokine therapy. *Mol Psychiatry* 2002; 7(5): 468–473.

25. Capuron L, Neurauter G, Musselman DL et al. Interferon-alpha-induced changes in tryptophan metabolism: relationship to depression and paroxetine treatment. *Biol Psychiatry* 2003 Nov 1; 54(9): 906–914.

26. Littrel JL. Taking the perspective that a depressive state reflects inflammation: implications for the use of antidepressants. *Front Psychol* 2012; 3: 297.

27. Campos AC, Fogaca MV, Scarante FF et al. Plastic and neuroprotective mechanisms involved in the therapeutic effects of cannabidiol in psychiatric disorders. *Front Pharmacol* 2017; 8: 269. doi: 10.3389/fphar.2017.00269.

28. Iseger TA, Bossong MG. A systematic review of the antipsychotic properties of cannabidiol in humans. *Schizophr Res* 2015; 162(1–3): 153–161.

29. Campos AC, Fogaca MV, Sonego AB, Guimaraes FS. Cannabidiol, neuroprotection and neuropsychiatric disorders. *Pharmacol Res* 2016; 112: 119–127.

30. Leweke FM, Piomelli D, Pahlisch F et al. Cannabidiol enhances anandamide signaling and alleviates psychotic symptoms of schizophrenia. *Transl Psychiatry* 2012; 2(3): e94.

31. Osborne AL, Solowij N, Weston-Green K. A systemic review of the effect of cannabidiol on cognitive function: relevance to schizophrenia. *Neurosci Biobehav Rev* 2017; 72: 310–324.

32. Reddy DS, Golub VM. The pharmacological basis of cannabis therapy for epilepsy. *J Pharmacol Exp Ther* 2016; 357(1): 45–55.
33. Devinsky O, Marsh E, Friedman D et al. Cannabidiol in patients with treatment-resistant epilepsy: an open-label intervention trial. *Lancet Neurol* 2016; 15(3): 270–278.
34. de Mello Schiar AR, de Oliveira Rebeiro NP et al. Antidepressant-like and anxiolytic-like effects of cannabidiol: a chemical compound of Cannabis sativa. *CNS & Neurological Disorders—Drug Targets* 2014; 13: 953–960.
35. Berhamaschi MM, Queiroz RH, Chagas MH et al. Cannabidiol reduces the anxiety induced by simulated public speaking in treatment-naive social phobia patients. *Neuropyschopharmacology* 2011; 36(6): 1219–1226.

chapter fifteen

Cannabis in palliative care

Betty Wedman-St. Louis

Contents

Although most people believe that death and dying are a natural part of the life cycle, we generally avoid planning or discussing end-of-life wishes that can be known and honored by surviving loved ones. The World Health Organization estimates that globally about 60% of all those who die would benefit from palliative care before death, and palliative care is not exclusively reserved for patients at the end of life [1]. Palliative care focuses on the amelioration of physical, emotional, psychological, and spiritual suffering that is supported through symptom management of patients facing life-limiting illness [2].

Primary palliative care outlines basic pain management and disease prognosis that leads to advanced care planning to provide comfort, dignity, and meaning at the end of life. Individuals have the right to know all the options available including treatment options, rights to refuse treatments, and when treatment withdrawal is desired.

Patients suffering from symptoms and the stress of illnesses such as cancer, congestive heart failure (CHF), chronic obstructive pulmonary disease (COPD), kidney disease, Alzheimer's, Parkinson's, amyotrophic lateral sclerosis (ALS), and other disorders can benefit from palliative care to handle pain, depression, appetite issues, difficulty sleeping, nausea, and anxiety.

Palliative care is a treatment available to anyone at any age living with a chronic illness long before the need for hospice. A brief description of the differences between hospice and palliative care follows.

Hospice

- End of life
- <6 months to live
- Comfort or relief

Palliative Care

- Any stage of illness
- As long as necessary
- Curative treatment can be pursued

Cannabis use in palliative care

The nonmedical use of cannabis has long dominated the media, which has led to significant debate about its medical use as legislation for cannabis use spreads across the United States. Healthcare professionals need to be aware of the legal as well as the pharmacological uses of cannabis [3]. The integration of cannabis-derived medications into medical use and proper dosing regimens has been the subject of numerous clinical trials [4–7]. The use of medical cannabis repeatedly indicates patients reporting an improvement in their quality of life from improved sleep, better appetite, and reduced depression to a reduction in opioid dose [8].

In palliative care, the focus is on individual choice, patient autonomy, empowerment, comfort, and quality of life. Mathre and Krawitz [9] describe cannabis use as an advocacy issue for patient rights because the use of cannabis supports the philosophy of comfort measures as an integrative approach. Many of the drugs used in palliative care are highly toxic with potentially lethal effects, whereas cannabinoids have low toxicity and no lethal dose [10].

As a healthcare professional, the emphasis should be on personal choice in treatment instead of a declaration that "the patient is breaking the law," but they must stay well informed about local regulations and document details of the discussion with patients and family. In addition, cannabis use, like any drug, must be assessed and monitored regularly. The Compassionate Investigative New Drug (IND) program of the Food and Drug Administration (FDA) for medical marijuana reported that cannabis can be a safe and effective medicine [11].

Pain and palliative care

Cannabinoid use for pain management is increasing, especially when conventional treatments have failed, particularly in terminal cancer and neurological disease [12]. Individual therapeutic trials are needed to determine benefit and dosing. Acceptance of cannabis use and the safety of cannabinoids in pain management and palliative medicine varies throughout Europe and among states within the United States [13–15]. Carter et al. emphasizes the need for long-term drug safety in palliative medicine and cites cannabis as a safer alternative than opioids [16].

Cannabinoids in palliative cancer care

S. K. Aggarwal, MD, PhD, points out that all cannabis-related medicinal products have yet to be integrated into healthcare because of "the gap between available scientific evidence on cannabis and cannabinoids, and current practices" [17]. The benefits of cannabinoid integrative medicine (CIM) have been recognized in nearly half of the United States and all of Canada, but it remains underutilized, especially in oncology patients.

Donald I. Abrams, MD, a hematologist-oncologist at San Francisco General Hospital, San Francisco, California, has observed that many cancer patients benefit from adding cannabis to their pain regimen. High doses of opiates administered by oncologists can alter a patient's cognitive function, which reduces communication and mobility skills. These patients can wean themselves down or off opiates by using cannabis [18].

AIDS and palliative care

Age may be one of the reasons people with AIDS are frequently users of medical marijuana [19]. According to the National Academy of Science, it may be because the generation with HIV grew up experimenting with marijuana. Because HIV attacks the immune system, it produces effects throughout the body and frequently triggers a wasting syndrome, nerve damage, and dementia. Cannabis can assist in the treatment of depression, nausea and vomiting from medications, and appetite improvement in addition to neuropathic pain as the disease progresses to AIDS.

Cachexia is seen in the late stages of almost every major illness but particularly in cancer and AIDS [20]. Scientists are treating cachexia as a condition driven by inflammation and metabolic imbalances that could be regulated with feeding to offset the wasting of muscles associated with AIDS and cancer [21].

ALS and palliative care

Palliative care physicians and healthcare professionals are becoming increasingly involved in the care of patients with amyotrophic lateral sclerosis (ALS) [22]. Cannabis has powerful antioxidant, anti-inflammatory, and neuroprotective effects, which can play a role in ALS [23]. In an ALS mouse study, cannabis administration prolonged neuronal cell survival and slowed the progression of the disease [24]. A survey of ALS patients who used cannabis reported that cannabis reduced symptoms of appetite loss, depression, pain, spasticity, and drooling [25].

A few words for consideration

Drs. S.K. Aggarwal and E. Russo provided the following statement in the Huffington Post, October 20, 2015, entitled Cannabis, Medical Science and Fundamental Human Rights [26].

> The criminalization of indigenous, traditional practices done without consultation of indigenous communities raises a number of human rights and development concerns. The ban on traditional uses of coca, opium, and cannabis was passed at a time when scant attention was given to cultural and indigenous rights and before the adoption of key international instruments and relevant jurisprudence protecting the right of all indigenous peoples to free and prior informed consent relating to issues that affect them, and to maintain traditional, religious, and medical practices, and to own, develop, control and use their real property and resources. Criminalization of drugs used for traditional and religious purposes likewise contradicts human rights protections for the traditional and religious uses of controlled drugs.

References

1. Stjernsward J, Clark D. Palliative medicine: A global perspective. In: Doyle D, Hanks G et al. (eds). *Oxford Textbook of Palliative Medicine*. 3rd ed. NY: Oxford University Press; 2005. pp. 1197–1224.
2. World Health Organization (WHO). *WHO Definition of Palliative Care*. Geneva, Switzerland: WHO; 2015. http://www.who.int/cancer/palliative/definition/en.
3. Green AJ, De-Vries K. Cannabis use in palliative care-an examination of the evidence and the implications for nurses. *J Clin Nurs* 2010; 19: 2454–2462.
4. Berlach DM, Shir Y, Ware MA. Experience with synthetic cannabinoid Nabilone in chronic noncancer pain. *Pain Med* 2006; 7: 25–29.
5. Howard J, Kofi A, Holdcroft A et al. Cannabis use on sickle cell disease: A questionnaire study. *Br J Haematol* 2005; 131: 123–128.
6. Amtmann D, Weydt P, Johnson KL et al. Survey of cannabis use in patients with amyotropic lateral sclerosis. *Am J Hospice Pallait Med* 2004; 21: 95–104.
7. Bagshaw SM, Hagen NA, Baker T. Medical efficacy of cannabinoids and marijuana: A comprehensive review of the literature. *J Palliat Care* 2002; 18: 111–122.

8. McCarberg BH. Cannabinoids: Their role in pain and palliation. *J Pain Palliat Care Pharmacother* 2007; 21: 3–19.

9. Mathre ML, Krawitz M. Cannabis series—The whole story. Part 4: The medicinal use of cannabis pre-prohibition. *Drug Alcohol Prof* 2002; 2: 3–7.

10. Bagshaw SM, Hagen NA, Baker T. Medical efficacy of cannabinoids and marijuana: A comprehensive review of the literature. *J Palliat Care* 2002; 18: 111–122.

11. Russo E, Mathre ML, Byme A et al. Chronic cannabis use in the compassionate investigational new drug program: An examination of benefits and adverse effects of legal clinical cannabis. *J Cannabis Therapeutics* 2002; 2(1): 3–57.

12. Peat S. Using cannabinoids in pain and palliative care. *Int J Palliat Nurs* 2010; 16(10): 481–485.

13. Krcevski-Skvarc N, Wells C, Hauser W. Availability and approval of cannabis-based medicines for chronic pain management and palliative/supportive care in Europe: A survey of the statics in the chapters of the European Pain Federation. *Eur J Pain* 2017; Nov 13. doi: 10.1002/ejp.1147.

14. Bonfa L, Vinagre RC, de Figueiredo NV. Cannabinoids in chronic pain and palliative care. *Rev Bras Anestesiol* 2008; 58(3): 267–279.

15. Hauser W, Fitzcharles MA, Radbruch L et al. Cannabinoids in pain management and palliative medicine. *Deutsches Arzteblatt Int* 2017; 114(38): 627–634.

16. Carter GT, Flanagan AM, Earleywine M et al. Cannabis in palliative medicine: Improving care and reducing opioid-related morbidity. *Am J Hosp Palliat Care* 2011; 28(5): 297–303.

17. Aggarwal SK. Use of cannabinoids in cancer care: Palliative care. *Curr Oncol* 2016; 23(Suppl 2): S33–S36.

18. Meuche G. The integration of cannabis in oncologic care. *Oncology Nurse Advisor* March 29, 2017. http://www.oncologynurseadvisor.com/side-effect-management/use-of-cannabis-in-cancer-care/article/647302.

19. Institute of Medicine. *Marijuana and AIDS. Marijuana As Medicine? The Science Beyond the Controversy.* Washington, DC: The National Academies Press, 2000. https://www.nap.edu/read/9586/chapter/7.

20. Lok C. Cachexia: The last illness. *Nature* 2015; 528: 182–183.

21. Dalton JT, Barnette KG, Bohl CE et al. The selective androgen receptor modulator GTx-024(enobosam) improves lean body mass and physical function in healthy elderly men and post-menopausal women: Results of a double-blind, placebo-controlled phase II trial. *J Cachexia Sarcopenia Muscle* 2011; 2(3): 153–161.

22. Karam CY, Paganoni S, Joyce N et al. Palliative care issues in amyotropic lateral sclerosis: An evidence-based review. *Am J Hosp Palliat Care* 2016; 33(1): 84–92.

23. Carter GT, Abood ME, Aggarwal SK et al. Cannabis and amyotrophic lateral sclerosis: Hypothetical and practical applications, and a call for clinical trials. *Am J Hosp Palliat Care* 2010; 27(5): 347–356.

24. Wendt P, Hong S, Witting A et al. Cannabinol delays symptom onset in SOD 1 (G93A) transgenic mice without affecting survival. *Amyotropic Lateral Scler Other Motor Neuron Disord* 2005; 6(3): 182–184.

25. Amtmann D, Weydt P, Johnson KL et al. Survey of cannabis use in patients with amyotrophic lateral sclerosis. *Am J Hospice Pallait Med* 2004; 21: 95–104.

26. Aggarwall SK, Russo E. Cannabis, medical science and fundamental human rights. *Huffington Post*, October 20, 2015.

chapter sixteen

What to expect at the cannabis dispensary

Betty Wedman-St. Louis

Contents

Dispensaries are the trusted source of quality medical cannabis for patients with reliable and accurate information on therapeutic use and research. Privacy and compassion are key elements in patient care whether they are alleviating their suffering, managing their disease, or restoring their health.

The patient and physician share the decision to discuss the risks and dosing issues prior to the patient arrival at the dispensary. Patients need to know that the dose and the frequency needs to be discussed with their physician throughout the treatment process with careful monitoring. A written treatment plan outlining the medicinal benefits cannabis may provide is required in some states with follow-up reviews at designated time periods.

Patient education should also include the discussion about standardized, laboratory tested products sold at a licensed dispensary versus "street" products. In addition, the risks of misuse and how to safeguard cannabis from children in the home needs to be included. Cannabis is not recommended for use during pregnancy and breastfeeding.

A Minnesota pharmacists study on medical cannabis knowledge and preparedness reported in Pharmacy and Therapeutics, November 2016 concluded that pharmacists needed more training and education on the regulatory and clinical aspects to provide patients information on the pharmacotherapy aspects of cannabis. Most respondents to the questionnaire were highly interested in filling in their knowledge gaps about cannabis as a medication.

Legalization of a once-illicit substance as a therapeutic agent calls for all healthcare providers to become knowledgeable in dosage forms, regulatory parameters, efficacy, and safety as well as medication interactions.

Visiting a dispensary

Arrange a visit to a local cannabis dispensary and look for these quality management guidelines:

- Are products labeled with strain and dose?
- Do products have child-resistant packaging or locked box for sale to safeguard all medications, including cannabis?
- Are edibles offered, and are they labeled with strain and dose?
- Is a patient verification system used to register each user?
- Are employees compassionate and well-trained?
- Are security systems in place—alarms, surveillance?
- Where are Certificates of Analysis kept for patients to verify their cannabis is safe?

Physicians need to consider whether cannabis is an appropriate treatment for their patient and weigh the risks and benefits associated with its use. They must caution all patients who engage in activities that require mental alertness that they may become impaired when using cannabis products containing delta 9-tetrahydrocanninoid (THC).

Dispensaries offer the patient and the physician the opportunity to initiate treatment with a prescribed amount of quality cannabis at a safe and effective dose. Trained and compassionate staff at the dispensary allow for titration of the dose to provide maximum benefit for symptom control.

When beginning cannabis therapy, patients are advised to immediately stop therapy if unacceptable or undesirable side effects occur such as disorientation, dizziness, loss of coordination, agitation, anxiety, rapid heartbeat, chest pain, low blood pressure/feeling faint, depression, and hallucinations. Some patients prefer to have a trusted family member or friend with them when they start therapy in case an adverse event should occur.

Interview—Giving Tree Dispensary in Phoenix, Arizona
with Lilach Mazor Power, Founder and Managing Director

The Giving Tree has 57 employees who are "passionate, talented and knowledgeable," according to Lilach Mazor Power. They have all participated in the "Giving Tree University" three-day training program followed by shadowing an experienced employee before assisting a new patient. Policies and procedures are required by the state, which includes

Health Insurance Portability and Accountability Act (HIPAA) compliance and the personal business ethos of patient satisfaction.

Security at the facility is monitored by cameras, alarms, and videos, along with security personnel on site. No security issues have been a problem in the past five years of business. Since purchases are cash-based, carrying large amounts of money may be a concern for patients, so security can be important.

Each patient coming to the Giving Tree is advised that their appointment will be at least 30 minutes, and they are free to bring family members so everyone can be introduced to the cannabis experience. A patient consultant gathers data about their symptoms, lifestyle, comfort level with cannabis, prior experience with cannabis, and what form of cannabis would suit their individual needs. Recommendations for the type of cannabis products available are made with a 100% guarantee for return if not satisfied. Patients are advised to start slow with small amounts of cannabis in their medicinal regime.

When asked about product safety, Ms. Power indicated they only use products from responsible growers and do not order any products where butane extraction has been used. Third-party independent laboratory results are available in the dispensary, and patients are encouraged to ask questions about growing and processing of their products.

The Growing Tree does not sell edibles because capsules provide a more accurate dosing regimen. They also have sublingual strips and sprays for those not selecting capsules.

When asked about the future of cannabis dispensaries, Ms. Power sees a growing market for recreational use if society can get past the "marijuana stoner" mentality and look at cannabis as an alternative to a "glass of wine" for relaxation. "People are becoming more open-minded to try cannabis because they are more knowledgeable," she concluded (Figures 16.1 through 16.3).

Interview—Liberty Health Sciences, Inc.
with George Scorsis, CEO and Director

Liberty Health Sciences, Inc. (formerly Chestnut Hill Tree Farm, LLC) is committed to delivering high-quality, clean, and safe pharmaceutical grade cannabis from its facility in Alachua, Florida. The company's largest shareholder is Aphria, Inc., a leading licensed producer of medical cannabis in Canada. Aphria Inc. also lends Liberty proprietary greenhouse growing techniques and licenses its medical brand. Liberty CEO and Director George Scorsis outlined the philosophy of patient-centered, compassionate education to ensure a quality and safe experience for each patient.

He described how Liberty dispensaries are going to be unique and draw from years of Canadian experience. Since most physicians have very

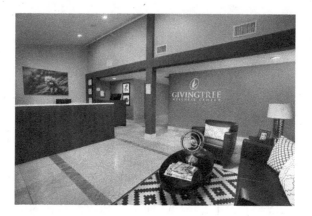

Figure 16.1 Giving Tree lobby.

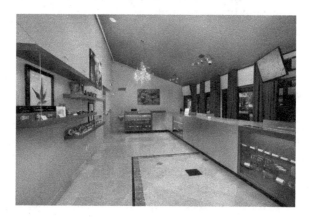

Figure 16.2 Giving Tree dispensary.

minimum knowledge about the endocannabinoid system and cannabis dosing, dispensaries will act as "cannabis education centers" with private rooms for patient education and seminars for medical staff. Mr. Scorsis outlined that both the medical staff and patients need knowledge about titration of the cannabis dose, dosing protocols, and guidelines for symptom management for a personalized care approach.

Mr. Scorsis candidly related an experience he had with a lady suffering from severe arthritis pain who was prescribed cannabis without any recommendations on titration of the dose or how cannabis is utilized in the body. Such lack of education can lead to poor patient outcome, which he wants to be sure does not happen at Liberty Health Sciences dispensaries.

To ensure high quality cannabis, they use a DNA hybrid strain with standard operating procedures to guarantee a pharmaceutical grade

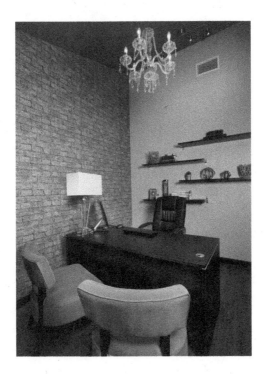

Figure 16.3 Giving Tree counseling office.

product. Third-party testing reconfirms safety and quality. Capsules, oils, and "proprietary devices" will be available in the dispensaries along with edibles that meet pharmaceutical dosing standards.

Mr. Scorsis believes collaboration between physicians, dispensary staff, and patients is essential to the success of a medical cannabis treatment program. Liberty Health Sciences will be using an EMR (electronic medical records) system to track patient usage and symptom management, as well as looking for interactions between cannabis and other drugs prescribed to the patient.

chapter seventeen

Cannabis nutrition

Betty Wedman-St. Louis

Contents

Cannabis has been described as an oral medicine since the Chinese treatise on pharmacology indicated Emperor Shen Nung in 2737 BCE used it as medicine [1]. Hindu texts in Atharva Veda also refer to oral consumption of cannabis as one of five sacred herbs [2]. Clay tablets from the Royal Library of Ashurbanipal, described as the first library in the world, also documents cannabis use as medicine [3].

In fact, cannabis has been used for medicinal purposes throughout the world including Assyria, Egypt, Greece, Rome, and the Islamic empire [4]. Arabs in the eleventh century used cannabis in a dried fruit, nuts, and honey mixture as a confection that became popular throughout northern Africa from Egypt to Morocco. A recipe is included for those wanting to try this ancient treat.

The Netherlands was the first country to legalize marijuana, but many populations throughout the world have been enjoying the health benefits of cannabis in their cuisine for thousands of years.

Cannabis is a nutritious plant that has been documented through the ages as a therapeutic botanical that benefits the body and the mind. Its ability to increase appetite makes it important in the wasting syndrome management of HIV/AIDS and cancer [5].

The effects of eating cannabis are less immediate than smoking because results can be sustained over hours instead of minutes—15 to 30 minutes for smoking and three to four hours for eating. The oral consumption effects are described as more relaxed, but care is needed to control portions to avoid overconsumption, which can result in a sick or confused state with the inability to move or talk four or five hours after ingestion. The remedy for overeating cannabis-infused food is to drink lemon juice in water and use CBD concentrate to offset the THC [6].

Professor Richard E. Schultes in his book, *The Plants of the Gods: Their Sacred, Healing, and Hallucinogenic Powers* [7], described eating hemp as a special gift of the gods or "food from the gods" because of its medical and religious status. Indian mythology reports deity Shiva eating cannabis leaves as his favorite food, thus being called Lord of Bhang (bhange is Sanskrit for hemp). Buddha was reported to survive for six years on one hemp seed a day during his quest for enlightenment [8].

Cannabis in the kitchen

The first known cookbook that included cannabis recipes was Alice B. Toklas's memoir discussing her role as lover, secretary, muse, and cook for Gertrude Stein [9]. It featured a hashish fudge recipe made from spices, nuts, dried fruit, and cannabis, which made it one of the most successful cookbooks of all time. Her cannabis brownie recipe was another hit in 1968 with the Peter Sellers movie, *I Love You, Alice B. Toklas*.

Medical marijuana as an herbal cure has been popular throughout the ages. Currently, cannabis has been hailed as beneficial in medical conditions ranging from asthma to multiple sclerosis and neurological conditions such as ALS and Parkinson's disease, but individuals have been prosecuted for bringing "dope-laden" dinners of stew, pot pies, and brownies to ailing family and friends. While current anti-marijuana laws have not stopped the cannabis cooking trend popular today, the 1996 passage of California's Proposition 215 has legalized medical marijuana and opened the door for more people to share their cannabis recipes. While the brownie remains popular at dinner parties—chocolate covers up the flavor of cannabis—our palates are moving to more creative edibles such as salad dressings, pizza, banana bread, and salsa.

Nutritive value of cannabis

An exact nutrition profile for *Cannabis sativa* L. has not been published, but its seeds and foliage are assumed to be equivalent to hemp, one of the most nutritious foods in the world with high-quality protein and essential fatty acids from in its seeds. Hemp seeds contain all eight essential amino acids and can be sprouted for easier digestibility when added to a salad or shake.

Hemp food consumption and drug testing

Hemp seed oil has been available at health food markets in the United States and Canada for several years, and Mary Enig, PhD, reports that toxicology journals state that sufficient cannabinoids are present to identify users when drug tested [10]. According to Leson and Pless, the food containing hemp seeds or oil of the hemp plant (*Cannabis sativa* L.) had a THC concentration sufficiently low to prevent positive drug screening from consumption of hemp foods [11]. A THC intake of 0.6 mg/day is equivalent to the consumption of about 125 mL hemp oil containing 5 mcg/g THC or 300 g of hulled seeds at 2 mcg/g. These amounts are "well below the 15 ng/mL confirmation cutoff used in federal drug testing programs," according to Leson and Pless.

Their study evaluated the daily ingestion of THC via hemp oil on urine levels of 11-nor-9-carboxy-Δ-9-tetrahydrocannabinol (THC-COOH) for four distinct daily THC doses. The doses were identified as comparable levels of hemp seed products consumed over four successive days in a 10-day period by 15 THC-naive adults (single daily doses ranging from 0.09 to 0.6 mg). Urine samples were collected prior to the first ingestion, on days 9 and 10 for the study period, and one and three days after the last ingestion. Gas chromatography–mass spectrometry (GC-MS) was used to analyze the urine samples.

This study can help reassure users of hemp users to be aware of dosing levels if they want to avoid prosecution for using an illicit substance.

Fatty acid composition of hemp oil

The fatty acid composition of the oil according to Dr. Enig is 6% palmitic acid, 2% stearic acid, 12% oleic acid, 57% linoleic acid, 2% gamma linolenic acid, and 19% alpha linolenic acid. Linoleic and alpha linolenic acids are the two fatty acids that nutrition research has indicated are essential for human health. Other fatty acids can be produced in the body from the essential fatty acids. J.C. Callaway at the Department of Pharmaceutical Chemistry in Kuopio, Finland reported a slightly different fatty acid profile: 5% palmitic acid, 2% stearic acid, 9% oleic acid, 56% linoleic acid, 4% gamma linolenic acid, and 22% alpha linolenic acid for a 84% polyunsaturated fatty acid total [12]. In addition, Callaway compared the fatty acid profiles of hemp seed to flax, rapeseed (canola), soy, corn, and olive oils.

The essential fatty acids in hemp seed oil make it an ideal source for energy production, oxygen transfer, hemoglobin production, membrane components, prostaglandin synthesis, growth, and cell division, according to Udo Erasmus, PhD, in *Fats that Heal, Fats that Kill* [13]. He further recommends hemp oil be substituted for other oils in food preparation except frying or high-heat uses. Hemp oil use in salad dressing, mashed potatoes, and mixed with olive oil is apparent in cannabis cookbooks and medical cannabis recipes such as those included in the appendix.

The nutritional composition of hemp seed as described by Callaway in 2004 [14] recognizes that its value as food is still limited, especially in the United States. Europe, Asia, India, and Russia have a long and varied use of the oil and seeds. Essential fatty acids found in hempseed oil have been anecdotally reported as important in acute and chronic conditions such as cuts, burns, skin disorders, and influenza [15]. Hemp seed oil has a direct impact on dietary essential fatty acid metabolism for immune regulation [16].

Essential fatty acids or fatty acids that are not made by humans must be obtained in the diet and are needed to enhance human health and development, especially when they are lacking from the diet [17]. Polyunsaturated fats are incorporated as phospholipids in cellular and organelle membranes [18], which maintain cell membrane fluidity within the central neuronal system. Diets with sufficient polyunsaturated fatty acids can lower arterial levels of LDL cholesterol and blood pressure in humans. Hempseed has the potential to benefit cardiovascular disease because of its excellent omega-3 and omega-6 fatty acid ratio [19].

Protein in hemp

Due to the decades-long prohibition against growing hemp in the United States, there are very limited studies to review the benefits of hemp foods. As Aiello et al. states "hemp seed is an underexploited non-legume protein-rich seed" [20]. Albumin and edestin are the two main proteins in hemp providing similar amino acid profiles as egg whites and soy.

Hempseed protein has significant amounts of sulfur-containing amino acids methionine and cystine [21].

Vitamins and minerals in hemp

Callaway [22] lists the nutritive value for vitamins and minerals in hempseed:

Vitamin E (total)	90 mg/100 g
α tocopherol	5 mg/100 g
γ tocopherol	85 mg/100 g
Thiamine	0.4 mg/100 g
Riboflavin	0.1 mg/100 g
Phosphorus	1160 mg/100 g
Potassium	859 mg/100 g
Magnesium	483 mg/100 g
Calcium	145 mg/100 g
Iron	14 mg/100 g
Sodium	12 mg/100 g
Manganese	7 mg/100 g
Zinc	7 mg/100 g
Copper	2 mg/100 g

Most of the world's hempseed is consumed by small birds as commercial birdseed exported from China and sold in the local pet store. Hempseed is preferred over rapeseed (canola) and flaxseed for animal feed because it does not contain antinutritional components and toxic glycosides found in flaxseed meal. Under moist and acidic conditions, an enzyme in flax releases prussic acid (i.e., hydrogen cyanide gas or HCN) from the glycoside [23]. The amount of HCN limits how much flaxseed meal can be fed to poultry and other animals [24].

Phytochemicals in hemp

Animal studies have shown the antioxidant effects of hempseed meal [25], and chickens fed hempseed products had significantly more omega-3 fatty acids [26,27]. While oil seeds are a main source of essential fatty acids and they contain considerable protein, small notice is given to the phytochemicals in their oil and de-oiled meal [28]. Fresh cold-pressed hempseed oil offers delicate flavors and the nutritional contribution of flavonoids found in the terpenes [29,30].

Natural ligands are another phenolic compound in *Cannabis sativa* L. Beta-caryophyllene is found in the oils of numerous spice and food plants along with being a major component in cannabis [31]. It inhibits lipopolysaccharide (LPS)-induced proinflammatory cytokine expression in peripheral blood and attenuates LPS-stimulated phosphorylation in monocytes, which is evidence of anti-inflammatory action. A multiple sclerosis patient study confirmed the effectiveness of hempseed with antioxidant properties in humans [32].

In addition to anti-inflammatory benefits from cannabis phenolics, Gertsch describes how cannabimimetic phytochemicals in the diet have modulated the endocannabinoid system to co-evolve with food selection and metabolic stress adaptation [33]. This intriguing concept of how ancient lipid genes of hunter-gatherers were modified by agriculture and its production of high-carbohydrate foods bears further exploration. The interplay between diet and the endocannabinoid system bring into focus why dietary cannabimimetic phytochemicals such as beta-caryophyllene need more research. "Never in the history of human diets have we consumed more carbohydrates and less phytochemicals than today" [33].

Possible allergic reactions

According to Callaway and Pate [34], no reports of allergic reactions have been reported, but because hempseed is technically a nut with albumin as its primary protein, people with nut and/or egg allergies should be cautious when adding hempseed foods to their diet. Stadtmauer [35] in 2003 presented a case about an allergic reaction when an individual consumed part of a restaurant meal that contained dehulled hempseed. Vidal et al. [36] accounted a bronchial asthma issue from a person who inhaled dust from hempseed while feeding a pet.

Taking a closer look at cannabinoids

The cannabis plant, like other botanicals, will have different properties based on where and how it is grown, the variety or strain used, and how it is processed for use. All cannabis plants are not created equal. Different crops from the same strain can equal different potency [37].

Of the more than 60 cannabinoids known, the most well recognized is delta-9-tetrahydrocannabinol or THC, which is known for its psychoactive properties. Leaves contain THCA, the acid form of THC, which has no psychoactive properties and are used raw in salads and juicing. High levels of THC are found in the bud, which is usually dried and used to create canna butter or canna oil.

Cannabidiol or CBD can be found in most varieties of cannabis in various amounts. Many times, it is concentrated into pure CBD products for use in pain management. CBD has a sedative effect and can be used with THC to reduce the psychoactive effects of delta-9-tetrahydrocannabinol.

Food preparation requires that the cook know the strain and its cannabinoid content (THC and CBD) to enhance the culinary experience. When buying a prepared product, the THC content should be labeled on the package. A THC content of 15%–20% is considered above average according to numerous growers and reflects top quality, so amounts used in recipes may need to be reduced. A current standard amount of THC is 10%; therefore, a 1000 mg dried cannabis sample would equal ~100 mg THC [38].

High temperatures and overcooking can destroy cannabis health benefits. Using a lower temperature for a longer period will produce a more biologically active product than cooking too quickly at a high heat. Terpenes start to evaporate at 70°F as they give off the pungent aroma characteristic of cannabis. Terpenes contribute anti-inflammatory benefits that are lost when temperatures reach 100°F [39].

Flavonoids, another anti-inflammatory component of cannabis, are destroyed between 270 and 350°F. These are the flavors that are retained in canna oil and canna butter [40].

Patients should be advised to select a supplier of organic cannabis to avoid pathogens and pesticides that result from the growing process.

Cannabis edibles

Food products containing cannabis extract, called edibles, are popular for both recreational and medical cannabis users. Edibles include baked goods, candies, gummies, chocolates, lozenges, and beverages that can be homemade or prepared commercially for dispensaries [41]. In 2014, Colorado reported 1.96 million units of edible medical cannabis-infused products and 2.85 million units of edible retail cannabis-infused products sold the next year, which accounted for about 45% of the total cannabis sales in the state [42].

In a national 2016 study of U.S. adults, 29.8% of the respondents who had ever used cannabis reported consuming it in edible or beverage form [43]. Additional research in California, Washington, Colorado, and Canada found 11 to 26% of medicinal cannabis users had consumed an edible cannabis product [44,45].

The demand for cannabis edibles is a new supply demand for the food industry. Five years ago, this market did not exist, and today over 40 million servings a year are being produced with an outlook of 600+ million servings by 2021 [46].

"The legal market for recreational cannabis undercuts the black market and its associated social harms and law enforcement costs," according to Francis J. Boero, PhD, CFS, managing partner at Gavenum LLC [47].

Consumers already purchase more than $155 million of hemp-based foods and supplements yearly, so the edible market will be an extension of the cannabis market [48].

Few research studies have been undertaken using actual cannabis-infused edibles. One study by Cone et al. featured cannabis users who received cannabis-infused brownies. Participants completed behavioral and physiological measures to evaluate drug effect, with peak responses occurring in three hours after ingestion and total dissipation of effects within 24 hours [49,50].

Huestis explained one of the chief advantages of edibles is the long duration [51]. Hollister et al. compared the effects of delta-9-THC in a chocolate cookie, which had longer-lasting and less intoxicating effects than smoking [52]. Another study of daily cannabis smokers who consumed THC orally reported a longer analgesic effect than smoking [53].

Edibles avoid issues of odor and stigma of use because they can be consumed like any other food. In addition, edibles are easier to transport, particularly to places where their use may not be legal, but despite the advantages of edibles, overconsumption can result in cognitive and motor impairment, sedation, agitation, anxiety, and even vomiting [54]. The cannabis overdose lasts only as long the period of intoxication, but that can be hours or days. Each consumer of cannabis edibles needs to be conscientious of their tolerance. A 10 mg edible will not be the same for a beginner and a regular user. Expectations may also influence effect. The time of day edibles are consumed can influence perception of uplifting and sedative quality. If alcohol has been consumed, an increase in the THC uptake and effect may be experienced.

Oral pharmacokinetics describe edibles as introducing cannabinoids through the gastrointestinal tract where THC is absorbed into the bloodstream and travels via the portal vein to the liver. Liver enzymes (primarily cytochrome P450) hydroxylates THC to form 11-hydroxytetrahydrocannabinol (11-OH-THC), and 11-OH-THC crosses the blood–brain barrier [55]. According to several studies, 11-OH-THC is more potent than delta-9-THC and appears in blood at higher quantities than delta-9-THC when it is ingested as compared to when it is inhaled [56–58]. Lack of consistency in edibles infused with cannabis and the delayed intoxication may cause users to consume a higher quantity than can be tolerated. Edible products are responsible for most healthcare visits related to cannabis intoxication [59].

Dosage estimations for homemade and retail products may not be accurate or exact. State laws require total milligrams of THC and the number of servings per package, but testing for accuracy is not considered. Hudak reports that many patients initially ate the suggested serving size but consumed the entire edible after not feeling any effects [60]. Furthermore,

Huestis et al. emphasize that body weight, metabolism, gender, and eating habits all can influence oral intoxicated states [61].

Colorado has developed a metric calculating dose equivalency across methods of cannabis delivery [62]. Laboratory analysis of edibles and smokable cannabis in Colorado suggests 1 mg THC contained in an edible produces a behavioral effect similar to 5.71 mg THC in smokable cannabis. Regulations in Colorado and Washington define a single serving of an edible as a unit containing no more than 10 mg of THC [63].

Patients, especially medicinal cannabis users, need to know the precise amounts and concentrations of THC and CBD in edibles to access the effects that consumption will produce. Despite the evidence that cannabidiol (CBD) content provides its own value, few manufacturers of edibles report the CBD content of their products. Some products reported to contain CBD may only contain trace amounts or none at all [63].

Inaccuracies in labeling and inconsistencies in formulation were reviewed in 2014 by investigative reporting in the Denver Post [64,65]. The reporters found that the actual THC content of retail edibles differed significantly from the amount claimed on the label. Because of these findings, Colorado instituted a requirement that THC concentration for recreational edibles be assessed and reported [66]. This was a mandated threshold testing only but not a measure of label accuracy and ensures that edibles do not contain more than 100 mg of THC per serving.

The need for additional regulations for edibles and accurate labeling is imperative if overdosing and accidental pediatric exposures are to be avoided. The lack of regulations has resulted in many families learning how to make their own edible cannabis products.

Another consideration in edible production beyond dosing and accurate labeling is appropriate testing for biological contaminants and pathogens. Cannabis products used in edible production need to be adequately tested not only for potency but also pesticides, heavy metals, mold, and residual solvents. Should a company discover a contamination issue after production of the edible, it should be destroyed or recalled to ensure public safety, but there are no federal guidelines or Food and Drug Administration (FDA) regulations.

Cooking with cannabis

Cooking with cannabis at home is a great way to customize medication needs while avoiding the premade, prepackaged cannabis-infused treats loaded with sugar, high fructose corn syrup, and other unhealthy ingredients that are sold at dispensary and boutique shops.

Many medical cannabis patients prefer to make their own snacks and meals to reduce boredom in taking their medication while also controlling the quantity and quality of what they are ingesting. Edibles also provide a better solution for those not wanting to smoke cannabis.

An increasing number of individuals are considering cannabis as a dietary staple. When cannabis is heated or decarboxylated, the health benefits of THCA (nonpsychoactive THC) is lost. Raw cannabis can be used in juicing and smoothie recipes to provide the nutrient benefits of THCA. Only fresh leaves should be used, and they should be consumed within three days of being cut and cleaned. Store the leaves in the refrigerator, and plan 10–15 leaves per beverage.

To obtain THC and CBD benefits from oral consumption, cannabis needs to be combined with fat for use in shakes, casseroles, and baked goods. Home extraction procedures are provided along with recipes for use. Numerous cookbooks are available, but a selection of recipes are provided in the Appendix for patient education purposes.

Decarboxylation

Cooking with cannabis requires decarboxylation to release the THC content in the leaves and buds. As stated above, raw cannabis contains THCA and CBDA, which are not psychoactive. The concentration of THCA and CBDA depends on the variety/strain of cannabis, growth history, and storage conditions of the dried product. These acid forms need to be heated or decarboxylated to release THC and CBD for metabolism in the human digestive tract. Complete activation of THCA to THC and CBDA to CBD occurs at 220°F. after 90 minutes. During this process, some volatile terpenes and flavonoids are lost. Here is a description of the home process, which provides a strong odor that can fill the house:

- Preheat oven to 220°F (110°C).
- Chop (not mince) leaves, flowers, and buds into small pieces and place evenly on baking sheet.
- Place baking sheet in oven for 45–50 minutes or until leaves are completely dried. Plant color gets medium brown shade (avoid overheating which can destroy some cannabinoids).
- Check by crumbling several leaves and remove from oven.
- Crush into coarse powder for making into canna oil, canna butter, canna-coconut oil.
- Store in air-tight glass container in cool dry place.

Decarboxylators are available for purchase by those who do not want to smell up the house or who may be worried the neighbors may report cannabis activity. Several patients have reported more consistent decarboxylation using the NOVA product available at ardentcannabis.com.

Guidelines for cannabis use in cooking

When cooking with cannabis, the most difficult aspect is getting the quantity of THC and/or CBD correct for the person. The strength of the strain used to make the canna oil or canna butter is the primary factor. A good rule of thumb is to begin using small amounts and gradually increase the amount of THC and/or CBD until desired results are achieved. Eating too much can bring unexpected consequences.

A guide to cooking was achieved from interviewing several cannabis culinary chefs in Colorado and California who recommended Drake's Marijuana handbook as their guide [67]. What may create a THC "buzz" for one adult person or CBD sustained pain relief in another can differ widely, so body weight is the first gauge used to judge beginning oral cannabis intake limits.

THC (recreational) use

Weight	Amount cannabis bud per person per meal
125–179 pounds (57–83 kg)	1/4 to 1/2 teaspoon (1.2 to 2.5 mg)
180–250 pounds (84–102 kg)	2/3 to 1 teaspoon (3.5 to 5 mg)
250+ pounds (102+ kg)	1 to 1 1/2 teaspoons (5 to 7.5 mg)

CBD (pain and nausea) medical use

Weight	Amount CBD concentrate per person per meal
125–179 pounds (57–83 kg)	1/8 teaspoon (0.5 mg)
180–250 pounds (84–102 kg)	1/4 teaspoon (1.2 mg)
250+ pounds (102+ kg)	1/2 teaspoon (2.5 mg)

Cannabis used in food is a far more effective method of pain relief than smoking, which can last 60 to 90 minutes, while CBD taken orally can last four to five hours.

Personalized nutrition approach to cannabis

Each person needs to experiment to identify what amount of THC and/ or CBD works for them. Labels on purchased edibles need to indicate percentage of THC and milligrams of THC or CBD. Homemade edibles also need to have the dose calculated. The source of the cannabis needs to be considered before calculating the dose [68–70]. A recommended daily dose of THC for a 150-pound adult is:

Source of Cannabis	Dose
Leaf or plant trim (10% THC)	0.25–1.5 g (1/4 to 1 1/2 g)
Bud (15%–20% THC)	0.125–0.75 g (1/8 to 3/4 g)
Kief/hash (high THC)	0.062–0.5 g (1/16 to 1/2 g)

Calculating cannabis dose

To estimate the THC dose of a recipe, the amount and the source of cannabis plus the number of servings is needed. One gram of cannabis = 1000 mg × 10% standard cannabis THC = 100 mg THC [71]. Kynon de Cesare, chief research officer at Steep Hill Labs, explains why actual calculations of THC, CBD, and various terpenes are difficult to achieve for an accurate analysis. Unless the cannabinoid (THC and/or CBD) are tested pre and post extraction, there is no way for home bakers to get an accurate calculation [72]:

The THCA (nonpsychoactive acid) is broken down during heating/decarboxylation yielding psychoactive THC. Then there is the inefficiency of butter and oil extraction to make canna-THC oil or canna-THC butter.

Lena Davidson, market relations and brand development for Seattle and Portland Botanica offices—one of Washington state's largest edible producers—indicates that butter and coconut oil are ideal extractors, but the only way to know how potent a homemade edible is would be to require analysis before eating [73]. Some estimates state 40 to 60% of the cannabinoids are present in the butter, while other estimates are as low as 30%. The best way to minimize variances is to know the THC potency before making the butter or coconut oil extraction. If the THCA is listed on the label, use the 0.88 conversion rate to determine THC.

Some calculation tips to remember:

1. Butter from the bottom of the batch will be different than butter from the top.
2. Measure amounts of canna butter used in recipes—don't guess.
3. Mix the batter well to get canna butter distributed throughout the bakery product.
4. Cut small, equal size portions.
5. 1 g dried cannabis = 6 mL cannabis oil.
6. A suitable new user dose of THC oil is 0.5–1.5 mL.

Canna butter calculation

1 cup butter (48 teaspoons)
1 ounce of dried cannabis 10% THC (28 g)
28 ÷ 48 = 0.5 g THC per teaspoon THC

Edible potency calculation [74]

1. 100 g 20% (high potency) cannabis or 200 mg THCA per 1 g flower
200 mg × 100 = 20,000 mg THCA

2. Convert THCA to THC 20,000 mg × 0.88 = 17,600 mg THC when extracted
3. Making canna butter = 60% efficiency 17,600 mg × 0.6 = 10,560 mg THC in canna butter
4. Want no more than 200 mg THC per brownie 10,560 mg ÷ 200 mg = 53 brownie servings made from recipe

Making cannabis THC products for use in recipes

CANNA-THC OIL

2 cups olive oil or vegetable oil
1 ounce of cannabis buds, finely ground, or 2 ounces of dried ground leaves

Heat in oil in heavy saucepan over low heat for two to three minutes. Add ground cannabis, stirring well to coat all cannabis. Simmer over low heat for 45 minutes. Remove from heat, cool, and strain to remove plant matter. Press well to extract all oil. Refrigerate for use within two months. May be used in salad dressings, sauces, and baked goods.

CANNA-THC BUTTER

1 cup unsalted butter
1 ounce of ground cannabis leaves or buds

Melt butter over low heat in saucepan. Avoid burning or scorching the butter. Add ground leaves or buds. Simmer 30–45 minutes over low heat. Butter will turn green color. Strain butter into a glass dish, pressing leaves/buds to squeeze out all the butter. Discard plant material. Refrigerate or freeze for use in recipes.

Note: Adding equal amounts of water to butter when making canna butter can help avoid burning and scorching, which can result in useless THC and poor taste.

CANNA-THC COCONUT OIL

14-ounce jar coconut oil
1 ounce of dried cannabis buds or 2 ounces of dried cannabis
  leaves

Fill large saucepan half full of water and add cannabis. Simmer over low heat for one hour. Add coconut oil. Cover and leave simmer 60–90 minutes. Mixture will be deep green. Remove from heat. Cover and let coconut oil mixture cool at room temperature. Strain mixture. Press plant matter to remove oil and water. Refrigerate oil and water in a glass jar for 24 hours. Separate solidified oil from water. Pat oil dry with paper towels. Melt canna-coconut oil in saucepan until liquid. Pour into glass jars for use in cooked vegetables, sauces, stews, soups, and shakes.

CBD oil production

CBD oil production requires careful selection of appropriate cannabis and hemp varieties. Choosing a genetic strain that is high in CBD improves yield and quality. Hemp strains are chosen to contain the lowest concentrations of THC and the highest concentration CBD. Because CBD is a by-product of hemp manufacturing of paper and clothing, patients like knowing that its production is less detrimental to the environment. Carbon dioxide extraction can be used to produce CBD oil but requires more equipment and skill than an ethanol or alcohol method. Carbon dioxide is forced through the plant material in a temperature- and pressure-controlled chamber, causing the cannabinoids to separate out of the plant matter where by they can be collected in different chambers [75]. This method results in a clean-tasting product but is more expensive.

Extracted CBD oil can be sold as oil or concentrated into a paste. Most people only need a dose the size of a grain of rice one or two times daily (~4 mg CBD) to relieve pain or anxiety in disorders such as multiple sclerosis and ALS.

CBD hemp oil is sold in different concentrations: 150 mg, 450 mg, 1500 mg.

CBD hemp oil paste is concentrated so it is absorbed slower in the mouth and is great to use in recipes because it is unflavored.

HOME EXTRACTION OF CBD OIL

Home extraction of CBD oil can produce a potent medical CBD oil using grain alcohol as the solvent and made in small batches as needed [76]:

30 g ground buds or 60–100 g dried trim from hemp
4 L grain alcohol

Combine hemp and 1 L of alcohol in large mixing bowl. Stir three to five minutes with a wooden spoon to extract resin. Filter liquid off using a sieve, squeezing out as much liquid as possible. Return hemp and another liter of alcohol to the mixing bowl. Stir five minutes to extract more CBD. Drain off alcohol in sieve again. Repeat process two more times.

Pour the strained liquid into a heavy saucepan, and heat to boiling. Let the alcohol evaporate while keeping heat just enough to bubble around the edges about 15–30 minutes. Keep stirring and scrape the sides of the saucepan with a spatula.

Transfer the concentrated oil into dosage container such as a plastic syringe or a small glass bottle with a lid. Dispense dosage needed by using toothpicks or small spoons. The CBD extract will be thick, and the quantity will be based on the quality of raw hemp used. (This procedure was observed at a patient's home).

Making CBD oil for use in recipes

CANNA-CBD OIL

2 cups olive oil or vegetable oil
1 g (100 mg) CBD hemp oil concentrate

Combine olive oil and hemp oil concentrate in a saucepan over low heat. Stir until well mixed. Pour into a glass bottle. Refrigerate until ready to use in salad dressing, baked goods, or sauces.

CANNA-CBD BUTTER

1 cup soft butter
1 g (100 mg) CBD hemp oil concentrate

Blend butter and hemp oil concentrate using a blender or a wire whip.
Place in a glass dish and use in recipes or as topping for vegetables.

CANNA-CBD COCONUT OIL

14-ounce jar coconut oil
2 g (200 mg) CBD hemp oil concentrate

Combine coconut oil and hemp oil concentrate in a saucepan over
low heat. Stir until hemp oil concentrate is dissolved. Pour back into
coconut oil jar, and store until ready to use in shakes, vegetables,
stews, and soups.

Recipes

Recipes for use of canna oils and butter are included in the Appendix.
They range from brownies, chocolate chip hemp cookies, pizza, macaroni
and cheese to banana bread, salsa, hot chocolate, and truffles. They are
provided to guide healthcare professionals in educating patients about
appropriate use of cannabis products.

Oral intake and emerging issues

One emerging issue is oral consumption and drug testing. Snack bars and
other foodstuffs were prepared from pressed hemp seeds and urine testing
for 24 hours after ingestion showed positive using EMIT immunoassay and
gas chromatography–mass spectrometry (GC-MS) [77]. Those individuals
eating two hemp seed bars showed increased immunoreactivity over those
eating only one. Individuals who ate three cookies made from hempseed
flour and butter screened positive at both 50 and 20-ng/mL cutoffs, while
hemp seeds alone did not demonstrate the presence of THC when tested by
GC-MS. Synergistic components in recipes may result in positive test results.

In another study of ingested marijuana-laced or THC brownies, a
substantial amount of THC-related metabolites were excreted over a period
of 3–14 days [78]. No positive results would be found from consuming pure
CBD foodstuffs.

State laws in Alaska, Colorado, Oregon, and Washington require edibles to be labeled with product information that includes risk factors associated with consumption [79,80], but female nonusers were more concerned about edibles than males in a focus group and compared them to drinks that could be spiked with drugs [81]. Male sentiment in that focus group centered around the attitude that if you can't handle edibles, don't use them.

Cannabis and pregnancy

Melanie C. Dreher, RN ,PhD, FAAN, Dean of the College of Nursing, University of Iowa, Iowa City, Iowa, outlines the use of cannabis in pregnancy [82]. Scientists explored a 1600-year-old tomb in Egypt and found cannabis in the abdominal area of a 14-year-old female who apparently died in childbirth [83]. Dreher goes on to state medical texts from the nineteenth century used cannabis to increase uterine contractions and reduce the pain of labor. Cambodian women who have just given birth are "given a glass of cannabis tea by the midwife before each meal to combat postpartum stiffness and to increase the milk supply of nursing mothers," Dreher writes.

Despite these historical and cultural accounts, little research has focused on the therapeutic value of cannabis in pregnancy and childbirth. Only the possible harmful effects of ingesting cannabis during pregnancy is reported. Early research on the effects of prenatal cannabis exposure was done on primates and small mammals to study the psychoactive THC exposure and how readily it crossed the placental barrier to the fetus. In nonhuman populations, it was concluded that THC did cross the placenta and was found in the fetal nervous system. It was also discovered in the milk of lactating animals, so cannabis was linked to neurological abnormalities, poor maternal weight gain, and lower birth weight [84,85].

Other studies in the 1980s and 1990s were inconclusive and contradictory about the influence of cannabis on pregnancy outcome. Moreover, legal and social sanctions against cannabis use have made it difficult in the United States to recruit subjects for research and accurately assess cannabis exposure during pregnancy.

Dr. Dreher describes a study where women in Jamaica smoke ganja (cannabis) or drink ganja tea throughout pregnancy and lactation. The comparison at three days of life for exposed and unexposed infants revealed no neurobehavioral effects from prenatal exposure, but by the end on the first month, there were significant differences. Cannabis users had infants more physiologically stable and socially responsive using the Brazelton Neonatal Assessment Scale [86].

The conservative approach of medical professionals in the United States to protect the unborn child is understandable, but restricting or eliminating cannabis use without good science is a disservice to pregnant women. The women in Jamaica used ganja/cannabis to increase their appetite, control and prevent nausea of pregnancy, and as a sleep aid and energizer. The role of cannabis to lift feelings of postpartum depression is another area for research.

The National Institute on Drug Abuse (NIDA) states that "more research is needed on how marijuana use during pregnancy could impact the health and development of infants" [87]. NIDA indicates no human research connects marijuana to mischarge but cites a primate study where it could be a factor. It also indicates that the potential of marijuana to negatively impact the developing brain has led the American College of Obstetricians and Gynecologists to recommend women be counseled against use of marijuana while trying to get pregnant, during pregnancy, and while breast feeding [88].

References

1. Huang KC. *The Pharmacology of Chinese Herbs*, second ed. CRC Press, 1998.
2. Bloomfield M. Hymns of the Atharva-Veda. *Sacred Books of the East*, vol. 42.
3. Lee C. Cachexia: the last illness. *Nature*. 2015; 528(7581).
4. Small E. *Cannabis—A Complete Guide*, vol. 277. CRC Press, 2017.
5. Davis M, Maide V, Daenenck P et al. The emerging role of cannabinoid neuromodulators in symptom management. *Supportive Care in Cancer*. 2006; 15(1): 63–71.
6. Caraceni P, Borrelli F et al. Potential therapeutic applications of cannabinoids in gastrointestinal and liver diseases: focus on Δ-9-tetrahydrocannabinol pharmacology. In: Di Marzo V, ed. *Cannabinoids* 2014. Wiley Blackwell, Hoboken, pp. 219–226.
7. Schultes RE, Hofmann A. *The Plants of the Gods: Their Sacred, Healing and Hallucinogenic Powers*. Healing Arts Press, 1979.
8. Pilcher T. *The Cannabis Cookbook*. Chartwell Books, 2007.
9. Toklas AB. *The Alice B Toklas Cookbook*. Harper & Brothers, NY, 1954.
10. Enig MG. *Know Your Fats—The Complete Primer for Understanding the Nutrition for Fats, Oils and Cholesterol*. Bethesda Books, 1993.
11. Leson G, Pless P. Evaluating the impact of hemp food consumption on workplace tests. *Journal of Analytical Toxicology*. 2001; 25(8): 691–698.
12. Callaway JC. Hempseed as a nutritional resource: an overview. *Euphytica* 2004; 140: 65–72.
13. Erasmus U. *Fats That Heal, Fats That Kill*. Alive Books, 1993.
14. Callaway JC. Hempseed as a nutritional resource: an overview. *Euphytica* 2004; 140: 65–72.
15. Deferne JL, Pate DW. Hemp seed oil. Both (n-3) and (n-6) fatty acids stimulate wound healing in rat intestine epithelial cell line. 1EC-6. *Am Soc Nutr Sci.* 1996; 29: 1791–1798.
16. Darshan SK, Rudolph IL. Effect of fatty acids of w-6 and w-3 type on human immune status and role of eicosanoids. *Nutrition* 2000; 16: 143–145.

17. Simopoulos AP. Omega-3 fatty acids in health and disease and in growth and development. *Am J Clinical Nutr.* 1991; 54: 438–463.
18. Oliwiecki S, Burton JL, Elles K et al. Levels of essential fatty acids in plasma red cell phospholipids from normal controls and patients with atopic eczema. *Acta Derm Venereol.* 1991; 71(3): 224–228.
19. Rodriguez-Leyva D, Pierce GN. The cardiac and haemostatic effects of dietary hempseed. *Nutr Metab (Lond)* 2010; 7: 32.
20. Aiello G, Fasoli E et al. Proteomic characterization of hempseed (Cannabis sativa L.). *J Proteomics* 2016; 147: 187–96.
21. Odani S and Odani S. Isolation and primary structure of a methionine and cysteine-rich seed protein of Cannabis sativa L. *Biosci Biotechnol Biochem* 1998; 12: 650–654.
22. Callaway JC. Hempseed as a nutritional resource: an overview. *Euphytica* 2004; 140: 65–72.
23. Matthaus B. Antinutritive compounds in different oilseeds. *Fett/Lipids* 1997; 99: 170–174.
24. Wanasundara PK, Shadridi F. Process-induced compositional changes of flaxseed. *Adv Exp Med Biol.* 1998; 434: 307–325.
25. Girgih AT, Alashi AM et al. A novel hemp seed meal protein hydrolysate reduces oxidative stress factors in spontaneously hypertensive rats. *Nutrients* 2014; 6(12): 5652–5666.
26. Neijat M, Suh M et al. Hempseed products fed to hens effectively increased n-3 polyunsaturated fatty acids in total lipids, triacylglycerol and phospholipid of egg yolk. *Lipids.* 2016; 51(5): 601–14.
27. Jing M, Zhao S, House JD. Performances and tissue fatty acid profile of broiler chickens and laying hens fed hemp oil and Hemp Omega TM. *Poult Sci* 2017; 96(6): 1809–1819.
28. Mediavilla V, Steinemann S. Factors influencing the yield and quality of hemp (Cannabis sativa L.) essential oil. *J Int Hemp Assoc* 1998; 5(1): 16–20.
29. ElSohy M. In: Grotenherman, F. & Russo, E., eds. *Chemical Constituents of Cannabis.* Harworth Press, Binghamton, NY, 2002, pp. 27–36.
30. Shukla VKS, Wanasundra PKJPD, Shahidi F. In: Shadi F, ed. *Natural Antioxidants: Chemistry, Health Effects and Applications.* AoCS Press, Champaign, IL, pp. 97–133.
31. Gertsch J, Leonti M, Raduner S et al. Beta-caryophyllene is dietary cannabinoid. *Proc Nat Acad Sci USA.* 2008; 105(26): 9099–9104.
32. Rezapour-Firouzi S, Arefhosseini SR et al. Activity of liver enzymes in multiple sclerosis patients with Hot-nature diet and co-supplemented hemp seed, evening primrose oils intervention. *Complement Ther Med.* 2014; 22(6): 986–93.
33. Gertsch J. Cannabimimetric phyochemicals in the diet-an evolutionary link to food selection and metabolic stress adaptation? *Br J Pharmacology* 2017; 174(11): 1464–1483.
34. Callaway JC, Pate DW. *Hempseed oil.* Hempseed NEW, indd 9/12/2008. www.finola.com
35. Stadtmauer G. Anaphylaxis to ingestion of hempseed. *J Allergy Clin Immunol.* 2003; 112(1): 216–217.
36. Vidal C, Fuilnte R, Iglesias A et al. Bronchial asthma due to the cannabis sativa seed. *Allergy* 1991; 46: 647–649.
37. Small E. *Cannabis—A Complete Guide.* CRC Press, 2017, pp. 212–214.

38. Holt S. *Hemp nutrition. The Cannabis Revolution- what you need to know.* Holt Institute of Medicine, Little Falls, NJ, 2016, pp. 137–146.

39. Casano S, Grassi G, Martini V et al. Variations in terpene profiles of different strains of Cannabis sativa L. *Acta Horticulturae*.2011; 925: 115–121.

40. Baser KHC, Buchbauer G, ed. *Handbook of essential oils: Science, technology, and applications.* CRC Press, Boca Raton, FL, 2010.

41. Barrus DG, Capogrossi KL et al. *Tasty THC: promises and challenges of cannabis edibles.* Methods Rep RTI Press, 2016. 10.37 68/rtipress.

42. Brohl B, Kammerzell R, Koski WL. *Colorado Marijuana Enforcement Division: Annual Update.* Colorado Department of Revenue, Denver, CO, 2015.

43. Schauer GL, King BA et al. Toking, vaping, and eating for health or fun: marijuana use patterns in adults, US, 2014. *American Journal of Preventive Medicine* 2016; 50(1): 1–8.

44. Pacula R, Jacobson M, Maksabedian EJ. In the weeds: a baseline view of cannabis use among legalizing states and their neighbors. *Addiction* 2016; 111(6): 973–980.

45. Murphy F, Sales P et al. Baby boomers and cannabis delivery systems. *Journal of Drug Issues.* 2015; 45(3): 293–313.

46. Grella CE, Rodriguez L, Kim T. Patterns of medical marijuana use among individuals sampled from medical marijuana dispensaries in Los Angeles. *Journal of Psychoactive Drugs.* 2014; 46(4): 263–272.

47. Boero FJ. Bring food science into the cannabis, hemp edibles conversation. www.IFT.org/Food-Technology/Perspective/2017/August/02/bring-food-science-into-the-cannabis-hemp-edibles-conversation.aspx

48. Hemp Industry Association. http://www.votehemp.com/PR/2017–4-14_2016_annual-retail-sales-for-hemp-products-estimated-at-$688million.html

49. Walsh Z, Callaway R et al. Cannabis for therapeutic purposes: patient characteristics, access, and reasons for use. *The International Journal on Drug Policy.* 2013; 24(6): 511–516.

50. Cone EJ, Johnson RE et al. Marijuana-laced brownies: behavioral effects, physiological effects, and urinalysis in humans following ingestion. *Journal of Analytical Toxicology* 1988; 12(4): 169–175.

51. Huestis MA. Human cannabinoid pharmacokinetics. *Chemistry & Biodiversity* 2007; 4(8): 1770–1804.

52. Hollister LE, Gillespie HK et al. Do plasma concentrations of delta-9-tetrahydrocannabinol reflect the degree of intoxication? *Journal of Clinical Pharmacology.* 1981; 21(8–9 Suppl): 171s–177s.

53. Cooper ZD, Comer SD, Haney M. Comparison of the analgesic effects of dronabinol and smoked marijuana in daily marijuana smokers. *Neuropsychopharmacology.* 2013; 38(10): 1984–1992.

54. Galli JA, Sawaya RA, Friedenberg FK. Cannabinoid hyperemesis syndrome. *Current Drug Abuse Reviews.* 2011; 4(4): 241–249.

55. Grotenhermen F. The toxicology of cannabis and cannabis prohibition. *Chemistry & Biodiversity* 2007; 4(8): 1744–1769.

56. Hall W, Solowj N. Adverse effects of cannabis. *Lancet* 1998; 352(9140): 1611–1616.

57. Bui QM, Simpson S, Nordstrom K. Psychiatric and medical management of marijuana intoxication in the emergency department. *The Western Journal of Emergency Medicine.* 2015; 16(3): 414–417.

58. Mura P, Kintz P et al. THC can be detected in brain while absent in blood. *Journal of Analytical Toxicology.* 2005; 29(8): 842–843.
59. Hollister LE. Structure-activity relationships in man of cannabis constituents, and homologs and metabolites of Δ 9-tetrahydrocannabinol. *Pharmacology.* 1974; 11: 3–11.
60. Hudak M, Severn D, Nordstrom K. Edible cannabis-induced psychosis: intoxication and beyond. *The American Journal of Psychiatry.* 2015; 172(9): 911–912.
61. Huestis MA. Human cannabinoid pharmacokinetics. *Chemistry & Biodiversity* 2007; 4(8): 1770–1804.
62. Monte AA, Zane RD, Heard KJ. The implications of marijuana legalization in Colorado. *JAMA* 2015; 313(3): 241–242.
63. Vandrey R, Raber JC et al. Cannabinoid dose and label accuracy in edible medical cannabis products. *JAMA* 2015; 313(24): 2491–2493.
64. Baca R. Tests show THC content in marijuana edibles is inconsistent. *The Denver Post.* Mar 8, 2014.
65. Orens A, Light M et al. *Marijuana equivalency in portion and dosage.* Colorado Department of Revenue, Denver, CO, 2015.
66. Brohl B, Kammerzell R, Koski WL. *Colorado Marijuana Enforcement Division: Annual Update.* Colorado Department of Revenue, Denver, CO, 2015.
67. Drake B. *Marijuana, a Cultivator's Handbook.* Ronin Publishing, Berkeley, CA, 1979.
68. Conrad C. *Hemp for Health: The Medicinal and Nutritional Uses of Cannabis Sativa.* Healing Arts Press, 1997.
69. Sicard C. How to Calculate THC Dosages for homemade edibles. www.hightimes.com
70. Edible Dosage Calculator. originalweedrecipes.com
71. Squibb S. How to calculate THC dosage in recipes for marijuana edibles. www.thecannabist.com
72. de Cesare K, Chief Research Officer, Steep Hill Labs, Inc. Interview.
73. Olsen-Koziol J. Learn about Botanica Seatle's mouthwatering line of cannabis edibles. Aug 9, 2017. RespectMyRegion.com
74. Konen B. ed. *Cooking with cannabis: how to make edibles.* https://www.leafy.com/news/science-tech/dosing-homemade-cannabis-edibles-why-its-nearly-impossible-to-cal
75. How is CBD oil made? herb.com
76. How to make your own CBD. www.cannabis.info/en
77. Fortner N, Fogerson R et al. Marijuana-positive urine test results from consumption of hemp seeds in food products. *J Analytical Toxicology* 1997; 21(6): 476–481.
78. Cone EJ, Johnson RE. Marijuana-laced brownies: behavioral effects, physiological effects, and urinalysis in humans following ingestion. *J Analytical Toxicology* 1988; 12(4): 169–175.
79. Gourdet C, Giombi KC et al. How four U.S. states are regulating recreational marijuana edible. *Int J Drug Policy.* 2017; 43: 80–90.
80. Kosa KM, Giombi KC et al. Consumer use and understanding of labeling information on edible marijuana products sold for recreational use in the states of Colorado and Washington. *Int J Drug Policy.* 2017; 43: 57–66.
81. Friese B, Slater MD et al. Teen use of marijuana edibles: a focus group study of an emerging issue. *J Prim Prev* 2016; 37(3): 303–309.

82. Mathre ML, ed. *Cannabis in Medical Practice—a legal, historical and pharmacological overview of the therapeutic use of marijuana.* McFarland & Company, Inc, Jefferson, NC, 1997, pp. 159–170.
83. Zias J, Stark H, Seligman J et al. Early medical use of cannabis. *Nature* 1993; 363(20): 215.
84. Day N, Sambamoorthi U, Taylor P et al. Prenatal marijuana use and neonatal outcomes. *Neurotoxicity and Teratology* 1991; 13: 329–334.
85. Fried PA. Marijuana use during pregnancy: consequences for the offspring. *Seminars in Perinatalogy* 1991; 15(4): 280–287.
86. Als H, Tronick E, Lester BM et al. The Brazelton Neonatal Assessment Scale (BNAS). *Journal of Abnormal Psychology* 1997; 5(3): 215–231.
87. Can marijuana use during and after pregnancy harm the body? National Institute on Drug Abuse. http://www.drugabuse.gov/publications/research-reports/marijuana/can-marijuana-use-during-pregnancy-harm-baby
88. Marijuana Use During Pregnancy and Lactation—ACOG. http://www.acog.org.Resources-and-publications/committee-opinions/committee-on-obstetric-practice/marijuana-use-during-pregnancy-and-lactation. Published July 2015.

chapter eighteen

Clinical recommendations and dosing guidelines for cannabis

Betty Wedman-St. Louis

Contents

Medical professionals need assurance that the cannabis products they are recommending have quality standards that are confirmed through reputable analysis to ensure they are providing patients safe and effective products. Whether over-the-counter cannabis products need to be held to the same quality standards as pharmaceuticals has yet to be determined. Research and consumer demand will help determine future requirements.

Medical personnel ordering cannabis products need to meet state requirements and ensure that the patient meets eligibility criteria for using cannabis. First-time patients arriving at a dispensary need assistance for registration, purchasing, and selecting products [1]. Discussion with the patient helps define what cannabis product(s) may be correct for them.

A chemotherapy patient's needs will differ greatly from a Parkinson's disease sufferer or a diabetic with neuropathy [2].

Cannabis products should be backed with a Certificate of Analysis verifying testing for potency, cannabinoid profile, microbial/pesticide/ mold residues, and heavy metals assessment. A batch number on the product can be traced and should be on each product.

Because of its status as a Schedule 1 substance, federal law prohibits physicians from prescribing cannabis, [3] so licensed physicians write recommendations instead of prescriptions [4].

Dosing rule of thumb

A general rule of thumb is dose low and slow, especially with edibles that may be the patient's choice for introduction to the cannabis market. Patient education needs to focus attention on a 5 mg product being consumed over an hour, not every 10 minutes. Edibles are more difficult to dose because time of day, liver metabolism, and whether consumed on an empty stomach can all effect symptom management and absorption, but Bunka [5] estimated

Smoking and vaping = ~30% absorption

Edibles = ~4 to 7% absorption depending on the fat level in the edible for cannabinoid availability

"No one dose fits all" according to Debra Kimless, MD, at the April 2017 Pittsburgh Cannabis Conference. "The dose needs to change with frequency of use and as children/adults age; they may need an increased dose for symptom management" [6]. With over 400 chemicals in the whole plant and not knowing what chemical is going to be effective, or what combination of chemicals are needed for synergistic benefit, patience and knowledge are required by the physician and the patient, Dr. Kimless stressed.

Personalized medicine

Cannabis use requires a personalized medicine regimen depending on the person and the condition. A patient's sensitivity to THC is a key factor determining the ratio (THC:CBD) and the dose plus frequency [7]. CBD is used to reduce or neutralize the intoxicating effects of THC. Patients with anxiety, depression, and pediatric seizure disorders may do best with a CBD dominant dose. Use of THC and CBD are considered to work best together in cancer and neurological diseases [8].

Body weight is frequently used as a guide in selecting an appropriate dose, especially for edibles containing THC, because overindulgence leads to a sleepy patient. Tolerance can build up over time, and the dose may need to be increased accordingly. The amount of ground cannabis powder dosing by body weight for edibles is:

125–175 pounds = 1/4 teaspoon
176–220 pounds = 1/2 teaspoon
221–290 pounds = 3/4 teaspoon

[Canna oil and canna butter are an easy way to add cannabis to meals. Cannabis peanut butter is easy to prepare and a good way for children and adults to consume CBD and/or THC. See Cannabis Nutrition chapter and recipes for more details].

Determining dosage [9]

- Decide format for cannabis use—spray, oil, edible.
- Find the ratio of THC to CBD that works for patient.
- Begin with low dose.
- Space out dose over 8–10 hours rather than single dose.
- Repeat same dose three to four days before increasing.
- Adjust ratio and dose as needed.

Dosing frequency tips [10]

- Inhalation five to six times daily
- Sublingual three to four times daily
- Ingestion two to three times daily

Specific disease recommendations

The Mayo Clinic reported dose recommendations based on scientific research, publication reviews, and expert opinion to provide healthcare providers with guidelines for therapy [11].

Amyotrophic lateral sclerosis: 10 mg THC orally per day
Cancer chemotherapy nausea: 5 mg/meter squared dronabinol orally one to three hours before chemotherapy, then every two to four hours after chemotherapy (10 mg per meter squared THC taken two hours before and four, eight, 16, and 24 hours after chemotherapy)
Cancer loss of appetite: 2.5 mg THC orally with or without CBD
Chronic pain: capsules or spray into mouth 2.5–20 mg THC
Eating disorders: 7.5–30 mg THC orally per day
Epilepsy: 200–300 mg CBD orally per day

Sleep disorders: 40–160 mg CBD orally

Multiple sclerosis: 2.5 mg dronabinol orally per day or 15–30 mg cannabis extract capsules orally in 5 mg doses or mouth spray Sativex containing 2.7 mg THC and 2.5 mg CBD eight sprays within three hours

Tourette's syndrome: capsules containing 2.5–10 mg THC daily

Glaucoma: 5 mg THC sublingually daily or 20–40 mg CBD sublingually

Possible side effects from THC products

Patients need to be educated about possible side effects of using THC cannabis products [12]:

Xerostomia (dry mouth), dizziness, nausea, vomiting

Fecal impaction or severe constipation

Interaction with prescription medications

Irritability or brain fog

Interaction with dietary supplements

Variety of cannabis products available [13]

Smoking: Small amount of dried cannabis flower in a pipe, a water pipe (bong) or rolled in paper ("joint") delivers instant relief, is fairly easy to regulate dosage, and is less expensive, but patients with pulmonary damage or asthma need not consider this option.

Topicals: Predominately CBD products that don't provide a "high" but primarily are used for localized pain.

Oral solutions: CBD oil, spray or concentrate, and THC oil in 1- or 2-ounce bottles.

Capsules: CBD and/or THC.

Vaporizing cartridge: Slim, ballpoint pen-size way to discreetly inhale delivering instant relief, but battery powered units need to be recharged to heat cannabis for release of medicinal compounds.
CBD 200–250 mg per cartridge
THC 500 mg per cartridge

Tinctures: Predominately CBD in assorted flavors in a small bottle for squirting or spraying under the tongue with ease in controlling dose plus faster action that from edibles.

Transdermal patches: Need to be applied to clean, dry, hairless skin (inner wrist or top of foot) to provide symptom management without smoking or eating. Most come in 10 mg dose but can be cut in half for reduced dose.

Suppositories: Cannabis extract for insertion in the rectum as an alternative to edibles that provides symptom relief quickly.

Edibles: Look on the label for potency and select childproof packaging

Hard candy	Chocolates
Chocolate chip cookies	Snickerdoodle cookies
Brownie bites	Krispy cereal bars
Fruit chews	Gummies

Combination of products with THC and CBD

Capsules—10 mg TBC + 10 mg CBD
Oral solution—10 mg THC + 10 mg CBD
Sublingual solution—10 mg THC + 10 mg CBD
Vaporizer cartridge—250 THCo + 250 CBD

Delivery of cannabis [14]

Smoking (leaves and buds): 0.5–1 g cannabis
   1 gram of flowers = 100–200 mg cannabinoids
   10% THC = 16 mg THC

[Doses of THC as low as 2.5–3 mg are associated with therapeutic benefit and minimal psychoactivity [15–17]].

Oral ingestion: 1 g THC = ~20 mg cannabinoids

[Various peer-reviewed studies in scientific and medical literature indicate that most people using smoked or ingested cannabis for medical purposes reported using between 10 and 20 g of cannabis per week, about 1–3 g of dried cannabis daily [18]].
   [A Netherlands study [19] reported the median dose of edibles was 1.5 g per day.]

Capsule: 0.1–0.5 g contains 10–50 mg cannabinoids (higher dose options
   can contain 25–100 mg cannabinoids)
Tinctures and Extracts
   Alcohol = 10–15 mg cannabinoids/mL
   Glycerin = 3–10 mg cannabinoids/mL
Patch = 12 mg cannabinoids

[There is no information available on dosing amounts for topical ointments, creams, lotions, balms, and salves.]
   The route of administration for cannabis affects the onset, intensity, and duration of the therapeutic effects of cannabis. Patients refer to

the relaxation and euphoria felt after consuming THC as a "high." When cannabis is smoked or vaped, it quickly diffuses to the brain producing effects within seconds to minutes. Blood levels usually reach the maximum within 30 minutes and then subside within one to three hours [20–22].

Eating does not produce effects for 30–120 minutes and can last five to eight hours. The slow action of oral ingestion is due to THC being absorbed in the intestines, transported to the liver, and converted into 11-OH-THC, which is a longer acting metabolite [23]. The intoxication effects from the delayed onset from edibles is a consequence of overconsumption [24].

Cannabis/THC side effects

Side effects of cannabis/THC use may be more of a nuisance and usually not a cause of concern but are directly related to dose, absorption, and the mindset of the patient. The potential for side effects include:

- Euphoria—a feeling of well-being or elation expressed as talkativeness, laughter, or quiet introspection that lasts about 20 to 30 minutes after inhaling THC.
- Drowsiness—feeling sleepy after use, which is usually dose related.
- Tachycardia or rapid heart rate—"heart pounding" can start 20 minutes after an inhalation dose and lasts about an hour, so patients with angina or cardiac issues should use caution.
- Increased appetite—commonly called "cannabis hunger" or munchies begins soon after use.
- Dry mouth frequently follows cannabis/THC use.

Acute symptoms of cannabis intoxication are the patient's sociability and sensitivity to colors, music, and lights. High levels of THC can cause the patient to experience panic attacks, paranoid thoughts, and hallucinations [25]. Gonzalez et al. [26] points out that chronic use of cannabis can trigger desensitization, which can render users tolerant to the THC effects.

Hypersensitivity to cannabis

The possibility of allergy to cannabis is real and can manifest as a gastrointestinal upset or rash. If a serious breathing problem is experienced, emergency care is needed. Individuals with chemical sensitivities should be encouraged to only use organically grown cannabis to avoid chemicals that may have been used in the growing process.

Cannabinoid-based medications

Three cannabinoid drugs have been licensed by the U.S. Food and Drug Administration:

- Dronabinol (marketed as Marinol) is synthetic delta-9-THC and indicated for nausea and vomiting associated with chemotherapy and to stimulate appetite in AIDS patients with wasting syndrome.
- Nabilone (marked as Cesamet) is a synthetic delta-9-THC prescribed for similar symptoms.
- Syndros is a liquid form of dronabinol.

Both dronabinol and nabilone are oral capsules and have a slow onset of action. They are available by prescription.

Cannabis and pregnancy

The American College of Obstetricians and Gynecologists recommend that obstetricians and gynecologists counsel women against using cannabis while trying to get pregnant, during pregnancy, and while breast-feeding.

Safety of cannabidiol

Cannabidiol (CBD) may have therapeutic value in an increasing number of diseases, from epilepsy to anxiety, depression, and inflammatory bowel disease [27]. No known biological pathway exists in the human body to convert CBD to THC, but an experimental study by Merrick et al. [28] found that cannabidiol may be converted into psychoactive cannabinoids delta-8-THC and delta-9-THC. Their conclusion centered around "the acidic environment during normal gastrointestinal transit can expose orally CBD treated patients to levels of THC and other psychoactive cannabinoids that may exceed the threshold for a positive physiological response." They issued a warning about oral use of CBD and recommended other delivery methods such as transdermal applications be developed [29].

According to Grotenhermen [30], the clinical data did not support the conclusion that other delivery systems were needed. High doses of CBD have not caused any psychological, psychomotor, or cognitive/ physical effects similar to THC dosing. Grotenhermen pointed out in his commentary that two of the six authors were paid consultants of Zynerba Pharmaceuticals, and another three of the six authors work for Zynerba Pharmaceuticals, which develops transdermal CBD preparations.

CBD interactions with other drugs

The safety of cannabidiol (CBD) even at high doses has been established in numerous clinical studies. Bergamaschi et al. [31] reviewed 132 original studies in 2011, with an update by Iffland and Grotenhermen in 2016 [32].

Drug interaction with CBD research has been limited, but in vitro studies had shown that CBD inhibits the ABC transporters P-gp (3–100 μM CBD) and Bcrp in leukemia cells [33] with implications for anticancer drugs that also bind to these transporters, but CBD was shown to not cause clinically relevant drug interactions. Further research is needed.

The cytochrome 450 complex enzymes are the primary drug metabolizing enzymes via the CYP3A4 enzyme. Drugs such as ketoconazole, itraconazole, ritonavir, and clarithromycin inhibit this enzyme, which can slow CBD degradation. Phenobarbital, rifampicin, carbamazepine, and phenytoin induce CYP3A4 causing reduced CBD availability [34]. Proton pump inhibitors and antiepileptic drugs (risperidone, pantoprazole, clobazam) are degraded via the P450 complex, and co-administration with CBD may alter bioavailability.

Consequently, human studies are needed to monitor CBD–drug interactions to ensure dosing and administration regimens.

Other clinical comments

Patients may be interested in volunteering for a cannabis study, with over 100 studies ongoing as of September 2017. Studies vary from seizure disorders to inflammatory bowel disease, anxiety, and substance use disorder.

Medical professionals can gain continuing education and mentoring at national and international conferences such as:

- IACM International Academy of Cannabinoids Medicine
- ICRS International Cannabinoid Research Society Annual Symposium
- AACM American Academy of Cannabinoid Medicine
- International Cannabis and Cannabinoids Institute
- Society for Cannabis Clinicians

References

1. Patient resources. United Patient's Group. www.unitedpatientsgroup.com/resources.
2. Cotte, S. First time cannabis patients. *World Medical Cannabis Conference & Expo*, April 22, 2017, Pittsburgh, PA.
3. Blaszczak-Boxe, A. Marijuana's history: How one plant spread through the world. *Live Science*. www.livescience.com/48337-marijuana-history-how-cannabis-traveled-world.html.

4. State medical marijuana laws. *National Conference of State Legislatures*. www. ncsi.org/research/health/state-medical-marijuana-laws.
5. Bunka, C. Topicals, tinctures, capsules, edibles. *World Medical Cannabis Conference & Expo*, April 22, 2017, Pittsburgh, PA.
6. Kimless, D. First time cannabis patients. *World Cannabis Conference & Expo*, April 21–22, 2017, Pittsburgh, PA.
7. Pacher, P., Batkai, S., and Kunos, G. The endocannabinoid system as an emerging target of pharmacotherapy. *Pharmacol Rev*, 2006; 58(3): 389–462.
8. Bushak, L. A brief history of medical cannabis: From ancient anesthesia to the modern dispensary. *Medical Daily*. www.medicaldaily.com/brief-history-medical-cannabis-ancient-anestesia-modern-dispensary-370344.
9. *Cannabis dosing*. www.projectcbd,org/cannabis-dosing.
10. Malka, D. Delivery and dosage of cannabis medicine. *Medical Marijuana—An educational symposium for Florida physicians*, June 3, 2017. www.slideshare.net/CannaHoldings/delivery-and-dosage-of-cannabis-medicine-by-deborah-malka-md-phd.
11. Marijuana (Cannabis sativa) dosing. Mayo Clinic. www.mayoclinic.org/drugs-supplements/marijuana/dosing.hrb-20059701.
12. Volkow, N.D. *The biology and potential therapeutic effects of cannabidiol*. National Institute of Health/National Institute on Drug Abuse. www.drugabuse.gov/about-nida/legislative-activities/testimony-to-congress/2016/biology-potential-therapeutic-effects-cannabibiol. Published June 24, 2015.
13. Patient resources. United Patient's Group. www.unitedpatientsgroup.com/resources.
14. Malka, D. Delivery and dosage of cannabis medicine. *Medical Marijuana—An Educational Symposium for Florida Physicians* June 3, 2017. www.slideshare.net/CannaHoldings/delivery-and-dosage-of-cannabis-medicine-by-deborah-malka-md-phd.
15. Health Canada Information for Health Care Professional: Cannabis (marihuana, marijuana) and the Cannabinoids, 2013.
16. Neuropathic Pain. *Canadian Medical Association Journal*, 182(14): E694–701.
17. Eisenberg, E. et al. The pharmacokinetics, efficacy, safety, and ease of use of a novel portable metered-dose cannabis inhaler in patients with chronic neuropathic pain: A phase 1a study. *Journal of Pain and Palliative Care Pharmacotherapy*, 2014; 28: 216–225.
18. Health Canada Information for Health Care Professional: Cannabis (marihuana, marijuana) and the Cannabinoids, 2013.
19. Hazekamp, A. et al. The medicinal use of cannabis: An international cross-sectional survey on administration forms. *Journal of Psychoactive Drugs*, 2013; 45(3): 199–210.
20. Fabritius, M., Chtioui, H., Battistella, G. et al. Comparison of cannabinoid concentrations in oral fluid and whole blood between occasional and regular cannabis smokers prior to and after smoking a cannabis joint. *Analytical and Bioanalytical Chemistry*, 2013; 405(30): 9791–9803.
21. Huestis, M.A. and Cone, E.J. Blood cannabinoids. I Absorption of THC and formation of 11-OH-THC and THCCOOH during and after smoking marijuana. *Journal of Analytical Toxicology*, 1992; 16(5): 276–282.
22. Abrams, D.I., Vizoso, H.P., Shade, S.B. et al. Vaporization as a smokeless cannabis delivery system: A pilot study. *Clinical Pharmacology and Therapeutics*, 2007; 82(5): 572–578.

23. Huestis, M.A. and Cone, E.J. Blood cannabinoids. I Absorption of THC and formation of 11-OH-THC and THCCOOH during and after smoking marijuana. *Journal of Analytical Toxicology*, 1992; 16(5): 276–282.

24. MacCoun, R.J. and Mello, M.M. Half-baked—The retail promotion of marijuana edibles. *New England Journal of Medicine*, 2015; 3729(11): 989–991.

25. Agrawal, A., Madden, P.A., Bucholz, K.K. et al. Initial reactions to tobacco and cannabis smoking: A twin study. *Addiction*, 2014; 109(4): 663–671.

26. Gonzalez, S., Cebeira, M., and Fernandez-Ruiz, J. Cannabinoid tolerance and dependence: A review of studies in laboratory animals. *Pharmacology Biochemistry and Behavior*, 2005; 81(2): 300–318.

27. Grotenhermen, F., Gebhardt, K., and Berger, M. *Cannabidiol*. Solothurn, Switzerland: Nachschatten Verlag, 2016.

28. Merrik, J., Lane, B., Sebree, T. et al. Identification of psychoactive degradants of cannabidiol in simulated gastric and physiological fluid. *Cannabis and Cannabinoid Research*, 2016; 1(1): 102–112.

29. Grotenhermen, F., Gebhardt, K., and Berger, M. *Cannabidiol*. Solothurn, Switzerland: Nachschatten Verlag, 2016.

30. Grotenhermen F. *Even High Doses of Oral Cannabidiol Do not Cause THC-Like Effects in Humans*. Nova Institut, Sept 2016.

31. Bergamaschi, M.M., Queiroz, R.H., Zuardi, A.W. et al. Safety and side effects of cannabidiol, a Cannabis sativa constituent. *Current Drug Safety*, 2011; 6(4): 237–249.

32. Iffland, K. and Grotenhermen, F. European Industrial Hemp Association (EIHA) review on: Safety and side effects of cannabidiol—A review of clinical data and relevant animal studies, 2016. www.eiha.org.

33. Bih, C.I., Chen, T., Nunn, A.V. et al. Molecular targets of cannabidiol in neurological disorders. *Neurotherapeutics*, 2015; 12(4): 699–730.

34. Iffland, K. and Grotenhermen, F. European Industrial Hemp Association (EIHA) review on: Safety and side effects of cannabidiol—A review of clinical data and relevant animal studies, 2016. www.eiha.org.

section three

Regulations & Standards

chapter nineteen

Cannabis identification, cultivation, analysis, and quality control

Betty Wedman-St. Louis

Contents

Marijuana and hemp are members of the Cannabaceae family along with hops (humulus) with flowers occurring on male and female plants. Leaves are a basic way to identify different species of cannabis [1].

Humans have dispersed cannabis worldwide over the past 10,000 years from Central Asia in the Himalayas to various habitats throughout the world. It can be found in fertile, moist farmlands, in open habitats, in waste areas, and in open woodlands along with the cultivation indoors and outdoors for recreational and medicinal use [2].

Cannabis raw material—stems, leaves, and flowers—can vary in color based on the variety and the environmental factors during the growing process, including light, water, nutrients in the soil, handling, and curing process. The color should be consistent throughout the sample with no gray or black, which could indicate mold [3].

Cannabis has a bitter and pungent taste, which has required producers of edibles to use highly flavored ingredients such as chocolate to mask the taste.

Cannabis in commerce

Breeding and selection have produced cannabis strains unique for either fiber or drug production. The dried inflorescence (flower head) along with the leaves and stems of the female plant are the most widely available commercial sources on the market. The most important cannabinoid in the U.S. market is THC, with breeding focusing on plants that produce high THC. Indoor growing due to law enforcement efforts to eradicate production has resulted in increased THC yields well above the usual 10% THC potency [4].

In the United States, the average percentage of THC in cannabis during the 1960s and 1970s was less than 1%. By the 1980s, the average THC concentration rose to about 3% [5], and since 1997, samples can be found with 8%–29% THC, during which time CBD concentrations have remained stable [6].

The European Union THC potency has an upper limit for cultivated cannabis with ranges from 1.1% (Hungary 2002) to 16.9% (Italy 1998), with no minimum or maximum THC–CBD concentration ratios legally mandated [7].

Cannabis is cultivated in over 170 countries, with North America providing the largest amount of herbal cannabis on the market [8]. The three primary sources of cultivated cannabis in the United States are: (1) federally legal material; (2) material regulated by select states; and (3) material that is traded illegally according to state or federal law.

Federally legal cannabis in the United States is produced by the Coy W. Waller Laboratory Complex of the University of Mississippi (UM) for research and medicinal use, since it is classified as a Schedule 1 controlled substance with growth, transport, and possession restricted. UM also receives cannabis samples seized by law enforcement and continues to supply cannabis to patients in The Compassionate Investigational New Drug program of 1978 [9].

Numerous states have allowed the medicinal use of cannabis with provisions for growing, processing, and using it. Colorado and Washington approved the nonmedical use of cannabis in 2014. State approval can vary from distribution at dispensaries to individuals allowed to grow their own cannabis. Cole indicates that federal regulators allow the use of medical cannabis as long as state regulations are followed, but federal drug policies indicate that states do not have a legal right to regulate cannabis [10]. Such inconsistency in regulations and enforcement policies have prevented many medical professionals from even recommending medicinal use of cannabis.

Most of the cannabis used in the United States is from illegal sources, with most of it being used for recreational purposes. According to Gettman, cannabis is grown in every U.S. state, and much of the illicit imports come from Mexico [11].

Cultivation

Cultivation of cannabis starts with selection of seed and clones for the desired strain and growing environment. Growth from seeds results in some male plants in the crop, but this can be avoided by starting with clones. Cross breeding of the two predominant species—sativa and indica—results in a hybrid known as "skunk" (75% sativa, 25% indica) to produce high THC concentrations from sativa and higher yields from indica [12].

All plants whether propagated from seed or clone must be identified—genus, species, variety, and chemo type—with traceability to ensure healthy production. Cuttings from female plants can be used for propagation to avoid male plants and prevent seed fertilization so more flowers and increased cannabinoids and resin are produced.

Soil, fertilization, and irrigation are important concerns in addition to climate control of light, humidity, and temperature, which are imperative for the cannabinoid profile and reduction of insect infestation or fungal contamination.

Harvest

Cannabinoids and terpenoids are produced and stored in the trichomes (tiny hairs that cover the bud) of the plant. The timing of harvest is based on cannabinoid content with THC content varying widely based on strain and the part of the plant used [13]. THC is highest (10%–12%) in the flower head, leaves average 1%–2%, stalks contain 0.1%–0.3% and roots no more than 0.03% with no cannabinoids in clean seeds [14]. For an optimum harvest, some growers perform analysis of the raw material daily to determine the peak THCA concentration or assess visually when at least ~75% of the stigmas turn brown and shrivel [15].

Post harvest handling

Cannabis plant material needs to be immediately processed after harvesting to reduce pest and fungal contamination along with preventing degradation of the active compounds. Buds are removed manually, and leaves can be removed by hand or with a trimming machine.

Chen and Majumder describe the drying process for preserving the medicinal compounds and reducing the risk of mold contamination. Drying can be done by either cutting the flowering tops from the plant or hanging the entire plant upside down in a shaded area. It takes 24–72 hours when drying the plant by hanging in a controlled temperature and humidity-controlled area [16].

After drying, the flower heads are placed in single-layer boxes, on breathable trays or screens to allow air flow in a well-ventilated area for the next three days. Temperature and humidity are consistently controlled to remove moisture and avoid drying too quickly so organoleptic properties are maintained. A final drying process occurs to allow complete drying of the flower head when placed in a closed glass container or plastic bag with regular opening every 12–24 hours for one to two weeks [17].

Storage

Once cannabis is properly dried, degradation of the cannabinoids is negligible if protected from air and light. Storage at 20°C is recommended, with several sources not recommending freezing [17].

Contaminants and adulterants

Several plant species have similar characteristics comparable to cannabis species—hibiscus, Japanese maple, Asian nettle, and false hemp—which can be used as a contaminant internationally [18]. These plant materials can be identified microscopically, so close examination is needed on plant materials. Other common contaminants are microbial (fungal and bacteria) and heavy metals. These contaminants occur during cultivation and storage [19,20].

Adulterants such as growth enhancers and pesticides are possible risks for cannabis users [21]. Banned substances and tiny glass beads (to increase weight) and other cholinergic compounds have been reportedly added to cannabis [22]. Synthetic cannabinoids named "spice" and "K2" can be sold as incense or smoking blends, which can produce a medical emergency and are dangerous [23].

Medicinal cannabis should be free of molds and bacteria, free of heavy metals contaminants, and void of pesticides and fungicides that could present a health issue for consumers. Dispensaries should maintain quality control standards to ensure purity and quality by independent lab testing and verification of Certificates of Analysis. Dispensary personnel need to be appropriately trained in processing and handling of cannabis products to ensure purity, quality, and identification of materials sold [24].

Constituents in cannabis

Over 750 different constituents have been identified in cannabis including terpenoids, noncannabinoid phenols, nitrogenous compounds, and other plant compounds. Cannabinoids are the most studied and well-known, but emerging research has suggested terpenoids are an important component in modulating cannabinoid responses [25]. Cannabinoids (CBs) are the compounds most commonly associated with the pharmacological activity of cannabis [26]:

Δ-9-tetrahydrocannabinol (THC) is the primary psychotropic with medicinal action

- Activates PPAR-y and TRPA1
- Analgesic via CB1 and CB2 agonism
- Antiemetic
- Anti-inflammatory
- Antioxidant
- Antipruritic, cholestatic jaundice
- Benefits duodenal ulcers
- Bronchodilatory
- Muscle relaxant
- Reduces Alzheimer's symptoms

Cannabidiol (CBD) is a nonpsychotropic with medicinal action

- Anandamide (AEA) reuptake inhibitor
- Analgesic
- Anticonvulsant
- Antidepressant in rodents
- Antiemetic
- Antifungal
- Anti-inflammatory
- Antagonizes effects of THC in humans
- Antioxidant
- Effective against methicillin-resistant Staphylococcus aureus (MRSA)
- Increase adenosine A2A signaling
- Proapoptotic against breast cancer cell lines
- Treatment of addiction
- Treatment of psychosis

Cannabichromene (CBC) is a nonpsychotropic with medicinal action

- Analgesic
- Anandamide reuptake inhibitor

- Anti-inflammatory
- Antimicrobial
- TRPA1 agonist

Cannabigerol (CBG) is a nonpsychotropic with medicinal action

- Analgesic via α-2 adrenergic blockade
- Anandamide reuptake inhibitor
- Antifungal
- Anti-inflammatory, antihyperalgesic
- Effective against MRSA
- GABA uptake inhibitor
- Reduces keratinocytes proliferation in psoriasis
- 5-HT1A antagonist, counters antiemetic effects of CBD
- TRPM8 antagonist
- TRPV1, TRPA1, and cannabinoid agonist

Δ-9-Tetrahydrocannabivarin (THCV) is a nonpsychotropic

- Antagonizes Δ-9-THC at low doses; acts as CB1 agonist at higher doses in mice
- Anticonvulsant
- Reduced food intake in mice
- Improved glucose tolerance, insulin sensitivity, and insulin signaling in vivo

Cannabidivarin (CBDV) is a nonpsychotropic

- Anticonvulsant in vitro and in vivo

Cannabinol (CBN) is a nonpsychotropic (by-product of Δ-9-THC oxidation)

- Decreases breast cancer resistant protein
- Effective against MRSA
- Reduces keratinocytes proliferation in psoriasis
- Sedative
- TYPV2 agonist for burn

β-Caryophyllene is nonpsychotropic sesquiterpene of essential oil

- Anti-inflammatory
- Antibiotic
- Antioxidant

- Anticarcinogenic
- Local anesthetic activity

Terpenoids are the essential oils produced by the cannabis plant. Over 200 have been extracted from cannabis with monoterpenoids and sesquiterpenoids dominating over di and triterpenoids, megastigmanes, and apocarotenoids [27]. The quality and quantity of terpenoids can vary between batches of the same seed source, with the biological profile of these compounds unknown beside the accepted benefit of providing aroma and possible modulation of the THC effects [28]. Maffei et al. report that terpenoids can provide anti-inflammatory, acetylcholinesterase inhibition, antioxidant, antibiotic, and antimutagenic activity [29].

Growing, drying, and harvesting conditions can significantly alter terpenoid trichome content. Ross and ElSohly demonstrated that freshly collected material had 0.29% v/w essential oil; one-week-old material air dried at room temperature and stored in a paper bag yielded 0.20% (loss of 31%); one-month-old cannabis yielded 0.16% (loss of 45%); three-month-old cannabis yielded 0.13% (loss of 55%) [30].

Monoterpenoids

Monoterpenoids are the predominate essential oil extracted from fresh plant material [30]. β-myrcene is recognized as the sedative, muscle relaxant with anti-inflammatory and analgesic properties [31]. Limonene is readily available and anxiolytic, anticarcinogenic, and a free-radical scavenger that is used to treat GERD (gastroesophageal reflux disease) and gallstones [31–34]. α-pinene is a widely available terpenoid in nature and is reported to have anti-inflammatory, bronchodilatory, and antibiotic properties [35–37]. Terpinolene has sedative and antispasmodic effects [38,39], while linalool (lavender) has anxiolytic, analgesic, and anticonvulsant properties [40–42].

Sesquiterpenoids

The primary sesquiterpenoid in cannabis is β-caryophyllene, with caryophyllene oxide being reported the volatile compound sensed by drug detection dogs that is present in all cannabis strains [43]. β-caryophyllene is the constituent in black pepper and cloves that offers anti-inflammatory, gastric cytoprotective, analgesic, and antimalarial properties [44–46].

Flavonoids

Over 29 flavonoids have been identified in cannabis [47–50] in two classes: flavones (vitexin, apigenin, isovitexin, luteolin, orientin) or flavanols (kaempferol, quercetin). Flavones have been shown to act as phytoestrogens [51].

Analysis and quality control

Cannabis was removed from the U.S. Pharmacopeia in 1942, so quality control analysis of this botanical has been neglected. Healthcare professionals and patients need to be assured about the quality and quantity of THC and CBD, the two primary active ingredients in cannabis. Gas chromatography (GC) has been the primary methodological technique used for federal regulatory and toxicology purposes, but there is a need for standardized and validated testing methodologies [52].

In 2010, the American Herbal Products Association (AHPA) formed a cannabis committee to address recommendations for regulators and best practices for laboratory analysis because without proper testing and standardization there would not be credibility for state and federal policymakers when considering legislation.

During a GC analysis, the cannabis sample moves through an oven which decarboxylates the tetrahydrocannabinolic acid found in the plant to the active form THC. Decarboxylation in the GC system varies based on temperature, geometry of the injector, and how effective the decarboxylation occurred, so standardization is essential to ensure accurate analysis [53].

High-performance liquid chromatography (HPLC) can provide quantification of the cannabinoids as both the acid (THCA, CBDA) and active forms (THC, CBD) [54]. Debruyne et al. compared analysis of a single cannabis specimen and got different quantitative peaks using different methods, so laboratory certification that employs a sampling protocol along with bioanalytical method validation is needed [55]. As Donald Abrams, MD, an integrative oncologist at the University of California and chief of hematology/oncology at San Francisco General Hospital stated, "the ability to ascertain potency and content of cannabis products sold in dispensaries is critical if we are able to allow patients to know what they are getting and for them to be able to re-assess strains that are effective for them" [56].

References

1. Clarke RC, Merlin MD. 2016. Cannabis taxonomy-the "sativa" vs "indica" debate. *Herbal Gram* 110;44–49.
2. 2014. *Cannabis Inflorescence-Standards of Identity, Analysis, and Quality Control.* Scotts Valley, CA: American Herbal Pharmacopoeia.
3. McPartland J. 2002. *Contaminants and Adulteration in Herbal Cannabis.* Binghamton, NJ: Haworth.
4. Mikuriya TH, Aldrich MR. 1988. Cannabis: Old drug, new dangers. The potency question. *J Psych Drugs* 20:47–55.
5. ElSohley MA, Holley JH, Lewis GS et al. 1984. Constituents of cannabis sativa L. XXV. The potency of confiscated marijuana, hashish and hash oil over a ten year period. *J Forsenic Sci* 29(2):500–514.

6. ElSohly MA, Ross SA, Mehmedic Z et al. 2000. Potency trends of delta-9-THC and other cannabinoids in confiscated marijuana from 1980–1997. *J Forensic Sci* 45:24–30.
7. UNODC. United Nations Office on Drugs and Crime. 2009. *Recommended Methods for the Identification and Analysis of Cannabis and Cannabis Products.* Vienna: United Nations Office on Drug and Crime. http://www.unodc.org.
8. EMCDDA. European Monitoring Centre for Drugs and Drug Addiction. 2008. *A Cannabis Reader: Global Issues and Local Experiences.* Lisbon: European Monitoring Centre for Drugs and Drug Addiction.
9. ProCon.org. 2014. Who are the patients receiving medical marijuana through the federal government's compassionate INDProgram? http://www.medical marijuana.procon.org/view.
10. Cole JM. 2013. *Guidance Regarding Marijuana Enforcement.* Washington, D.C.: US Dept of Justice.
11. Gettman J. 2006. Marijuana production in the United States (2006). *Bull Cannabis Reform.* http://www.drugscience.org/archive/bcr2mjcropsreport_2006.pdf.
12. UNODC. United Nations Office on Drugs and Crime. 2009. *Recommended Methods for the Identification and Analysis of Cannabis and Cannabis Products.* Vienna: United Nations Office on Drugs and Crime. http://www.unodc.org/documents/scientific/ST-NAR-40-Ebook.pdf.
13. Potter D. 2009. *The Propagation, Characterisation and Optimisation of Cannabis Sativa L. as a Phytopharmaceutical.* London: King's College London.
14. UNODC. United Nations Office on Drugs and Crime. 2009. *Recommended Methods for the Identification and Analysis of Cannabis and Cannabis Products.* Vienna: United Nations Office on Drugs and Crime. http://www.unodc.org/documents/scientific/ST-NAR-40-Ebook.pdf.
15. UNODC. United Nations Office on Drugs and Crime. 2009. *Recommended Methods for The Identification and Analysis of Cannabis and Cannabis Products.* Vienna: United Nations Office on Drugs and Crime. http://www.unodc.org/documents/scientific/ST-NAR-40-Ebook.pdf.
16. Chen GH, Majumdar AS. 2006. Drying of herbal medicines and tea. In Mujumdar AS, ed. *Handbook of Industrial Drying.* 3rd ed. CRC Press, Boca Raton.
17. Clarke RC. 1981. *Marijuana Botany: An Advanced Study, The Propagation and Breeding of Distinctive Cannabis.* Berkeeley, CA: Ronin.
18. UNODC. United Nations Office on Drugs and Crime. 2009. *Recommended Methods for the Identification and Analysis of Cannabis and Cannabis Products.* Vienna: United Nations Office on Drugs and Crime. http://www.unodc.org/documents/scientific/ST-NAR-40-Ebook.pdf.
19. McLaren J, Swift W et al. 2008. Cannabis potency and contamination: A review of the literature. *Addiction* 103:1100–1109.
20. McPartland J. 2002. *Contaminants and Adulteration in Herbal Cannabis.* Binghamton, NJ: Haworth.
21. McPartand JM, Pruitt PP. 1999. Side effects of pharmaceuticals not elicited by comparable herbal medicines:the case of tetrahydrocannabinol and marijuana. *Altern Therap* 5:57–62.
22. McPartland J. 2002. *Contaminants and Adulteration in Herbal Cannabis.* Binghamton, NJ: Haworth.

23. NIDA. National Institute Drug Abuse. 2012. Spice (synthetic marijuana) http://www.drugabuse.gov.

24. APHA. American Herbal Products Association. 2013a. *Recommendations to Regulators: Cannabis Dispensing Operations.* Silver Springs, MD: American Herbal Products Assoc.

25. Russo EB. Taming THC: Potential cannabis synergy and phytocannabinoid-terpenoid entourage effects. *Brit J Pharmacol* 2011; 163:1344–64.

26. Upton R et al. ed. 2014. *Cannabis Inflorescence Cannabis spp. Standards of Identity, Analysis and Quality Control.* Scotts Valley, CA: American Herbal Pharmocopoeia.

27. Hillig KW. 2004. A chemotaxonomic analysis of terpenoid variation in cannabis. *Biochem System Ecol.* 32:875–91.

28. Fischedick JT, Hazekamp A et al. 2010. Metabolic fingerprinting of Cannabis sativa L. Cannabinoids and Terpenoids for chemotaxonomic and drug standardization purposes. *Phytochemistry* 71:2058–2073.

29. Maffei ME, Gertsch J et al. 2011. Plant volatiles: Production, function and pharmacology. *Nat Prod Report* 28: 1359–80.

30. Ross SA, ElSohly MA. Cannabis sativa L. *J Nat Prod* 59:49–51.

31. DoVale TG, Furtado EC et al. 2002. Central effects of citral, myrcene and limonene constituents of essential oil. Chematypes from Lippa alba (Mill.) NE Brown. *Phytomedicine* 9:709–14.

32. Elson CE, Maltzman TH et al. 1997. Anti-carcinogenic activity of d-limonene during the initiation and promotion/progression stages of DMBA-induced rat mammary carcinogenesis. *Carcinogenesis* 9:331–2.

33. Malhotra S, Suri S, Tuli R. 2009. Antioxidant activity of citrus cultivars and chemical composition of citrus karna essential oil. *Planta Med* 75:62–4.

34. Sun J. 2007. D-limonene: safety and clinical applications. *Altern Med Review* 12:259–64.

35. Gil MI, Jimenez J et al. 1989. Comparative study of different essential oils of Burpleurum gibraltaricum Lamarch. *Die Pharmazie* 44:284–7.

36. Falk AA, Hagberg MT et al. 1990. Uptake, distribution and elimination of alpha-pinene in man after exposure by inhalation. *Scand J Work Environ Health* 16:372–8.

37. Kose EO, Deniz IG et al. 2010. Chemical composition, antimicrobial and antioxidant activities of the eseential oils of Sideritis erythrantha Boiss. and Heldr.(var.erythrantha and var. cedretorum PH Davis) endemic in Turkey. *Food Chem Toxicology* 48:22960–5.

38. Ito K, Ito M. 2013. The sedative effect of inhaled terpinolene in mice and its structure-activity relationship. *J Nat Med* 67:833–7.

39. Riyazi A, Hensel A et al. 2007. The effect of the volatile oil from ginger rhisomes (Zingiber officinale), its fractions and isolated compounds on the 5-HT3 receptor complex and the secretoninergic system of the rat ileum. *Planta Med* 73:355–62.

40. Souto-Maior FM, de Carvalho FL et al. 2011. Anxiolytic-like effects of inhaled linalool oxide in experiemental mouse anxiety models. *Pharmacol Biochem Behav* 100:259–63.

41. Peana AT, De Montis MG et al. 2004. Effects of (-)-linalool in the acute hyperalgesia induced by carrageenan, L-glutamate and postaglandin E2. *Eur J Pharmacol* 497:279–84.

42. Karlaganis G. 2002. *SIDS initial assessment report for SIAM 14: Linalool.* Berne: UNEP No CASN: 78-70-6.
43. Stahl E, Kunde R. 1973. Die Leitsubstanzen der Haschisch-Suchhunde. Leading substances for hashish narcotic dog. *Kriminalistik* 9:385–8.
44. Basile AC, Sertié JA et al. 1988. Anti-inflammatory activity of oleoresin from Brazilian copaifera. *J Ethnopharmacol* 22:101–9.
45. Tambe Y, Tsujiuchi H et al. 1996. Gastric cytoprotection of the non-steroidal anti-inflammatory sesquiterpene, beta-caryophyllene. *Planta Med* 62:469–70.
46. Campbell WE, Gammon DW et al. 1997. Composition and anti-malarial activity in vitro of the essential oil of tetradenia riparia. *Planta Med* 63:270–2.
47. Clarke MN, Bohm BA. 1979. Flavonoid variations in cannabis. *Bot J Linnean Soc.* 79:249–57.
48. ElSohly MA, Slade D. 2005. Chemical constituents of marijuana: the complex mixture of natural cannabinoids. *Life Sci.* 78: 539–48.
49. Ross SA, ElSohly MA et al. 2005. Flavonoid glycosides and cannabinoids from pollen of Cannabis sativa L. *Phytochem Anal* 16:45–48.
50. Vanhoenacker G, Van Rompaey PD et al. 2002. Chemotaxonomic features associated with flavonoids of cannabinoid-free cannabis (Cannabis sativa sybsp sativa L.) in relation to hops (Humulus lupulus L.). *Nat Prod Lett* 16:57–63.
51. Sauer MA, Rifka SM et al. 1983. Marijuana: interaction with the estrogen receptor. *J Pharmacol Exp Ther* 224(2):404–7.
52. ElSohly MA, Ross SA, Mehmedic Z et al. 2000. Potency trends of delta-9-THC and other cannabinoids in confiscated marijuana from 1980–1997. *J Forensic Sci* 45:24–30.
53. UNODC. United Nations Office on Drugs and Crime. 2009. *Recommended Methods for the Identification and Analysis of Cannabis and Cannabis Products.* Vienna: United Nations Office on Drugs and Crime. http://www.unodc.org/documents/scientific/ST-NAR-40-Ebook.pdf.
54. Swift W, Wong A et al. 2013. *Analysis of Cannabis Seizures in NSW.* Australia: Cannabis potency and cannabinoid profile. PLOS One 8:e70052.
55. Debruyne D, Albessard F et al. 1994. Comparison of three advanced chromatographic techniques for Cannabis identification. *Bull Narc* 44:109–121.
56. Stafford L. 2012. The growing industry of medical cannabis analysis. *Herbal Gram* 94:21–23.

chapter twenty

Commercial cultivation of cannabis

Ashley Vogel

Contents

Laboratory manager alternative medical enterprises

Cannabis may be grown outdoors, in greenhouses, or indoors. Indoor and greenhouse growing may be in soil or by hydroponics. Many considerations go into choosing a growing method. Outdoor growing utilizes Mother Nature for light, temperature, and humidity, while indoor growing utilizes expensive equipment to control the environmental conditions. Indoor growing media may be different based on grower preference for indoor cultivation; for example, soil and hydroponics. While hydroponics assists with a faster growth rate than in soil, its cost is significantly greater. The downfall for growing plants in soil is the root system, which will eventually outgrow the container, resulting in transplanting. Thus, the facility and the equipment requirements for outdoor growing are minimal compared to those for indoor cultivations. Mother Nature provides nearly all the resources, with commensurate lessening of monetary requirements. For greenhouse growing, a facility constructed with materials to allow natural sunlight to reach plant is required with fans for air circulation. Greenhouse growing takes the concept of growing indoors but utilizing Mother Nature for natural light [1].

Growing season

Cannabis may be grown outdoors through about four to six months of the year, starting in spring and ending in fall or early winter, whereas indoor growing can be conducted any time with proper environmental controls. The environmental conditions and growth cycle for the plant remain the same regardless of the cultivation being indoor, outdoor, or a greenhouse, though indoor growing can expedite the growth cycle to harvest to eight weeks for sativa dominate and 12 weeks for indica dominate plants and can result in yields larger than those of outdoor growing.

Environment and plant yield

Outdoor growing can result in very large plants that can reach several meters tall. Indoor plants may reach up to 1–2 m tall, depending on space requirements. However, one benefit of indoor growing can be yields of multiple crops per year from a multitude of plants due to environmental controls as opposed to one crop per year from the same plant outdoors. However, many people believe the best option for growing cannabis is to do so in a greenhouse. The natural light will heat the greenhouse facility and create an ideal growing environment for the plant. The plants do not require as much water as with outdoor and indoor growing due to the increased humidity in the environment. Though humidity and temperature are contributors to mold growth, they are easily controlled by ventilation. In a greenhouse, adverse weather in the cooler climates no longer becomes an issue for outdoor cultivation sites.

Outdoor growing

Mother Nature contributes to the plants through natural sunlight and fresh air, which minimizes the amount of artificial resources needed to maintain healthy plants. Different strains are successful with outdoor grows and usually produce many seeds [1]. Basic grower requirements for a successful outdoor cultivation are the quality of the light, soil, and water sources. Well-irrigated soil with a pH of 6.5 is ideal for growing cannabis outdoors. Natural fresh water is the best source for watering plants, but ensure the soil is not too moist from the natural source, as it will cause root rot. Components such as sand and vermiculite can be added to the soil to aid with water retention and loss. As the fall season approaches, frost may be a factor that could harm plants. The best way to protect plants from frost and wind is to cover them until the weather changes. The plants need direct sunlight for at least four hours every day from mid-morning through the afternoon. An outdoor cultivation can produce mature flower in approximately three months, starting in late springtime after the last frost of the year. This timeline will give the flowering plants shorter amounts of daylight during August and September [1]. Outdoor high-density grows typically place plants 6 inches apart. High-density grows yield more product per harvest, but heavy branch will lead to the constant need for crop work and crop maintenance. Orchard-style grows have larger spacing between plants and yield less per square foot; however, less maintenance and crop work is needed through the plant's growth cycle. Equipment needed for an outdoor grow is mostly restricted to the crop work needed to maintain healthy plants. In the case that a frost may occur, covering plants protects them from frostbite.

Indoor growing

Indoor growing allows certain growing efficiencies at the expense of considerable facilities and equipment. Other complications are mold, algae, pests, and mineral deficiencies. Many of these issues can be avoided by having the proper protocols in place to ensure well-ventilated areas and robust nutrient systems. Lighting, watering, and nutrition are key elements for healthy cannabis plants. Indoor environmental conditions are controlled through the high-intensity lamps, HVAC, and CO_2-emitting equipment. By manually controlling these conditions, cannabis has the opportunity to be better quality than outdoor grown cannabis. Hydroponics and soil are the two growth mediums that are used in indoor cultivations. Hydroponics is costlier but can expedite the growth rate for the plants. By using hydroponics, plants can be watered daily, and issues such as root rot and excess minerals in the soil are no longer applicable. Soil is a more economical option for indoor growing and can be less maintenance. Ultimately, the growers experience and understanding of the plant helps in the decision in utilizing hydroponics or soil as a growth medium. The ideal temperature range for cannabis plants is from 24°C to 30°C. Temperatures outside this range tend to decrease cannabis potency.

The light cycle changes as the plant continues to mature, starting at 16–24 hours of light at the seedling stage to 8 hours of light right before harvest. Growing cannabis indoors utilizes many different light sources such as fluorescent, light-emitting diode (LED), and high-intensity discharge lighting (metal halide or high-pressure sodium), depending on the room size and ventilation. Maximum exposure to quality light in a range of 16–24 hours will optimize the amount the amount of photosynthesis that occurs in the cannabis plant. The lighting source should be a sufficient distance to ensure that the entire plant canopy is illuminated even as the plant grows. As the plants continue to grow, watering and fertilizing frequency increase to accommodate the larger root system.

During vegetation, there can be as many as four plants per square foot. After vegetation, each plant requires approximately 1 square foot for growth. The square footage needed for a facility should be considered when establishing production goals equipment for purchase. Too many plants in one area will cause air flow issues and compromise the quality of the cannabis.

Indoor grow facilities should be built according to the appropriate fire and safety code required by local building officials. Other requirements needed for indoor grow facilities are lights, HVAC system, fans for air circulation, and CO_2-emitting equipment.

Greenhouse growing

Greenhouse growing is a hybrid between outdoor and indoor growing, providing some efficiencies after a one-time investment in the greenhouse structure. Greenhouse growing is a hybrid of indoor and outdoor growing by combining the large yields from outdoor and the high quality from indoor. Greenhouse structures can be constructed of various materials but should have the ability for sunlight to penetrate. Greenhouse growing utilizes natural sunlight for the lighting and temperature controls of the facility. Most greenhouses still need high-intensity lamps and shades to offset the seasonal effects of daylight as well as air circulation and heaters if the temperature gets too cold for the plants.

As in indoor and outdoor growing, basic grower requirements for a successful greenhouse cultivation are the quality of the light, soil, and water sources. Many of the same technique are used for growing cannabis, but some resources (light) may be less costly when compared to indoor growing. Sunlight is utilized for greenhouse growing; however, high-intensity lamps and shades may also be utilized for greenhouse growing. The techniques remain consistent from indoor growing when considering soil and hydroponics as a growth medium. Temperature ranges for cannabis are consistent with indoor, outdoor, and greenhouse growing. The biggest difference is how the temperature is controlled. For greenhouses, ventilation is used in the case that the temperature was too hot, and heaters are used when temperature are too cold.

The sun is utilized as the light source for greenhouse growing. High-intensity lamps are utilized for additional light or shades to provide coverage from too much light. In the case that the sun heats the greenhouse too much, air ventilation should be utilized to lower the temperature. Seasonal constraints are less of a factor for greenhouse growing than that of outdoor growing. Light sources and shades are used when the daylight hours are not optimal for the growth phase of the plant. Temperatures are controlled with air conditioning and heaters to keep the ambient environment controlled.

The acreage needed for greenhouse growing is similar to that of indoor growing. Each plant requires approximately 2–3 square feet for growth. Square footage is an important factor when determine production capabilities. Overcrowded plants have additional health and growth issues that can reduce quality and cannabinoid potency. The greenhouse will not require all the same equipment as indoor facilities; however, basic fire and safety codes should still be met in the building process. The lighting and shading needs will correspond to the season. Temperature controls will also adjust throughout the year with seasonal, climate changes.

Growth cycle

Cannabis is an annual plant that can reach up to 5 meters in height and has an extreme dependence on environmental conditions. The four components that affect the growth of cannabis are light, temperature, air circulation, and humidity. The ideal growing environment for cannabis is sunny, well-irrigated soil that is rich in nutrients. The different growth phases of cannabis are germination, seedling, vegetative, pre-flowering, and flowering. Growing conditions range depending on the growth stage the plant is in.

Cannabis is a dioecious plant, and the gender resemblance is identical before the pre-flowering stage. As the days become shorter, the female cannabis flower starts to mature, entering the flowering stage, and a hormone reaction occurs creating compressed clusters containing resin sacs (also known as trichomes). The male cannabis flowers produce pollen, which is used to fertilize the female plant. The male plant stops shedding pollen after two to four weeks and dies. Fertilized female flowers produces ripe seeds after three to eight weeks and then dies. If the female flower is not fertilized, the female plant will continue to produce trichomes in hopes of "catching" pollen, which leads to higher cannabinoid potency. Unfortunately, if the plant is stressed for too long trying to reproduce without pollen present, the plant will hermaphrodite, causing male and female reproductive components on the same plant. The plant will then reproduce and create seeds. For cultivation growing, the technique of sinsemilla ("without seed") is ideal. It removes male plants to prevent uncontrolled fertilization of the female flower. Fertilized female flower has a lower potency of cannabinoids in the resin sacs due to the reallocation of natural energy used to produce seeds rather than more flower [2].

Germination

Germination occurs when the protective coating from the seed cracks due to various environmental factors and the root and seed leaves form. Cannabis germinates in three to seven days and continues to grow at a strong rate by establishing a root system and increasing the number of stems and leaves as the days begin to lengthen from longer light exposure. This is known as the vegetative stage. The germination process can be bypassed by cloning from a mother plant.

Cloning

Cloning is an asexual reproduction technique for taking cuttings from a healthy mother plant and starting the growth phase in the vegetative stage. A cutting from a mother plant should be 2–3 inches in length from the internode of a branch. Different sterilization and hormone solutions are used to ensure the new cutting is viable without disease. Growth mediums for clones are the same as indoor growing, soil or hydroponics. Clones need a humid growing environment, and growers typically utilize a "clone dome" with no more than 24 clones in each dome. To ensure the genetic material of the plant is as close to the parents as possible, many commercial growers will clone the plant to generate new offspring.

Seeding and grafting techniques

Seeding is another way of growing cannabis from germination phase. Seeds vary in color and size; for example, indica seeds tend to be darker and have stripes. Hardness is another quality of healthy seeds, since cracked seeds allow pests and disease to compromise the plant. It is important to pick good seeds as the genetics contributes to the health of the plant.

Interbreeding

Natural selection and growing conditions have affected the content of cannabis throughout the years. Once humans understood the dividends the plant could offer, they genetically manipulated through breeding. This culminated in a superior product. Sexual reproduction of male and female plants generates seeds. The seeds contain genetic material from the parents; however, many of the seeds have varying traits as well. The variances may alter physical characteristics, terpenes, or cannabinoid content. Most breeders grow the seeds and determine which female plants should be kept. Breeding can bring the genetic material of different plants into offspring, creating a hybrid that caters to specific preferences.

Nondrug and drug plants

Cannabis cultivation began in Central Asia, eventually moving throughout Eurasia. Initially humans cultivated Cannabis for hemp production. Ropes, baskets, and clothing were made from the tall, fibrous, nondrug plant. Eventually, a genetic mutation caused cannabis plants to produce the phytocannabinoid THC, later leading to different species and subspecies of cannabis. C. sativa and C. indica can be categorized based on the leaf characteristic (narrow or broad), cannabinoid profile (high or low THC), and the ancestry of the plant. Narrow-leaf hemp varieties are thought to originate in Europe (low THC), narrow-leaf drug varieties are from South Asia (high THC), broad-leaf hemp from East Asia (low THC), and broad-leaf drug varieties are from Afghanistan (high THC) [3].

Whole plants and isolates

The major isolates from cannabis that are popular today are THC and CBD. These cannabinoids are separated from the whole plant extract to provide the effects of pure THC or CBD. Whole plant extracts can have 400 different components, some of which are cannabinoids, terpenes, and other aromatic compounds. The whole plant extracts have more diversity in the therapeutic properties than just a single cannabinoid. The terpenes, cannabinoids, and other aromatic compounds work synergistically to create the entourage effect.

Harvesting and yield

Once the cannabis flower is mature, it is then harvested and cured. Determining if the plant is mature enough for harvest depends on the subspecies of the plant (indica or sativa), if the cultivation is indoor or outdoor, and the type of desired high for the end product. During the end of the life cycle, cannabis trichomes (resin sacs containing cannabinoids) mature from a cloudy, white appearance to clear or amber brown. This indicates that the cannabinoids have reached their highest potency potential, and the plant is ready for harvest. The longer the trichomes "ripen," the more THC they contain; however, allowing the trichomes to ripen too long results in degradation of THC to CBN (mostly amber trichomes) and affect yields [4].

Single-plant timeline

Single-plant timeline is typical of outdoor grows. The best time to harvest is in the fall when the daylight has reduced to 12 hours. Since cannabis is an annual plant, the plant has one grow cycle for the year, ending in the fall, and dies after seeding. The seeds are the next generation of offspring that germinate in the spring.

Harvesting schedule

Determining when to harvest plants depends on the subspecies of cannabis and if the grow is indoor, outdoor, or a greenhouse. The THC degrades into CBN if the plant continues to grow, causing a lower potency of THC and a different effect for the end user. Because growing conditions change cannabinoid potency, the best method to determine the harvest schedule is to monitor the plant closely. Mature trichomes change color, and if too ripe, they become black. Another sign of plant maturity is yellowing fan leaves. These leaves eventually fall off, preparing the plant for the next phase of the lifecycle.

Drying

Drying cannabis is an important control measure to be taken to ensure the cannabis is ready for human use. There are two different technique utilized in industry, air drying and freeze drying. When harvesting cannabis, a separate area for drying is recommended with ventilation and a consistent temperature of around 21°C. Drying helps promote a high potency in cannabinoids for certain strains of cannabis. The most common method of air drying is to suspend the plant upside down and allow air to circulate throughout the area. The flower should be checked daily to ensure that mold and mildew does not start to grow in the humid environment. Once the cannabis flower has reached a moisture content range of 45%–55%, it can be cured to promote the preservation of terpenes and cannabinoids. Curing is the last step to enhance the flavor of the cannabis before reaching the consumer. The best method for curing is to store the flower in an airtight, light-resistant container at room temperature, from seven days to months [5]. Freeze drying works by utilizing dry ice to uptake the moisture from the plant and disperse the moisture as humidity in the environment. This technique requires the plant material to be fresh, and it dries the material within a couple of days. Cannabis should have moisture content of 45%–55% before removing from packaging in light-resistant, airtight containers.

Extraction

Flower, trim, or both can be utilized for extractions to create hash oil; however, finer and more consistently ground product (flower and/trim) used yields higher results. There are many different techniques used to create concentrates, such as hydrocarbon (yielding butane hash oil [BHO]), supercritical liquid (utilizing carbon dioxide [CO_2]), and ethanol (yielding ethanol hash oil [EHO]). Although many consumers have preferences for the extraction method, hydrocarbon (butane, propane, etc.) has the potential to be the most dangerous. Butane hash oil, CO_2, and EHO require a closed-loop extraction apparatus, where extraction time, temperature, and pressure ranges depend on the eluent (the solvent used to extract the cannabis) and the desired end product. EHO can be manipulated in different products, such as sugar wax, shatter, crumble, and Rick Simpson oil (RSO). RSO does not require a closed-loop system, as this process of extracting cannabis is a long soak in ethanol and then removal of the excess ethanol to result in a dark green product that may be used for in capsules. The extraction technique involving supercritical liquid CO_2 causes undesirable components (lipids and chlorophyll) to be extracted along with the cannabinoids. The best way to remove all the lipids and chlorophyll is to "winterize" the extract by soaking in ethanol at negative temperatures. Regardless of the extraction technique, the extract must be purged of excess solvent and heated. The end products should be tested for residual solvents, which ensures safe limits of butane, propane, or ethanol in the product. Each state has different legal solvent limits that must be met for release to sell.

Decarboxylation

All cannabinoids contain an acid component when present in cannabis flower. Partial decarboxylation occurs through drying and curing flower; however, to complete remove the carboxyl group (COOH) of the cannabinoid, the product must be heated over time. For best results, decarboxylation should occur at approximately 105°C for 30–45 minutes. Decarboxylation can be performed at lower temperatures to preserve the terpene content of the product. In result of lower temperatures, the length of time the product decarboxylates increases.

THC: CBD ratio adjustment

Through natural selection and breeding, the cannabinoid content of cannabis genetically manipulated to create a superior product. There are many different THC:CBD cannabinoid ratios, such as 10:1, 1:1, and 1:20. THC is known to be the psychoactive component, with a sedative, antinausea, appetite-improvement, anti-insomnia, and pain-relieving effect for most users. Strains that are known for high yields of THC are Girl Scout Cookies, Kosher Kush, and Bruce Banner. High-CBD strains are Charlotte's Web, ACDC, and Death Star, which have properties to suppress inflammation, epileptic seizures, and the THC's euphoric effect. Formulations with THC and CBD as a 1:1 ratio work synergistically (also known as the entourage effect) to create a relaxed, antianxiety feeling without as much of a euphoric effect. Strains popular for this ratio are Sweet and Sour Widow, Pennywise, and Cannatonic.

Analysis

Analyzing cannabis for cannabinoid potency or terpenes is the best way to determine the content of the plant. Many states require products to be tested by a third party prior to releasing the batch for sale. Standardized analysis is important because of the high variability of cannabinoid products, as demonstrated by a recent study by Elzinga et al. [6]. A number of product samples (494 in total) were obtained from patients in California and were tested for cannabinoid concentration and terpenes, with no less than eight strain replicates for 35 different strains. The principal component analysis (PCA) results indicated that cannabinoids were responsible for the strain differentiation and that most strains did not cluster, resulting in high variation of chemical composition. These results suggest that flower yields are mostly affected by growing conditions and that the subspecies of cannabis is not related to the cannabinoid content but rather the genetics [7].

Standards

In the pharmaceutical industry, many products are tested at several different stages of manufacturing to ensure transparent quality and safety of the product. Cannabis should be held to the same standards by ensuring that the cannabinoid potency, pesticide and residual solvent limit, terpene content, and microbial contamination are acceptable by state regulations. All states with a medical cannabis program have different criteria for acceptable product specifications and labeling of the product.

Certificate of analysis (COA)

A Certificate of Analysis (COA) is an easy way to review test results from responsible companies selling cannabis and cannabis-infused products.

Packaging and labeling

Packaging and labeling requirements are different according to the state in which the cannabis is sold. At a minimum, the strain type, fertilizers/salts used, and batch information should be listed. Many states also require warnings and test results for the product.

Shelf life and storage
Regardless of the type of cannabis product, all cannabis and cannabis-infused products should be protected from light and warm temperatures, which degrade cannabinoid potency. Cured flower has a longer shelf life of up to six months.

References
1. Riley R. *Growing Elite Marijuana.* Infinity Publishing, 2016.
2. Thomas BF and ElSohly MA. *The Analytical Chemistry of Cannabis: Quality Assessment, Assurance, and Regulation of Medicinal Marijuana and Cannabinoid Preparations.* Elsevier/RTI International, Amsterdam, Netherlands, 2016.
3. Small E. Evolution and classification of Cannabis sativa (marijuana, hemp) in relation to human utilization. *Bot. Rev,* 2015; 81: 189–294.
4. Riley R. *Growing Elite Marijuana.* Infinity Publishing, 2016.
5. Riley R. *Growing Elite Marijuana.* Infinity Publishing, 2016.
6. Elzinga S, Fischedick J, Podkolinski R et al. Cannabinoids and terpenes as chemotaxonomic markers in cannabis. *Nat. Prod. Chem. Res,* 2015; 03: 181.
7. Elzinga, S, Fischedick J, Podkolinski R et al. Cannabinoids and terpenes as chemotaxonomic markers in cannabis. *Nat. Prod. Chem. Res,* 2015; 03: 181.

chapter twenty one

Quality assurance in the cannabis industry

Robert W. Martin

Contents

As the cannabis industry emerges and matures in North America, it becomes relevant to consider quality assurance principles. Unfortunately, the scientific literature offers little guidance in this area, as most of the necessary science was never performed due to federal restrictions. Hazekamp [1] reported quality differences between legal and illicit cannabis in the Netherlands, showing legal cannabis significantly cleaner using the measures reported. Almost all previous U.S.-based scientific publications regarding cannabis fall into one of two categories: the first, Schedule I bias (automatically assuming cannabis an herb with no value to humans) and the second, unsubstantiated fear generation caused by the former. Both categories of studies offer weak support at attempts to vilify or prove cannabis a causative origin to a myriad of maladies and illnesses [2–7]. Many of these studies were federally funded or performed by government forensic laboratories, openly willing to spread these negative impressions with apparent zeal.

The federal marijuana farm in Mississippi has contributed very little to our understanding of quality principles, as evidenced by articles in Science [8] and The Washington Post [9]. Both articles compare the weaker strains of the government-grown cannabis to more potent strains commonly distributed in the Colorado and California markets and thus not representative. Since cannabis remains a Schedule I designation, there is not much the government agencies can do but stand by, while others are forced to fill in the gaps of knowledge needed to build a safe and clean industry.

In 2010, laboratories in California began forming to address the growing interest for potency testing [10]. Commercial architecture formed around the understanding of price per milligram of active ingredient, and the U.S. testing industry was born. Broader quality testing for microbiological, chemical residues, and residual solvents evolved over time as a response to more medical patients being supplied this alternative medicine [10]. Controversy arose regarding the selection of quality measures within the industry as there were no significant scientific studies regarding the quality of cannabis in the scientific literature, and as a result, many states selected the strictest measures possible blanketing potency, microbiological, pesticide, residual solvents, aflatoxins, heavy metals, and, in some cases, radiation levels [11–15].

State regulators are mandating quality testing prior to any risk assessments. It is therefore recommended that cannabis regulators follow strict guidelines before selection of legitimate quality measures. First, each measure must be **achievable**; that is, it must be measurable using a recognized analytical method or protocol. Second, it must be **reproducible**; the measure must be measurable by methods without great variation. Third, it must be **easy to understand**; the measure must be translatable to those without scientific training. Fourth, it must be **affordable**; measures must exist in rational business planning without negative economic impact. Finally, they must be **scientifically valid**; the principles the measure is based upon must be supported by high probability of occurrence and not just random, precipitous events. This AREAS principle offers an understanding of the probability of a contaminant being present on plants or production products. The higher the probability, the greater the need to test while the lower the probability the lesser need. The following discussion follows this logic protocol.

Microbiological testing

Microbiological testing is important as medical patients are using this alternative medicine. Under normal growth conditions, the presence of bacterial species on cannabis is very limited, with post-harvest handling being the primary source of potential contamination [16]. Survey-plating techniques for aerobic bacteria followed by subsequent pathogen (*E. coli*, coliform, and *Pseudomonas*) analyses provides salient information regarding contamination sources and satisfactory safety testing [17]. Bacterial testing that allows an understanding of bacterial loads and potential risk organisms and satisfies the requirements for AREAS designation and approval. Today, many techniques and methods are available for identifying bacterial contaminations, results are easy to translate, relatively affordable, and scientifically valid.

Taylor [18] presented a survey-based report in Chicago at the Interscience Conference on Antimicrobial Agents, describing a *Salmonella* outbreak on cannabis in Michigan and Ohio using plasmid fingerprinting technologies. As such, the published work of Taylor et al. [19] has never been verified and is likely not substantiated due to poor experimental design, loose assumptions regarding cannabis usage, low sample size, lack of peer review, and results based upon uncertain plasmid markers. With plasmid fingerprinting contributing many false positives and difficulty due to protocol contaminations, these techniques have been replaced by refined polymerase chain reaction (PCR) methods that are much more reliable. Sound microbiological verification of this organism occurring on cannabis remains elusive due to the lack of scientific studies. It is questionable whether this organism should be singled out as a potential quality marker. Results from our studies clearly show no positive identifications in over 50,000 samples tested [16]. Testing for this organism fails to satisfy the AREAS requirements for QA measure selection.

Fungal species cause a great deal of spoilage to cannabis, and testing should be considered an important quality measure. No discourse on fungal activity on cannabis would be complete without a mention to McPartland [20–24]. These works serve as comprehensive reviews of the previous works regarding a wide range of microbiological diseases purportedly associated with cannabis. Aside from suggesting harvested plants remain dry, McPartland's work presents long lists of human pathogens unsubstantiated by proper scientific method or experimentation and do little to further our understanding of quality assurance.

Important spoilage organisms in cannabis include *Botrytis cinerea* or gray mold that occurs in periods of high moisture while plants are in anthesis and the common powdery mildews *Erysiphe sp. and Podosphaera sp.*, the bane of green house and indoor grow situations [25]. High humidity and cool temperatures promote the rapid growth of these fungi. These organisms account for most fungal contaminations on living cannabis and are not human pathogens and primarily results in loss of yield to the grower.

Aspergillus spp. have been reported occurring on cannabis, with most studies relating to terminally ill patients succumbing to aspergillosis in their final hospice situations [26–34]. While tragic and sad, these reports are extremely infrequent compared to the wide use of this alternative remedy. These organisms are ubiquitous and are more commonly found on moist substrata, rich in carbohydrates such as peanuts and corn. Llewellyn and O'Rear [28] cite their repeated difficulties in culturing *Aspergillus sp.* on plant material without copious amounts of water. Since *Aspergillus* is rarely found on commonly processed cannabis, physicians are recommended to guide their patients away from water pipes and other water-related smoking devices. As the great majority of cannabis is dry cured and is found to be less than 10% moisture [16], the probability of *Aspergillus* contamination remains remote.

Detailed scientific studies are needed to confirm this issue regarding *Aspergillus* contaminations. Where survey fungal testing meets the AREAS requirements, the testing for *Aspergillus* and subsequent aflatoxins clearly does not. Survey fungal testing meets the requirements for QA measure selection as many techniques and methods are available for identifying fungal contaminations, results that are easy to translate, relatively affordable, and scientifically valid. Methods utilized include Petri plating, PCR, and matrix-assisted laser desorption/ionization (MALDI).

Pesticide analysis

Pesticide analysis for food and other consumables are set by the U.S. Environmental Protection Agency (EPA), the U.S. Department of Agriculture (USDA), and the Food and Drug Administration (FDA) along with individual state regulatory regulations [34]. Allowable levels have been suggested for food items commercially available within the United States [35]. Currently, there are no approved pesticide levels in place for cannabis at the federal level. Many states have begun the systematic approach of listing groups of pesticides as guidance, but there is not very much known about actual usage by cannabis growers. Sullivan et al. [36] determined that selected pesticides were carried via smoke to the consumer, verifying the danger of pesticides in cannabis. The fact that pesticides should be monitored is not questioned; however, the selection of pesticides is problematic [37]. There are literally thousands of pesticides available on the commercial market. Selection of the types used in the cannabis industry becomes very problematic because all possible pesticides cannot logistically be tested. Usage data from the industry becomes essential in understanding the proper guidance for pesticide regulation. Regarding AREAS determination, wide regulatory selections of pesticides and infinitely low detection levels create the need for regulations that are affordable and rational.

Potency testing

Potency testing is an integral part of cannabis quality testing. Strength of dosage and process design calls for an accurate determination of the active cannabinoid compounds present. Economic decisions are often based upon cannabinoid measurement. Analysis is typically performed by either gas chromatography fitted with a flame ionization detector (FID) or liquid chromatography using high-performance liquid chromatography (HPLC) using pharmaceutical-grade standards. The HPLC methods enable quantification of the acid forms of the cannabinoids such as: THC-A and

CBD-A. Other methods based on infrared (IR) technologies have been recently developed to measure cannabinoids based upon comparisons with databases of previously measured samples. These methods are considered reference tools rather than analytical tools due to the lack of standards and loss of sample individuality. Potency testing meets the AREAS requirements for QA measure selection as many techniques and methods are available for accurately measuring cannabinoids, results are easy to translate, relatively affordable, and scientifically valid.

Heavy metals

Heavy metals remain poorly understood in the cannabis world. Most studies relate hemp strains of dubious origin grown on contaminated soils then diagnosed with atomic absorption for the presence of several heavy metals such as arsenic, nickel, cadmium, mercury, and lead [38–41]. Citterio [42] suggest that most heavy metal ions accumulate in the root tissues rather than above-ground tissues. With inherent variability in both plant material and atomic absorption spectroscopy (AAS) methods, it is difficult understand the true nature of heavy metals in cannabis given this limited information. It is generally known that cannabis cultivated in North America is grown in nutrient replenished or well-maintained soils rather than contaminated alternatives; therefore, much of the comparison drawn from outside the United States is difficult to consider [25]. Scientific study on various commercial strains grown on typical North America soils under commercial grow conditions are needed to truly understand the relevance of this analysis, and this data is needed to determine whether this protocol meets the AREAS requirements.

The manufactures of cannabis concentrates created interest in residual solvent testing as a means of differentiating their products against their competitors. Combined with an already growing fear of any Schedule I material, it is now matured into regulatory language. The great majority of laboratories utilize static headspace sampling and gas chromatography to achieve their results. By and large, most concentrate manufacturers utilize butane, ethyl alcohol, and CO_2 and are widely accepted and practiced throughout the industry. Butane, apart from its freezing effects, is a nontoxic and safe compound [43]. However, state agencies have relegated sometimes 20 or more solvents, many of them known to be very hazardous (i.e., benzene, ethyl ether, methanol, naphtha, trichloroethylene, and chloroform) that are rarely, if ever, utilized within the industry. Regulatory limits set by different agencies are very confusing as well. The Occupational Safety and Health Administration (OSHA) dictates n-butane under 800 ppm and is accepted by California, whereas Colorado requires under 50 ppm. Some regulatory agencies often lump very different solvents together, essentially approving both benzene and butane under 40 ppm

[11–14]. To compound the difficulty, collection and handling of headspace samples is ultrasensitive, and samples may easily off-gas resulting in wide ranges of variability. Egerton et al. [45] showed the presence of intrinsic solvents created in the plant tissues, which further complicate residual solvent testing.

Snow and Slack [46] reviewed the popularity of headspace analysis using gas chromatography and reported an increase in static headspace analysis in several industries, including biological, pharmaceutical, medical, and food. Other than Egerton et al. [44], this author can find no references where concentrates of cannabis have been studied scientifically for the atmospheric release of solvents during their manufacture or consumption. Scientific study on various concentrates (waxes, oils, tinctures, distillates) produced commercially are needed to truly understand the need for this analysis, and this data is needed to determine whether this protocol meets the AREAS requirements

A closing note regarding variation. As a laboratory operator in the cannabis industry, I am confronted daily with clients and colleagues who fail to fully understand the nature of variability. Most often our lab is supplied with a single cannabis sample to perform an array of analyses where many commercial decisions are then made. When expected numbers aren't generated, a second sample is often supplied, generating a predictably different number from the first. I mention predictable because of the nature of variability inherent in the system. Horowitz [47] reviews the nature of variability in his seminal work; therefore, I won't belabor his points here as they should be well known. In the cannabis industry, variability begins within the plant. No two leaves or flowers contain the exact amount of the any compound being analyzed, whether it is produced by the plant or exists as residue. Variability is further affected by the type of sampling protocol utilized to collect samples from the plant. If processed further, this processing creates new variability, and finally, when prepped and analyzed, there is analytical variation within each laboratory measured by International Organization for Standardization (ISO) accreditation protocols. The answer is to increase the numbers of samples, create meaningful sampling protocols, understand loss factors in processing, and ISO certification for laboratories, all things designed to understand and control the inherent variability in this unique system.

References

1. Hazekamp, A. An evaluation of the quality of medicinal grade cannabis in the Netherlands. *Cannabinoids* 2006; 1(1): 1–9.
2. McGlothlin, W. *Epidemiology of Marihuana Use*. Rockville, MD.: National Institute of Drug Abuse, 1976: 38–52. (National Institute of Drug Abuse Research Monograph Series no. 14.)

3. Rey, J. M., and Christopher C. T. Cannabis and mental health: More evidence establishes clear link between use of cannabis and psychiatric illness. *BMJ: British Medical Journal* 2002; 325(7374): 1183–1184.

4. Allen, J. H. Cannabinoid hyperemesis: Cyclical hyperemesis in association with chronic cannabis abuse. *Gut* 2004; 53(11): 1566–1570.

5. Thacore, V. R., and Shukla, S. Cannabis psychosis and paranoid schizophrenia. *Archives of General Psychiatry* 1976; 33(3): 383–386.

6. Mathers, D. C. and Ghodse, A. H. Cannabis and psychotic illness. *The British Journal of Psychiatry* 1992; 161(5): 648–653.

7. Donald, P. J. Marijuana smoking—possible cause of head and neck carcinoma in young patients. *Otolaryngology-Head and Neck Surgery* 1986; 94(4): 517–521.

8. Price, M. Government pot is less potent than commercial pot, questioning dozens of scientific studies. *Science* N.p., 11 November 2016.

9. Ingraham, C. and Chappell, T. "Analysis|Government marijuana looks nothing like the real stuff. See for yourself." The Washington Post. WP Company, 13 March 2017.

10. Association of Commercial Cannabis Laboratories website http://www.cacannabislabs.com.

11. Marijuana Labeling, Concentration Limits, and Testing. Oregon Secretary of State Archives Division. May 31, 2017.

12. Department of Revenue Marijuana Enforcement Division, Medical Marijuana Rules. 1 CCR 212-1. Code of Colorado Regulations.

13. Department of Revenue Retail Marijuana Code 1 CCR 212-2. Code of Colorado Regulations.

14. WAC 314-55-102: Quality assurance testing. Washington State Legislature. November 21, 2013.

15. NAC453A.658. Sample testing; disposal of samples; standards; laboratory test results; grounds for disciplinary action. Nevada Administrative Code.

16. Martin, R. W. et al. Microbiological implications of commercial Cannabis in N. California. Unpublished data, currently in review, 2017.

17. Tortorello, M. L. Indicator organisms for safety and quality—uses and methods for detection: minireview. *J AOAC Int* 2003; 86: 1208–1217.

18. Taylor T. N. et al. Centers for Disease Control (CDC). Salmonellosis traced to marijuana—Ohio, Michigan. *MMWR Morbidity and Mortality Weekly Report* 1981; 30: 77–79.

19. Taylor, T. N. et al. Salmonellosis associated with marijuana. *The New England Journal of Medicine* 1982; 306(21): 1249–1253.

20. McPartland, J. M., and Pruitt, P. L. Medical marijuana and its use by the immunocompromised. *Alternative Therapies in Health and Medicine* 1997; 3: 39–45.

21. McPartland, J. M. Cannabis pathogens XII: Lumper's row. *Mycotaxon* 1995; 54: 273–280.

22. McPartland, J. M. A review of Cannabis diseases. *Journal of the International Hemp Association* 1996.

23. McPartland, J. M. Contaminants and adulterants in herbal cannabis. In: Grotenberman F and Russo E, eds. *Cannabis and Cannabinoids—Pharmacology, toxicology, and therapeutic potential.* Binghamton NY. Haworth Integrative Healing Press, 2001, 337–343.

24. McPartland, J. M. Cannabis as repellent and pesticide. *Journal of the International Hemp Association* 1997; 4(2): 87–92.

25. Cervantes, J. *Marijuana Horticulture: The Indoor/Outdoor Medical Growers Bible*. Vancouver, B.C.: Van Patten, 2007.

26. Chusid, M. J., Gelfand, J. A., Nutter, C., and Fauci, A. S. Letter: Pulmonary aspergillosis, inhalation of contaminated marijuana smoke, chronic granulomatous disease. Annals of internal medicine U.S. National Library of Medicine, May 1975. 09 Aug. 2017.

27. Kagen, S. L., Kurup, V. P., Sohnle, P. G., and Fink, J. N. Marijuana smoking and fungal sensitization. *Journal of Allergy and Clinical Immunology* 1983; 71: 389–393.

28. Llewellyn, G. C. and O'Rear, C. E. Examination of fungal growth and aflatoxin production on marihuana. *Mycopathologia* 1977; 62: 109–112.

29. Llamas, R., Hart, D. R., and Schneider, N. S. Allergic bronchopulmonary aspergillosis associated with smoking moldy marihuana. Chest. U.S. National Library of Medicine, June 1978.

30. Hamadeh, R., Ardehali, A., Locksley, R. M., and York, M. K. Fatal aspergillosis associated with smoking contaminated marijuana, in a marrow transplant recipient. *Chest* 1988; 94: 432–433.

31. Szyper-Kravitz, M., Lang, R., Manor, Y., and Lahav, M. Early invasive pulmonary aspergillosis in a leukemia patient linked to aspergillus contaminated marijuana smoking. *Leukemia & Lymphoma* 2001; 42: 1433–1437.

32. Gargani, Y., Bishop, P., and Denning, D. W. Too many mouldy joints—marijuana and chronic pulmonary aspergillosis. *Mediterranea Hematology Infectious Diseases* 2011; 3: e2011005.

33. Remington, T. L., Fuller, J., and Chiu, I. Chronic necrotizing pulmonary aspergillosis in a patient with diabetes and marijuana use. *Canadian Medical Association Journal* 2015; 187(17): 1305–1308.

34. Cescon, D. W., Page, A. V., Richardson, S., Moore, M. J., Bourne, S., and Gold, W.L. Invasive allergic bronchopulmonary aspergillosis associated with marijuana use in a man with colorectal cancer. *Journal of Clinical Oncology* 2008; 26(13): 2214–2215.

35. Chemical Contaminants, Metals, Natural Toxins & Pesticides Guidance Documents & Regulations. http://www.FDA.gov 2017.

36. Sullivan, N., Elizinga, S., and Raber, J. C. Determination of pesticide residues in cannabis smoke. *Journal of Toxicology* 2013.

37. Federal Insecticide, Fungicide, and Rodenticide Act (FIFRA). 2017. http://www.EPA.gov.

38. Linger, P., Mussig, J., Fischer, H., and Kobert, J. Industrial hemp (Cannabis sativa L.) growing on heavy metal contaminated soil: Fibre quality and phytoremediation potential. *Industrial Crops and Products* 2002; 16(1): 33–42.

39. Eboh, L. O., and Thomas, B. E. Analysis of heavy metal content in cannabis leaf and seed cultivated in Southern part of Nigeria." *Pakistan Journal of Nutrition* 2004; 4(5): 349–351.

40. Zerihun, A., Chandravanshi, B. S., Debebe, A., and Mehari, A. Levels of selected metals in leaves of cannabis sativa L. cultivated in Ethiopia. *SpringerPlus* 2015; 4(1): n. pag. Web.

41. Aina, R., Sgorbati, S., Santagostino, A., Labra, M., Ghiani, A., and Citterio, S. Specific hypomethylation of DNA is induced by heavy metals in white clover and industrial hemp. *Physiologia Plantarum* 2004; 12(3): 472–480.

42. Citterio, S. et al. Heavy metal tolerance and accumulation of CD, Cr, Ni by Cannabis sativa L. *Plant and Soil* 2003; 256(2): 243–252.

43. Occupational safety and health guideline for n-butane. US Dept. of Labor/ US Dept. of Health and Human Services, 1992.
44. Haken, J. K. Head-space analysis and related methods in gas chromatography. *Journal of Chromatography* 1984; A301: 309.
45. Egerton, D., Fischedick, J., Hicks, A., Gypsy, T., and Clark, J. Endogenous solvents in cannabis extracts. *Poster Presentation AOCS Annual Meeting* Rosen Shingle Creek Resort, Orlando, FL, 2017.
46. Snow, S. H., and Slack, G. C. Head-space analysis in modern gas chromatography. *Trends in Analytical Chemistry* 2002; 21(9–10): 606–617.
47. Horowitz, W. Evaluation of analytical methods used for regulation of foods and drugs. *Analytical Chemistry* 1982; 54(1): 67–76.

chapter twenty two

Cannabis microbiome
Bacteria, fungi, and pesticides

Betty Wedman-St. Louis

Contents

Analytical science is rising to the challenges of cannabis analysis beyond cannabinoid identification. The presence of bacteria and fungi in medical and recreational Cannabis sativa poses a real threat to patients. As this industry moves toward greater regulation and detection, cannabis testing of microbiological contaminants is critical to ensure a safe and effective product.

Plant-associated microbes may provide benefits as well as risks. The microbiome of cannabis leaves and flowers include bacteria and fungi residing on the exterior surfaces as well as within the plant tissues [1]. Microbes on the exterior surfaces can result from dusts, liquids, or aerosols used in growing and production while residues inside the plant gain entry via the roots [2,3].

The cannabis microbiome has been shown to have several endophytic (internal) fungi species including Penicillium citrinum, Penicilllium copticola, and several Aspergillus species [4,5]. An investigation of the fungal microbiome in several dispensary-derived cannabis products identified numerous species including some toxigenic Penicillia and Aspergilli [6]. The Penicillia species have not been reported as infectious, but several cases of serious or fatal pulmonary aspergillosis-associated cases have been reported in marijuana smoking immunocompromised patients [7].

Other microbiome problems related to cannabis have been identified. An outbreak of salmonellosis across several states in the 1980s was reported [8,9], and the Denver Department of Environmental Health issued warnings about Clostridium botulinum in 2016 [10]. As Olga Shimelis of Millipore Sigma expressed at the Pittcom Conference, March 9, 2017, mycotoxins can be a major concern in cannabis plants because of the suspected carcinogens causing acute and chronic toxicity [11]. Aflatoxins are a naturally occurring mycotoxin produced by Aspergillus flavus and Aspergillus parasiticus. Aflatoxin B1 is considered the most toxic, but the presence of B2, G1 and G2 should also be considered. High moisture content and high temperatures have been associated as favorable conditions for growth.

State cannabis testing regulations vary widely with some states imposing no testing standards while others have adopted the United States Pharmacopeia (USP) and American Herbal Pharmacopeia (AHP) guidelines [12,13]. Some states, including New York and Hawaii, specify testing for Aspergillus, Klebsiella, Pseudomonas, Streptococcus, Mucor, and Penicillium. There is a lack of research to support the effectiveness and validity of microbial testing protocols, and no studies have been reported on beneficial endophytes on the Cannabis sativa microbiome [14].

Pesticide problems

Jack Cochran, chair of the Analytical Testing and Sampling Schemes at the Emerald Conference [15], outlined the numerous pesticides found in cannabis provided by the Pennsylvania State University police. Contaminants included triazole fungicides, pyrethroid, organochlorine, organophosphorus, and a pesticide synergist, piperonyl butoxide [16]. He went on to say which pesticides could be safely used on cannabis, what pesticides to test for in cannabis and cannabis products, but what the maximum levels of pesticides allowed should be has not been determined [17].

The number of pesticides proposed for testing is limited and designated by individual states [18,19]. Cochran believes that pesticide testing is on a limited scale while laboratories validate their methods and assess the high cost of equipment needed to complete testing in a LC-MS/MS or GC-MS/MS purchase.

The Cannabis Safety Institute evaluated toxicity, availability, and use rational to compile a list of over 120 compounds for testing, which includes pesticides that can be monitored using GC (gas chromtography) [20].

Health Canada added new terms and conditions for two licensed medical marijuana companies that were caught with banned chemicals in their products and now require regular testing for pesticides [21]. The pesticide myclobutanil is banned for use on products that are smoked (tobacco and cannabis) because it emits hydrogen cyanide when heated. A former employee had witnessed it being sprayed on plants. The company knew Health Canada did not test for banned pesticides, and when federal inspectors visited the facility, an employee hid the chemical inside the ceiling tiles of the offices to evade detection, according to reporter Grant Robertson of The Globe and Mail.

Health Canada plans to expand its testing regimen, a senior official told the newspaper, by subjecting all 38 federally regulated Canadian companies to random spot checks for banned pesticides. The companies are required to test regularly for mold and bacteria, but random spot checks for pesticides such as myclobutanil, a known carcinogen, hardly seems adequate to provide confidence for medical cannabis consumers.

Testing medical cannabis for quality

According to Meredith Cohen, a reporter for the Baltimore Sun, a group of doctors in Columbia, Maryland, plan to open a medical marijuana testing facility so they can be sure about the quality of cannabis sold for medical purposes. The State of Maryland is still deciding what contaminants to include in testing regulations. Since cannabis is becoming an accepted therapy in cancer treatment, epilepsy, and other medical conditions, physicians need assurance that it will not pose any contamination threat to their sick patients [22].

Quality control analysis

Growers and dispensers need to invest in accurate analysis of their cannabis products as a matter of public safety. Michelle Sexton, ND, a clinical cannabis researcher at Bastyr University in Redmond, Washington, states that much of the cannabis market is grown indoors making it a target for fungal infection and pest infestation. "The potential profit and cost of growing indoors then necessitates using chemical warfare to bring a crop to market. If you consider that there are legitimately ill patients accessing this medicine- such as patients with cancer, HIV, neurodegeneration, liver disease, kidney dysfunction, and more—it is an imperative to hold those who grow and dispense cannabis as medicine to high standard of quality control [23]."

Steve De Angelo, executive director of Oakland's Harborside Health Clinic dispensary, told HerbalGram that accurate analysis allows the dispensary to label its products with potency information and "enables patients to more effectively self-titrate their cannabis intake" plus "identify a particular cannabinoid profile that works best for them" [23]. The American Herbal Products Association has published a guidance on microbiology and mycotoxins that can be helpful for growers and dispensaries [24].

Validity of cannabis testing

The phytochemical content of each cannabis plant, even within the same strain, can differ from plant to plant. Storage time can affect a product's potency. Adequate sampling of an entire harvest needs to be performed, and guidelines for appropriate range calculations can be developed.

Challenges face the laboratories in the era of legalizing cannabis. Staying ahead of contaminate and adulterants detection is paramount. Ensuring accurate and complete data for regulators, growers, dispensaries, and patients is critical.

References

1. Turner TR, James EK, Poole PS. The plant microbiome. *Genome Biol.* 2013;14(6):209.
2. Compant S, Clement C, Sessitsch A. Plant growth-promoting bacteria in the rhizo and endosphere of plants: Their role, colonization, mechanisms involved and prospects for utilization. *Soil Biol Biochem.* 2010;42(5):669–678.
3. Winston ME, Hampton-Marcell J, Zarraonaindia I et al. Understanding cultivar-specificity and soil determinants of the cannabis microbiome. *PLUS One.* 2014;9(6):e99641.
4. Gautam A, Kant M, Thakur Y. Isolation of endophytic fungi from Cannabis sativa and study their antifungal potential. *Archives of Phytopathology and Plant Protection.* 2013;46(6):627–635.
5. Kusari P, Kusari S, Spitellar M et al. Endophytic fungi harbored in Cannabis sativa L.: Diversity and potential as biocontrol agents against host plant-specific phytopathogens. *Fungal Divers.* 2013;60(1):137–151.
6. McKernana K, Spangler J, Zhang L et al. Cannabis microbiome sequencing rveals several mycotoxic fungi native to dispensary grade cannabis flowers. *F1000 Res.* 2015;4:1422.
7. Gargani Y, Bishop P, Denning DW. Too many mouldy joints—marijuana and chronic pulmonary aspergillosis. *Mediterr J Hematol Infect Dis.* 2011;3(1):e2011005.
8. Taylor DN, Wachsmuth IK, Shangkuam YH et al. Salmonellosis associated with marijuana: A multistate outbreak traced by plasmid fingerprinting. *N Engl J Med.* 1982;306(21):1249–1253.
9. Centers for Disease Control (CDC). Salmonella traced to marijuana- Ohio, Michigan. *MMWR Morb Mortal Wkly Rep.* 1981;30(7):77–79.
10. Health DDOE. *Special Concerns Associated with Marijuana Extractions, Concentrations, Infusions, and Infused Foods.* Public Health Inspections Division, Washington, DC., 2016.
11. Shimelis O. Contaminants testing in marijuana: Pesticides, mycotoxins and residual solvenets. Pittcom, March 9, 2017.
12. McKernan K, Spangler J, Helbert Y et al. Metagenomic analysis of medical cannabis samples; pathogenic bacteria, toxigenic fungi, and beneficial microbes grow in culture-based yeast and mold tests. *F1000Res* 2016;5:2471.
13. Marcu J. Cannabis inflorescence cannabis spp. Standards of Identity, Analysis, and Quality Control. American Herbal Pharmacopoeia. 2013.

14. McKernan K, Spangler J, Helbert Y et al. Metagenomic analysis of medical cannabis samples; pathogenic bacteria, toxigenic fungi, and beneficial microbes grow in culture-based yeast and mold tests. *F1000Res* 2016;5:2471.
15. *Third Annual Emerald Conference*, San Diego, California, USA. Feb 2–3, 2017.
16. Cochran J. The pesticide problem- to keep cannabis consumers safe, tests for pesticide residue must use multiple methods. *Analytical Scientist*. Feb 2017. www.theanalyticalscsientist.com.
17. United States Environmental Protection Agency, Pesticide Use on Marijuana. Jan 27, 2016. http://bit.ly/2kce4Y7.
18. Oregon Administrative Rules, Oregon Health Authority, Public Health Division, Chapter 333, Cannabis Testing, OAR 333-007-0400, Exhibit A, Table 3, Pesticde Analytes and Their Action Levels. http://bit.ly/2110Q1z.
19. The Commonwealth of Massachusetts Executive Office of Health and Human Services, Department of Public Health, Bureau of Health Care Safety and Quality, Medical Use of Marijuana Program, Exhibit 5, Minimum Analysis Requirements for Residues of Pesticides and Plant Growth Regulators Commonly Used in Cannabis Cultivation. http://bit.ly/21wOgGe.
20. Voelker R, Holmes M. Pesticide Use on Cannabis. Cannabis Safety Institute, June 2015. http://bit.ly/21lyfWeU.
21. Robertson G. Two medical marijuana companies face new rules after banned pesticide use. The Globe and Mail. Feb 9, 2017.
22. Cohn M. Doctors seek to open lab to test medical cannabis for quality. Baltimore Sun. June 26, 2016.
23. Stafford L. The growing industry of medical cannabis analysis. *Herbal Gram.* 2012;94:21–23.
24. Guidance on microbiology & mycotoxins. American Herbal Products Association 2003, revised 2012. www.ahpa.org.

chapter twenty three

Cannabis testing
Taking a closer look

**Scott Kuzdzal, Robert Clifford,
Paul Winkler, and Will Bankert**

Contents

The cannabis industry is growing exponentially, and the use of marijuana for medical purposes is being adopted across the United States. The role of testing laboratories has become crucial to the process of increasing knowledge about cannabis. Scientists testing for potency, heavy metals, pesticides, etc., assure the safety of cannabis products.

Current U.S. cannabis research, policy, and law

Cannabis has demonstrated health benefits since ancient times. While less than 6% of today's studies on marijuana analyze its medical benefits, publications to date indicate that cannabis shows great promise for the treatment of many diseases and symptoms. However, patients with cancer and severe pain, for example, have been blocked from these benefits since the mid-twentieth century when federal regulations were enacted that prohibited the use, sale, and distribution of marijuana due to its psychoactive properties.

A partial listing of reported health benefits of cannabis in the scientific literature and news reports (but not approved by the FDA) includes:

- Appears to have powerful antitumor properties
- Reduces pain associated with chemotherapy
- Treats glaucoma by lowering intraocular pressure
- Decreases symptoms of epileptic seizures
- Reduces brain damage after a stroke
- Relieves discomfort from arthritis
- Lessens side effects from hepatitis C treatments
- Treats inflammatory bowel disease
- Slows progression of Alzheimer's and other neurodegenerative diseases
- Improves symptoms associated with lupus
- Shows promise in eliminating Crohn's disease
- Reduces pain in multiple sclerosis
- Helps fight obesity by increasing metabolism
- Reduces frequency and severity of concussions
- Helps reduce muscle spasms
- Reverses the carcinogenic effects of tobacco use
- Decreases anxiety and improves appetite

Since the 1960s, scientific research has been undermined in many countries because medical marijuana research has been blocked, primarily due to concerns with safety and efficacy. The U.S. Drug Enforcement Agency (DEA) stated in 2011 that marijuana has "no accepted medical use" and should, therefore, remain illegal under federal law. They ruled this even though marijuana has demonstrated medical benefits for many medical disorders and symptoms and contrary to a patent (US 6630507 B1, published in October 2003) issued to the United States as represented by the Department of Health and Human Services claiming "...cannabinoids useful in the treatment and prophylaxis of wide variety of oxidation associated diseases, such as ischemic, age-related, inflammatory and autoimmune diseases." Furthermore, there are many synthetic THC and cannabis-based drugs that have been FDA approved.

Strict scheduling and law enforcement actions have made it more difficult for researchers to obtain marijuana samples for scientific studies than LSD, MDMA, heroin, and cocaine. In June, the Drug Policy Alliance and the Multidisciplinary Association for Psychedelic Studies released a report titled "The DEA: Four Decades of Impeding and Rejecting Science." Citing case studies from 1972 to the present, this report claims the DEA suppressed research on the positive benefits of marijuana for medical use.

In 1999, the Institute of Medicine published a report determining that cannabinoids may play a role in treating pain and recommended that the medical community better establish the safety and efficacy of marijuana. More recently, 30 members of the U.S. Congress sent a letter to the Health and Human Services secretary demanding an end to the federal monopoly on marijuana research so that more studies can be performed by U.S. researchers.

Mainstream acceptance of cannabis has increased steadily over the past decade in the United States. Twenty-eight states and the District of Columbia have legalized or decriminalized marijuana in some form. Eight states and the District of Columbia have legalized marijuana for recreational use. Maryland has approved bills making medical marijuana accessible to patients and decriminalizing possession of limited amounts of the drug. In several states, criminal penalties have been eliminated for small amounts of marijuana. As the medical and recreational uses of cannabinoids increase both in the United States and globally, the need for improved quality control testing also increases.

Despite increasing acceptance of cannabis, political opposition and the illegal nature of cannabis research have forced marijuana growth and distribution to operate in an underground environment. Even in states where recreational and medical marijuana is legalized, the federal government opposition and scheduling of marijuana by the DEA as a Class I drug under the Controlled Substances Act forces industry pioneers to remain shrouded in a cloak of secrecy. These unregulated operations and channels have hampered quality assurance.

On a 2014 tour of medicinal marijuana businesses in Oregon, Shimadzu Scientific Instruments marketing managers learned all aspects of the cannabis industry and key differences between recreational and medical marijuana grow operations. For recreational marijuana operations, the focus is on high-volume yields, and plants are "shocked" into fast growth conditions to increase output. In some medical marijuana grow facilities, however, the plants are nurtured under more natural growth conditions to generate better medicines. The extraction processes are developed to enable higher yields of beneficial phytocannabinoids, including cannabigerol (CBG), cannabidiol (CBD), cannabinol (CBN), and terpenoids.

Chemistry and biomedical properties of cannabis

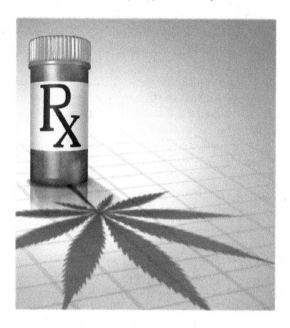

Cannabis plants contain more than 480 compounds that have been identified to be unique to cannabis, including over 144 cannabinoids. Cannabis also contains approximately 140 terpenes, which are more widespread in the plant kingdom. While tetrahydrocannabinol (THC) is the most abundant active component in cannabis, cannabidiol (CBD) and cannabinol (CBN), a degradation product of THC, are commonly measured in cannabis samples. CBD, a nonpsychoactive compound, has been shown to reduce convulsions, inflammation, nausea, and anxiety and has even eradicated tumors in some patients. (*Note:* The cannabinoid(s) recommended for specific medical conditions have not been approved by the FDA.)

Cannabis constituents and pharmacological characteristics

The graphic provides a partial listing of cannabinoid pharmacological characteristics. Recreational marijuana growers, primarily interested in high THC content are less concerned with the CBD, CBC, CBG, CBN, and CBGA profiles, whereas these compounds may be beneficial to biomedical marijuana patients with specific diseases or symptoms. Formulating effective homeopathic remedies by blending oils from various marijuana strains results in natural remedies with advanced healing properties.

As an example, when modern medicine failed to help Charlotte Figi, a young patient who was suffering from an advanced form of epilepsy known as Dravet syndrome, Charlotte's parents found a video online about a California boy with Dravet syndrome who was being successfully treated with cannabis. At a few months old, Charlotte showed signs of the disease. At 5 years old, she could hardly walk or talk and was restricted to a wheelchair while experiencing over 300 grand mal seizures per week. After a twice-daily regimen of cannabis oil, Charlotte, now 9 years old, is not only walking—she can ride a bicycle. She is talking, feeds herself, and is down to only a few seizures per month, mostly while sleeping. This miraculous treatment was featured on CNN News in the segment, "Charlotte's Web." Seeking similar outcomes, hundreds of families with children battling epilepsy have moved to medical marijuana legal states in search of natural cannabis cures.

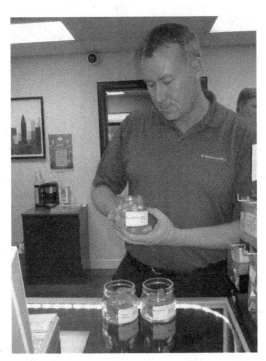

Cannabis consumption and delivery

Moving to medical marijuana states is simply the first step for patients. After establishing residency, patients must obtain a recommendation letter from a qualifying doctor to receive a medical marijuana (MMJ) card. With this letter or card, patients can enter a MMJ dispensary and select from many forms of marijuana-based products. They can choose from different strains of marijuana, varying widely in THC potency.

Smoking is an expedient method of consuming marijuana, but some experts argue that smoking can cause lung and respiratory problems and reduce bioavailability of some constituents. Marijuana plants naturally contain the acid forms of THC and CBD, known as tetrahydrocannabinolic acid (THCA) and cannabidiolic acid (CBDA). During smoking, heat converts THCA and CBDA into their more potent, nonacid forms, THC and CBD. This is referred to as decarboxylation.

Vaporizers provide a means of more gently heating the cannabis. Doing so releases more medicinal components of the marijuana and reduces the amount of noxious chemicals. Due to the volatility of cannabinoids, they vaporize at a temperature much lower than the combustion temperature of plant matter. Vaporization usually heats the sample to 150–200°C. This is sufficient to evaporate off the cannabinoids and terpenes but not to combust the sample into more carcinogenic compounds such as benzopyrene. The active compounds aerosolize and are inhaled without the production of smoke.

It is important to note that when marijuana products are smoked, combustion sterilizes cannabis from various mold and bacterial spores (including Aspergillus, Penicillium, Cladosporium, Alternaria, Yeasts, and E. coli). Migration to vaporization, however, puts immunocompromised cancer and HIV patients at increased risk for bacterial infections. Several states now require testing in this area.

Most MMJ patients prefer to consume edibles or beverages that have been created using butters and oils derived from plant extracts. Extracts high in THC are used to produce cookies, brownies, candies, gummies, etc. The effects of cannabis ingestion differ significantly from smoking or vaporizing, and the time it takes for therapeutic benefits to begin takes much longer. This delayed onset, coupled with high THC concentrations present in some edibles, puts consumers at greater risk of THC overdosing. Emergency room visits related to overconsumption of edibles are on the rise, and there are growing concerns over infants and children gaining access and overdosing on THC-infused edibles that look identical to candy.

Edibles are preferred by patients experiencing pain or sleep disorders but may exacerbate problems for patients with nausea and vomiting. Cannabis is rarely consumed raw; heating is used to convert the organic acids (THCA and CBDA) into their more potent nonacid forms, THC and CBD. Other cannabis products include tinctures, tonics, topicals, teas, soda, hash, and wax.

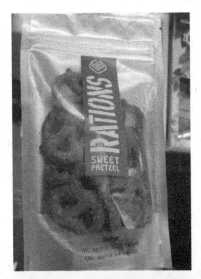

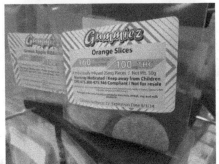

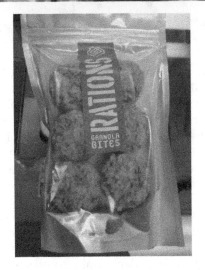

Towards personalized cannabis therapies

The premium products in medical marijuana dispensaries are products high in THC, but as described previously, it is actually the various CBD, CBN, CBG, and CBC compounds that appear to have enhanced health benefits. As research into cannabis treatments grows, much more will be known about the mechanisms of action of cannabinoids and terpenes.

Organic biomedical farms are pioneering new approaches for natural cannabis remedies and formulating cannabis oil blends in response to patient outcomes, delivering a personalized cannabis treatment approach for each patient. These growers tailor the plant growth, flower maturity, and signature genetics for maximum potency and purity. By fostering a relationship between the grower and the patient's needs, cannabis genetics can be tailored to accommodate health needs.

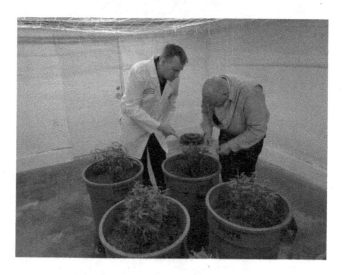

There are a growing number of cannabis oil success stories, including Elkan, now 10 years old, living in Oregon. Elkan suffered from severe autism, including attention deficit disorder (ADD), attention deficit hyperactivity disorder (ADHD), pervasive development disorder (PDD), and sensory processing disorder (SPD). Elkan also had trouble speaking, suffered intense leaky bowel syndrome symptoms, and needed to be physically restrained three to four times per week because he would start flailing around. In a 2014 interview with Elkan's mother, Laura, she commented that, "Elkan's doctors were not sure why all pharmaceuticals other than Ritalin were showing no benefit whatsoever." Nothing seemed to work, and most pharmaceuticals only exacerbated his symptoms. Elkan began taking a blend of natural CBD oils, and after just three months, he can now speak, does not experience leaky bowel syndrome symptoms, and does not need to be restrained. "It's unbelievable!" Elkan's mother added, "Now that Elkan is taking just one CBD oil formulation, he no longer has these symptoms and episodes."

Cannabis analytical testing

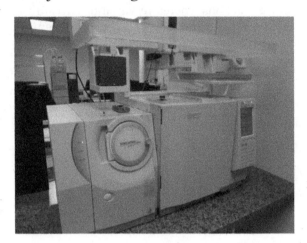

Cannabis growers and dispensaries benefit tremendously from testing performed at independent laboratories. The testing determines potencies, reduces the risk of contamination, and improves product quality. Routine cannabis testing services include cannabinoid potency, screening/ determination of terpenes, aflatoxins, heavy metals, molds, bacteria, pesticides, herbicides, and residual solvents.

Cannabinoid potency testing

Cannabis plants manufacture cannabinoids that determine the overall effect and strength of the strain. Depending on the way cannabis is grown, the number of cannabinoids produced can vary. Most labs quantitate levels of at least three major cannabinoids: THC, CBD, and CBN and their different forms (carboxylated versus decarboxylated). Some labs employ gas chromatography (GC), in which the sample is vaporized under heat. Both GC-FID and GC-MS are commonplace. Because intense heating is used in GC, any THCA present in the natural sample is converted to THC, and labs report this value as "THC total."

Other labs use high-performance liquid chromatography (HPLC) to determine the amount of cannabinoids present. Because HPLC does not require heating, testing by this method provides a more accurate determination of carboxylated or decarboxylated forms present in the sample. Potency testing accompanied with proper product labeling is needed to ensure that customers know exactly how much of the cannabinoids they are consuming.

The typical THC potency ranges from 5 to 25% in plant materials and edibles but can run much higher from concentrated oils. There are no established standard methods for chopping samples, homogenizing them, and performing extractions. Therefore, variations in cannabis potency can easily exceed 20%. Potency testing will improve as chemical standards of known potency become more readily available.

Shimadzu's "Cannabis Analyzer for Potency," based on the integrated HPLC i-Series, is suited to meet the challenges of cannabis potency testing. It can quantitatively analyze up to 11 cannabinoids in less than 10 minutes: delta 9-THC, delta 8-THC, THCA, THCV, CBD, CBDA, CBDV, CBN, CBG, CBGA, and CBC.

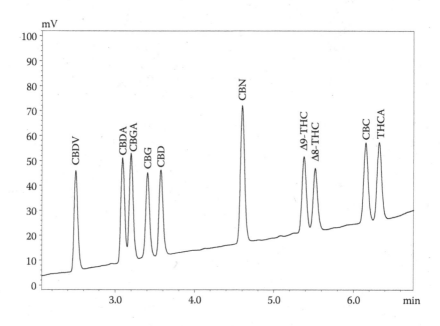

Pesticides and herbicides

The analytical detection of pesticides in cannabis remains challenging. Pesticides are used in commercial cannabis grow operations to kill mites that thrive on cannabis plants. Female mites lay over 2 million eggs per day at 90°F. They are mutating throughout the cannabis industry with resistance to some pesticides. Thrips (tiny, slender insects with fringed wings), aphids, and root gnats are common indoor pests. Spider mites, caterpillars, and grasshoppers threaten greenhouse growers. Halyomorpha halys, also known as the brown marmorated stink bug, is a voracious eater and has an affinity for cannabis plants. With so many insects threatening cannabis plants, it is no wonder there are an equal number of pesticides available to eliminate them.

With an enormous number of pesticides available in the commercial marketplace, no lab can test for all of them. The number of pesticides required for testing varies from state to state, ranging from zero to proposed rules in California for 66 pesticides. Organizations such as AOAC International are evaluating methods with more pesticides. Shimadzu's high-sensitivity LCMS-8050 triple-quadruple liquid chromatograph mass spectrometer can analyze 211 pesticides in cannabis dry product in less than 12 minutes. Because the pesticide list varies from state to state and country to country, and is subject to change, the addition of a GC-MS/MS may be required for complete pesticide analysis. Choose the triple quadrupole GSMS-TQ8050 with AOC-6000 autosampler for volatile pesticides, pesticides that are difficult to analyze by electrospray ionization (ESI), and other problematic pesticides, such as Captan, Chlordane, Chlorfenapyr, Cyfluthrin, Cypermethrin, Dichlorvos, Parthion Methyl, and Pentachloronitrobenzene (Quintozine), difficult to analyze by LC-MS/MS.

Residual solvents

Residual solvents are leftover chemicals from the process used to extract cannabinoids and terpenes from the cannabis plant. The solvents are evaporated to prepare high-concentration oils and waxes. Sometimes the evaporation process does not remove all solvents. Common solvents for such extractions included ethanol, butane, propane, and hexane. Since these solvents are not safe for human consumption, it is important to verify their absence, so consumers can be guaranteed a safe, chemical-free product.

Heavy metal testing

Heavy metals can be found in soil and fertilizers. As cannabis plants grow, they take up metals from the soil. Heavy metals are a group of metals considered to be toxic and include lead, cadmium, arsenic, and mercury. Laboratory testing helps to ensure cannabis products are free from toxic concentrations of these hazardous metals. There are several ways to determine trace metals in plant materials, all requiring an acid digestion. However, the inductively coupled plasma mass spectrometry (ICP-MS) method provides the sensitivity to measure low levels of these toxic metals without the need for additional sample preparation or purchase of additional expensive sample introduction accessories.

Terpene profiling

Terpenes are produced in the trichomes (where THC is produced) and give cannabis its distinctive flavor and aroma. Terpenes also act as essential medicinal hydrocarbon building blocks, influencing the overall homeopathic effect. From the pine odor of pinene to the citrus-like smell of limonene, the characterization of terpenes and their synergistic effect with cannabinoids is easily achieved using chromatography.

Cannabis can manufacture over 120 different terpenes depending on the age of the plant, climate, weather, and even time of day when harvested. The characterization of terpenes and their synergistic effect with cannabinoids is key for identifying the correct cannabis treatment plan for patients with pain, anxiety, epilepsy, depression, cancer, and other illnesses.

Terpene profiling is best done using gas chromatography (GC). GC is the only accurate way to identify and quantify terpenes. Some laboratories also use GC-MS with headspace for the profiling of terpenes since they are reported to have a synergistic effect with cannabinoids, referred to as the "entourage effect."

Moisture content

Moisture can be extremely detrimental to the quality of stored cannabis products. Dried cannabis typically has a moisture content of 10%–12%. A moisture content above 12% is prone to mold growth. Medical marijuana users may be immune deficient and are highly vulnerable to the effects of mold, so constant moisture monitoring is needed.

Mycotoxins analysis

Since cannabis has a high moisture content, long-term storage of the material can allow for fungal growth known as mold. Mycotoxins are a toxic secondary metabolite of mold. Aflatoxins are a subset of mycotoxins that are found in soils and decaying vegetation. Regulatory bodies have placed restrictions on the allowable limits present in food. Recreational and medical cannabis must be properly screened for microbial contamination. Traditional mold and bacteria testing with petri dishes is being replaced with quantitative real-time polymerase chain reaction (qPRC) platforms. Matrix-assisted laser desorption/ionization (MALDI) based microorganism identification may be useful as a qualitative technique to certify the presence or absence of various microorganisms. MALDI could also compete with genomics testing for cannabis strain typing. Mycotoxins (aflatoxin) can be detected using Shimadzu LC-MS/MS systems.

Considerations for future cannabis testing

The cannabis industry and cannabis testing are in their infancies. As the need for better quality control continues and standardization is introduced, it is likely that lower limits for the various cannabis contaminants will be established, and regulations will be introduced. Mass spectrometry will likely play a greater role in quantitation as detection levels are lowered and confirmatory tests are required. The health benefits of terpenes present in cannabis may also provide a fertile area of scientific research. CBD, CBG, and other compounds appear to have a synergistic relationship with each other as well as with various THC forms and terpenes. This field needs much more investigation to determine mechanisms of action, bioavailability, and health benefits.

With an increase in cannabis products, there comes an increase in public safety, such as "drugged driving." Law enforcement need new, low-cost methods for rapid salivary, breath-based, and/or finger-stick screening of individuals who appear to be under the influence of marijuana. Also, better packaging and labeling is needed to reduce accidental infant and child exposures, especially for candy-like, medicinal marijuana edibles.

A stronger integration of testing labs with grow operations, extractions, dispensaries, customers, and physicians is required to ensure that requisite cannabis product information is made more readily available. All-in-one business management software solutions are essential for the cannabis industry and will enable "cannabusiness" to run efficiently with automated inventory tracking, seed-to-sale reporting, financial accounting, grow management, and quality control.

Cannabis testing is not just a growing U.S. market. Sativex™, a synthetic, pharmaceutical version of cannabis, has been approved for use in 25 countries as a treatment for muscle spasm pain in multiple sclerosis patients. Marinol®, a synthetic THC product, has been FDA approved to treat nausea and vomiting associated with cancer chemotherapy in patients who have failed to respond adequately to conventional treatments. The FDA also approved Marinol® to treat appetite loss associated with weight loss in people with AIDS. Idrasil™ is a physician prescribed "medical cannabis in a pill." Unlike Marinol, which is a synthetic form of a single cannabinoid (THC) only, Idrasil is an all-natural cannabis plant extract containing the full spectrum of naturally occurring cannabinoids from cannabis. CBD oils can be purchased legally from Amazon.com and many other sources.

As more cannabis-based or synthetic cannabinoid drugs and homeopathic medicines enter the marketplace, and as more states legalize medical and/or recreational marijuana, the need for cannabinoid testing and standardization will continue to grow. The U.S. cannabis industry is projected to be a $44 billion industry by 2020, with rapid growth expected in all aspects of cannabis business, including personalized cannabis oil therapies that will benefit more people.

Suggested reading

American Herbal Pharmacopoeia. *Cannabis Inflorescence, Standards of Identity, Analysis and Quality Control*, Scotts Valley, CA, 2013.

An archaeological and historical account of cannabis in China. *Econ Bot*, 1974; 28: 437–438.

Bernstein, S.H. The cannabinoid acids: Non-psychoactive derivatives with therapeutic potential. *Pharmacol Ther*, 1999; 82: 87–96.

CNN Health. 7 Uses for Medical Marijuana. 2014. http://www.businessinsider.com/health-benefits-of-medical-marijuana-2014-4?op=1.

Joy, J.E., Watson, S.J., and Benson, J.A. Jr. (eds). Marijuana and Medicine: Assessing the Science Base. Division of Neuroscience and Behavioral Health Institute of Medicine, National Academy Press, 1999. Washington, DC.

Rudolf, B. Chemistry and analysis of phytocannabinoids and other cannabis constituents. In ElSohly, M.A. (ed). *Chapter 2 in Forensic Science and Medicine: Marijuana and the Cannabinoids*. Humana Press, Inc.

Sativex for relieving persistent pain in patients with advanced cancer (Spray III). ClinicalTrials.gov, 2011.

Schepp, D. Legal marijuana: A $44 billion business by 2020? CBS Moneywatch. http://www.cbsnews.com/news/legal-marijuana-a-44-billion-business-by-2020.

chapter twenty four

Legal aspects of cannabis

Vijay S. Choksi and Betty Wedman-St. Louis

Contents

Historical legal background of cannabis

The history of the cannabis plant is still debatable. Some scholars believe the first traces of the plant derive from ancient China, while others hypothesize the origins stem from ancient India. It is generally accepted that early humans recognized the medicinal, psychoactive, and industrial components of the cannabis plant. While growing in popularity in Asia and spreading to Africa, Europe, and finally migrating to the United States, cannabis was viewed as a plant with many useful applications from ship sails to rope. In colonial America, the plant was known for its industrial application of hemp fibers, and the psychoactive effects were merely secondary to its industrial use.

It wasn't until 1909 at the 13-nation international opium conference in China that drug trading became an issue due to the opium crisis. The purpose of the conference, which was registered in the League of Nations Treaty Series on January 23, 1922, was to control the export of cannabis along with coca and opium [1]. To the disfavor of the United States, the restrictions on imports were not as prohibiting as anticipated, which led to the signing of the International Convention relating to Dangerous Drugs by the League of Nations in Geneva on February 19, 1925. It completely banned exporting Indian hemp to countries such as the United States that had prohibited its use. The U.K. banned cannabis a few years later in 1928.

This convention eventually led to The Single Convention of Narcotic Drugs of 1961, which resulted in an international treaty responsible for shaping drug policy of nations throughout the world—including the U.K. Misuse of Drugs Act of 1971 and the U.S. Controlled Substances Act of 1970. The Single Convention of Narcotic Drugs of 1961 categorized narcotics into schedules and prohibited the use and production of certain drugs except under specific license for research and medical treatment. Today, U.S. government officials often cite that reforming marijuana laws would require a modification of the treaty.

Although several U.S. states enacted bans on cannabis between 1911 and 1930, marijuana was not included in the Harrison Act of 1914, which regulated opium and derivatives of the coca plant [2]. Fear of "marihuana" (cannabis) began in the 1920s and 1930s as Mexican immigrants increased, and the Federal Bureau of Narcotics encouraged states to adopt the Marihuana Tax Act as a means to criminalize the production and use of cannabis. It was passed in 1937, requiring federal registration of cannabis dealers with taxation on sales along with penalizing users of cannabis with a fine and imprisonment [3].

Today, federal criminal law prohibits the supply and use of cannabis with exceptions for medicinal and scientific purposes. The U.S. government relies on state and local authorities to enforce criminal law related to cannabis use. In 2014, more than 1.5 million arrests for drug law violations (about 30,000 made by DEA) with evidence of racial, social, and economic disparities in the arrests and penalties [4].

U.S. stance on "marijuana"

The U.S. government is currently undergoing a transformation since the public view of marijuana has changed drastically on the aftermath of Nixon's era "war on drugs." Today, more than 29 states including the District of Columbia have enacted some form of medical marijuana laws, and eight states have enacted through constitutional amendment recreational ("adult use") marijuana. Nonetheless, the remnants of The Single Convention of Narcotic Drugs still live through the Controlled Substances Act of 1971 (CSA). The CSA is a federal statute that established U.S. drug policy and was put into place by President Nixon. It organizes various drugs according to their medicinal value and potential abuse, where 5 is the lowest and 1 is the highest. Cannabis was designated as a Schedule I and remains to this day with its categorization of a Schedule I substance. Although the restrictions on a federal level have remained constant, the treatment of marijuana on a state level has seen volatility beginning in 1996 with California's Proposition 215.

The shift in the treatment of marijuana cannot be solely attributed to one event but instead is comprised of a generational shift in view where the current younger generations have an ability to influence politicians and older generations about the potential medical applications of the plant. Today, cannabis is the most popular illicit drug in the United States [5]. In 2015, the Center for Behavioral Health Statistics and Quality (CBHSQ) estimated 22.2 million of 265 million Americans 12 years of age or older reported having used cannabis in the past month of the study [6]. Azofeifa et al. [7] indicated a marked increase in the senior population (over 55 years) who reported using cannabis, while Burns et al. [8] noted an inversion of age ratios in cannabis users. In 2002, more than three times as many youths as older adults were using cannabis daily, but by 2011, 2.5 times more adults were daily users than youth.

The legal categorization of marijuana throughout the world is still largely dictated by the International Opium Convention of 1925. As of 2017, Austria, Bangladesh, Cambodia, Canada, Chili, Columbia, Costa Rica, the Czech Republic, Germany, India, Jamaica, Mexico, the Netherlands, Portugal, South Africa, Spain, Uruguay, and some U.S. jurisdictions have the least restrictive cannabis laws, while China, France, Indonesia, Japan, Malaysia, Nigeria, Norway, the Philippines, Poland, Saudi Arabia, Singapore, South Korea, Thailand, Turkey, Ukraine, the United Arab Emirates, and Vietnam have the strictest cannabis laws [9].

Although the United States has slowly opened up to a more tolerant stance concerning cannabis, marijuana is still regarded as a Schedule I substance and, therefore, is barred from federal research since it has no medicinal value. Cannabis is not included in most medical school curriculums, but the University of Maryland School of Pharmacy will begin offering a medical cannabis course along with the University of Vermont College of Medicine's Department of Pharmacology.

Nationwide, 89% of people in the United States think marijuana should be allowed for medicinal use, according to a 2016 Gallop poll. Even the esteemed Mayo Clinic says marijuana has possible benefits for people with chronic pain, epilepsy, seizures, glaucoma, Crohn's disease, and nausea due to cancer treatment [10].

Legal status of cannabis and cannabidiol in U.S. law

In the United States, federal and state laws regarding the medicinal use of cannabis (marijuana) and cannabidiol (CBD) are in conflict and have led to confusion for patients and healthcare professionals. Many cannabis and CBD products are available in dispensaries and Internet markets despite no Food and Drug Administration approval of efficacy and safety.

The Controlled Substance Act (CSA) of the U.S. Drug Enforcement Agency (DEA) controls manufacturing and distribution of substances classified in one of five categories based on medical effectiveness and abuse potential [11].

A **Schedule I** drug meets three criteria: (1) having a high potential for abuse, (2) having no currently accepted medical use in treatment in the United States, and (3) having a lack of accepted safety for use of the drug or other substance under medical supervision.

A **Schedule II** drug is accepted for medical use in the United States and has a high potential for abuse that may lead to severe psychological or physical dependence. Schedule II substances include opioids (e.g., oxycodone) and stimulants (e.g., methylphenidate). Opium and cocoa leaves are Schedule II because approved medications such as morphine were already on the market in 1970 when the CSA was enacted [12].

Schedule III—V substances are medically accepted for use but have lower abuse potential, adequate and well-controlled studies prove efficacy, and have a known chemistry with scientific evidence to validate use.

According to Mead, CSA criteria for classification of cannabis as Schedule I has been upheld in federal courts (Alliance for Cannabis Therapeutics v. DEA, 15 F.3d 1131 [D.C. Cir. 1994]). FDA approval of a product is sufficient to establish its "currently accepted medical use," but state laws authorizing use of cannabis for medical purposes do not satisfy this statutory standard (DOJ, DEA, Denial to Initiate Proceedings to Reschedule Marijuana, 21 C.F.R. 40552 at p. 40567 [July 8, 2011]).

A rescheduling of cannabis to a Schedule II substance initiated with the National Cancer Institute's reported use of cannabis (Cannabis sativa) in cancer treatment announced on March 17, 2011. Since it contradicted the federal government position and the Department of Health and Human Services (HHS)—which oversees the National Institutes of Health and the National Cancer Institute—a behind-the-scenes debate ensued regarding politics and public health [13]. On August 11, 2016, the DEA denied two marijuana rescheduling petitions because the DEA and the FDA found that marijuana has no currently accepted medical use and a high potential for abuse [14].

The prescription cannabinoid Marinol (synthetic dronabinol/THC) in sesame oil encapsulated in a soft gelatin is a FDA-approved substance with a Schedule II listing in 1985 upon FDA approval. Fourteen years later, by petition from the manufacturer, Marinol received Schedule III status (64 Fed Reg. 35928 [July 2, 1999]; 21 CFR Section .1308.13 [g][1]), but THC in any other form remains a Schedule I (21 CFR Section .1308.11 [d][31]). Nabilone (Cesamet), another synthetic cannabinoid, was a Schedule II substance after FDA approval in 1985 (52 Fed. Reg. 11042 [April 7, 1987]) and remains at that status [15].

According to Mead, the DEA and the FDA will continue to identify cannabis as a substance with "no currently accepted medical use" until more vigorous safety and efficacy data is produced, or until Congress enacts legislation to change abuse data and what is "accepted medical use" [15].

Decriminalization of cannabis possession and use

State and local governments maintain their own set of laws that regulate the supply and use of cannabis with a reduction of penalties for use-related acts (i.e., personal possession) referred to as decriminalization or depenalization [16]. Today, 21 states and the District of Columbia have decriminalized possession of small amounts of cannabis [17,18].

Medical cannabis laws

In 1996, California passed Proposition 215, allowing individuals suffering from various chronic illnesses to be able to use whole plant cannabis, which legalized medical cannabis. Medical cannabis laws and policies are now available in 29 states and the District of Columbia. Some states are more restrictive than others through limiting access for certain illnesses or conditions or by limiting production and distribution [19].

Nonmedical adult recreational cannabis

In 2010, California attempted to legalize recreational cannabis for adult use (nonmedically needed) but failed, while Colorado and Washington state passed initiatives in 2012. By 2014, Alaska and Oregon had approved recreational cannabis, and California, Maine, Massachusetts, and Nevada followed in 2016 [20].

The U.S. government has not challenged these state laws on recreational cannabis despite the possibility of invoking the supremacy clause of the U.S. Constitution [21]. The 10th Amendment affirms that the federal government cannot force a state to criminalize an act under state law [22]. By legalizing, regulating, and taxing recreational cannabis, penal provisions and sanctions prohibiting and criminalizing unauthorized cultivation, possession, and distribution was repealed at the state level.

Legalization and impact on public health

The public health impact of cannabis legalization remains controversial [23]. Advocates for legalization contend that it will provide for safer use with more efficient use of law enforcement resources. Opponents cite the adverse effects and increased use leading to:

- Increased adolescent access to cannabis [24,25]
- More pediatric ingestion of edible cannabis products [26]
- Increased motor vehicle accidents [27]
- More addiction among adolescents [28]
- Reduced cognitive function [29–31]
- Psychosis-like effects of paranoia and disorganized thinking [32]

As the legal status of cannabis rapidly changes, healthcare professionals need to become increasingly aware of public health issues related to cannabis use.

CBD versus other cannabis products

The cannabis plant contains over 100 cannabinoids, with THC and CBD being the predominant ones [33]. Tetrahydrocannabinol (THC) activates endogenous receptors CB1 and CB2, with CB1 causing the psychoactive properties identified with THC. Cannabidiol (CBD) does not activate CB1 and CB2 as studies by El-Alfy et al. [34] and Rosenberg et al. [35] have shown.

Lacking a standard definition of "medical marijuana," "high CBD" or "low THC" products may contain any number of cannabinoids, with high CBD products containing more than other medical marijuana products and THC levels ranging from 0.3 to 5% according to state law [36]. Furthermore, cannabidiol is a derivative or component of marijuana (as are other cannabinoids), which is a Schedule I substance (21 USC 803) [37].

The cultivation of hemp, a variety of cannabis with low cannabinoid content, has increased the awareness of CBD. European and Canadian hemp producers have been extracting CBD from hemp resins that the Controlled Substance Act has exempted, according to Mead [38,39]. Cannabidiol (CBD) is usually only found in the flowering buds of the hemp plant. Other parts of the hemp plant can be used as food. The seeds are ground for protein powders and used in cereals and bread. Seed oils are used in salad dressings, cosmetics, and dietary supplements [40].

Under the U.S. Food, Drug and Cosmetic Act, any product is considered a drug if it is to be used in diagnosis, cure, mitigation, treatment, or prevention of a disease, so in February 2015 and 2016, FDA sent warning letters to CBD sellers indicating their products were misbranded as nutraceuticals or dietary supplements [41,42].

Review of the warning letter sent to Brandon Nolte, Healthy Hemp Oil in Austin, Texas, outlines FDA's violations in the marketing found on the website:

- "Cannabidiol has been proven to be a powerful natural remedy against inflammatory diseases, chronic pain, and anxiety without known side effects..."
- "New and emerging research suggests that CBD may also be a potent natural remedy for a wide range of other ailments, including heart disease...diabetes..."
- "Scientific studies have shown potential health benefits for people with: anxiety disorders, stress, nausea" [43].

The warning letter continued outlining webpage content like the one entitled "Cannabidiol Cancer Research":

- Numerous recent studies have verified that cannabidiol exhibits some inhibitory effects on several types of cancer including breast cancer, colon cancer, certain types of brain tumors, leukemia, and others.'
- "CBD has been shown to render certain cancerous cells more susceptible to chemotherapy agents."
- CBD has been shown to induce programmed cell death in breast cancer cells.

As Robert T, Hoban, Esq., managing partner at Hoben & Feola LLC, states in *Nutraceuticals World*, these FDA warning letters put a "chill in the CBD marketplace" [44]. The FDA attack on the CBD industry was declared intentional by the manufacturers and distributors who classified it as a lack of understanding about the differences between hemp and marijuana. The FDA had not made any determination that CBD products are illegal or in violation of the Controlled Substance Act (CSA). The Ninth Circuit Court in 2004 established that the sale, production, and distribution of CBD oils/products derived from imported raw material industrial hemp are not in violation of the CSA (Hemp Industry Association v. DEA, 357 F.3d 1012 [9th Cir. 2004]).

More confusion in the hemp versus cannabis legalities occurred with the 2014 Farm Bill, Section 7606 of the U.S. Agricultural Act 2014 (7 USC 5940). The Farm Bill authorizes the growing and research of industrial hemp provided state law allows the growth and cultivation of Cannabis sativa L. with a THC concentration of <0.3%. Individual interpretation of the Farm Bill by states resulted in the U.S. Department of Agriculture, the Department of Health and Human Services (DHHS), and the DEA issuing a statement reviewing the cultivation, marketing, and research requirements for hemp [45].

In a recent federal court ruling, U.S. v. McIntosh, No. 15-10117 (9th Cir. Ct. App) August 16, 2016, states that the Department of Justice (DOJ) and the DEA cannot extend resources to interfere with state implementation of its medical marijuana law, including prosecuting individuals acting in compliance with the state law [46].

Cannabis research

As states have legalized cannabis for medical and recreational use, the federal government has not legalized cannabis and continues to enforce restrictive policies and regulations on research into the health benefits and harmful effects. Limited research in the United States has left patients and healthcare professionals without the information they need to make informed decisions regarding the use of cannabinoids. Even the National Academy of Sciences acknowledged this as a public health risk [47].

The elaborate regulations and review process for basic and clinical researchers wanting to obtain cannabis or cannabinoids for research purposes—for treating a medical condition or achieving therapeutic benefit—must obtain approvals from federal and state institutions, which is a daunting experience. This bureaucracy surrounding research of a Schedule I drug has led to discouraged researchers and limited knowledge about cannabis treatment potentials [48].

Furthermore, cannabis for research purposes is available only through the National Institute on Drug Abuse (NIDA) Supply Program [49] and has been sourced at the University of Mississippi since 1968. The varieties and potencies of cannabis available to researchers is limited and not comparable to what patients have available at dispensaries [50].

Funding is another limiting factor for cannabis research. The National Institute of Health spending in 2015 for cannabinoid research totaled $111,275,219 [51], accounting for only 16.5% ($10,923,472) for research on investigating therapeutic properties of cannabinoids.

Research barriers have resulted in limited evidence about the therapeutic effects of cannabis. In the absence of adequately funded cannabis research, patients may be unaware of viable treatment options, and healthcare providers are inadequately informed on prescribing effective treatment options.

Who is trained to prescribe medical marijuana?

A recent national survey of U.S. medical school curriculum deans, residents, and fellows at Washington University in St. Louis indicated that physicians-in-training lack preparation to prescribe medical marijuana [52].

Senior author of the survey, Laura Jean Bierut, MD, commented, "Medical education needs to catch up to marijuana legislation. Physicians-in-training need to know the benefits and drawbacks associated with medical marijuana so they know when or if, and to whom, to prescribe the drug" [53]. The survey also included a curriculum database review and found that only 9% of medical schools reported teaching students about medical marijuana. With even more states on the cusp of legalizing medical marijuana, physician training should adapt to encompass this new reality of medical practice.

References

1. League of Nations Treaty Series, vol 8, 188–239.
2. Musto DF. *The American Disease: Origins of Narcotic Control*. Oxford University Press, NY, 1999.
3. Booth M. *Cannabis: A History*. St. Martin's Press, NY, 2005.
4. Austin W, Ressler RW. Who gets arrested for marijuana use? The perils of being poor and black. *Applied Economics Letters*. May 4, 2016;1–3.
5. Wilkinson ST, Yarnell S, Radhakrishnan R et al. Marijuana legalization: Impact on physicians and public health. *Annu Rev Med*. 2016;67:453–466.
6. CBHSQ. Key substance use and mental health indicators in the United States: Results from the 2015 national survey on drug use and health. *Substance Abuse and Mental Health Services Administration*. 2016.
7. Azofeifa A, Mattson ME, Schauer G et al. National estimate of marijuana use and related indicators- National Survey on Drug Use and Health, United States, 2002–2014. *Morbidity and Mortality Weekly Report*. 2016;65(SS-11):1–25.
8. Burns RM, Caulkins JP, Everingham SS et al. Statistics on cannabis users skew perceptions of cannabis use. *Front Psychiatry* 2013;4:138.
9. Seven countries you don't want to get caught with drugs in. *The Good Drugs Guide*. March 21, 2009.
10. Legal pot use on the rise—29 states now allow medicinal use. *AARP Bulletin*. Jan–Feb, 2017.
11. U.S. Drug Enforcement Administration. The Controlled Substance Act. Jan 22, 2002. www.justice.gov/dea/pubs/csa/823.
12. Mead A. The legal status of cannabis (marijuana) and cannabidiol (CBD) under U.S. law. *Epilepsy Behavior*. May 2017;70:288–291.
13. Stafford L. Update: U.S. Government Institution Acknowledges Medicinal use of cannabis. *Herbal Gram* 2011;91:20–23.
14. Drug Enforcement Administration. Denial of petition to initiate proceedings to reschedule marijuana. *81 Fed Reg*. 2016;53699.
15. Mead A. The legal status of cannabis (marijuana) and cannabidiol (CBD) under U.S. law. *Epilepsy Behavior*. May 2017;70:288–291.
16. The Health Effects of Cannabis and Cannabinoids: The current state of evidence and recommendations for research. National Academy of Sciences; 2017.
17. Caulkins JP, Kilmer M, Kleiman RJ et al. Considering marijuana legalization 2015. http://www.rand.org/content/dam/rand/pubs/research_reports/RR800/RR864/RAND_RR864.pdf.

18. Caulkins JP, Kilmer B, Hawken A et al. *Marijuana Legalization: What Everyone Needs to Know*. Oxford University Press, NY, 2016.

19. The Health Effects of Cannabis and Cannabinoids: The current state of evidence and recommendations for research. National Academy of Sciences; 2017.

20. NORML. Election 2016—Marijuana Ballot Results. http://norml.org/election-2016.

21. The Health Effects of Cannabis and Cannabinoids: The current state of evidence and recommendations for research. National Academy of Sciences; 2017.

22. Garvey T, Yeh BT. State legalization of recreational marijuana: Selected legal issues. *Congressional Research Service*, Jan 13, 2014. http://fas.org/sgp/crs/misc/R43034.pdf.

23. Wilkinson ST, Yarnell S, Radhakrishnan R et al. Marijuana legalization: Impact on physicians and public health. *Annu Rev Med*. 2016;67:453–466.

24. Thurstone C, Lieberman SA, Schmiege SJ. Medical marijuana diversion and associated problems in adolescent substance treatment. *Drug Alcoh Dep*. 2011;118(2–3):489–492.

25. Salomonsen-Sautel S, Sakai JT, Thurstone C et al. Medical marijuana use among adolescents in substance abuse treatment. *J Am Acad Child Psychiatry* 2012;51(7):694–702.

26. Wang GS, Roosevelt G, Heard K. Pediatric marijuana exposures in a medical marijuana state. *JAMA Peditar* 2013;167(7):630–633.

27. Volkow ND, Baler RD, Compton WM, Weiss SR. Adverse health effects of marijuana use. *N Engl J Med* 2014;370(23):2219–2227.

28. Hall W, Degenhardt L. Adverse health effects of non-medical cannabis use. *Lancet* 2009;374(9698):1383–1391.

29. Pope HG, Gruber AJ, Hudson JI et al. Cognitive measures in long-term cannabis users. *J Clin Pharmacol* 2002;42(11 Suppl):41s–47s.

30. Bolla KI, Eldreth DA, Matochik JA et al. Neural substrates of faulty decision-making in abstinent marijuana users. *Neuro Image* 2005;26(2):480–492.

31. Schweinsburg AD, Nagel BJ, Schweinsburg BC et al. Abstinent adolescent marijuana users show altered fMRI response during spatial working memory. *Psychiatry Res* 2008;163(1):40–51.

32. Radhakrishnan R, Wilkinson ST, D'Souza DC. Gone to pot-a review of the association between cannabis and psychosis. *Front Psychiatry* 2014;5:54.

33. Fellermeier M, Eisenreich W, Bacher A et al. Biosynthesis of cannabinoids. *Eur J Biochem* 2001;268:1596–1604.

34. El-Alfy AT, Iveey K, Robinson K, Ahmed S et al. Antidepressant-like effect of delta-9-tetrahydrocannabinol and other cannabinoids isolated from cannabis sativa L. *Pharmacol Biochem Behav* 2010;95:434–442.

35. Rosenberg EC, Tsien RW, Whalley BJ et al. Cannabinoids and epilepsy. *Neurotherapeutics* 2015;12:747–768.

36. Mead A. The legal status of cannabis (marijuana) and cannabidiol (CBD) under U.S. law. *Epilepsy Behavior*. May 2017;70:288–291.

37. Mead A. The legal status of cannabis (marijuana) and cannabidiol (CBD) under U.S. law. *Epilepsy Behavior*. May 2017;70:288–291.

38. Vantreese VL. Hemp support: Evolution in E U regulation. (Paris, France: Institute National de la Recherche Agronomique. Unite Sol et Agronomie de Renne-Quimper). *J Ind Hemp* 2002.

39. Health Canada. *About Hemp & Canada's Hemp Industry*. Health Canada, Ontario, Canada, 2017.

40. Hemp Industries Association. Hemp industries association publishes statement in response to misbranding of cannabidiol products as "hemp oil". In: *HIA Statement Clarifies Production of Hemp Oil vs. Cannabidiol Products and Calls for Clarification in Marketplace among CBD Manufacturers*. Hemp Industries Association, Summerland, CA, 2014.

41. U.S. Food and Drug Administration. *Warning Letters and Test Results*. U.S. Food and Drug Adminstration, Silver Springs, MD, 2015.

42. U.S. Food and Drug Administration. *Warning Letters and Test Results*. U.S. Food and Drug Adminstration, Silver Springs, MD, 2016.

43. HealthyHempOil.com 2/1/16. Warning letter. http://www.fda.gov/1CEC1/EnforcementActions/WarmingLetters/2016/ucm484968.htm.

44. Hoban RT. FDA "chills" cannabidiol marketplace. http://www.nutraceuticalsworls.com/blog/blogs-and-guest-articles/2016-02-22/fda-chills-cannabidiol-maketplace/52030.

45. Department of Agriculture. Statement of principles on industrial hemp. In: Services DoHaH, Administration FaD, editors. 81 Federal Register, Washington, DC, 2016;53395.

46. Mead A. The legal status of cannabis (marijuana) and cannabidiol (CBD) under U.S. law. *Epilepsy Behavior*. May 2017;70:288–291.

47. *The Health Effects of Cannabis and Cannabinoids: The Current State of Evidence and Recommendations for Research*. National Academy of Sciences, 2017.

48. Nutt DJ, King LA, Nichols DE. Effects of Schedule I drug laws as neuroscience research and treatment innovation. *Nature Reviews Neuroscience* 2013;14(8):577–585.

49. NIDA 2016. NIDA's Role in Providing Marijuana for Research. http://www.drugabuse.gov/drugs-abuse/marijuana/nidas-role-in-providing-marijuana-research.

50. Stith SS, Vigil JM. Federal barriers to cannabis research. *Science* 2016;352(6290):1182.

51. NIDA 2016. NIH Research on Marijuana and Cannabinoids. http://www.drugabuse.gov/drug-abuse/marijuana/nih-research-marijuana-cannabinoids.

52. Evanoff AB, Quan T, Dufault C et al. Physicians-in-training are not prepared to prescribe medical marijuana. *Drug and Alcohol Dependence* Nov 1, 2017;180:151–155.

53. Prescriptions For Medical Marijuana: Education Lags Legislation. Pain Week. www.painweek.org/news_posts/prescriptions-for-medical-marijuana-education-lags-legislation.html.

Appendix A: Glossary

Bhang is an Indian term for cannabis flowers and leaves and can also be used to describe the milk drink, bhang lassi.

Bud of cannabis plant is the growth area producing a stem, flower or leaf.

Butane hash oil (BHO) is a type of cannabis concentrate made using butane as the primary solvent. Using this type of extraction, THC content can be as high as 80%–90%, making it popular with patients suffering from chronic pain and sleep disorders. It needs to be tested for purity to be sure that traces of butane, pesticides, or other contaminant residues are not in the oil.

Cannabis is a flowering plant that has a wide range of industrial and medical uses. The three variations of cannabis plants are: Cannabis ruderalis, Cannabis indica, and Cannabis sativa.

Cannabidiol (CBD) is one of over 80 chemical substances known as cannabinoids from the cannabis plant and is the second most abundant constituent of the plant. CBD is known as the nonpsychoactive cannabinoid.

- Cannabidiolic acid (CBDA) is the main form of CBD in the cannabis plant which is changed from the acidic form to CBD when decarboxylated
- Cannabidivarin (CBDV) differs from CBD by substitution of a pentyl (5 carbon) for propyl (3 carbon) sidechain and is being investigated in seizure control
- Cannabichromene (CBC) research indicates it has anti-inflammatory, antiviral effects
- Cannabinol (CBN) is a weak CB1 and CB2 agonist
- Cannabigerol (CBG) is a competitive CB1 antagonist
- Cannabigerovarin (CBGV) is a TRPV agonist

Cannabinoids are a diverse chemical family including natural and synthetically produced substances with a wide variety of effects in the body from relaxation to intoxication.

259

Cannabinoid receptors are sites in the human body that are known as CB1 and CB2. CB1 receptors are found mainly in the brain (and in the liver, kidneys and lungs), while CBS receptors are found primarily in the immune system.

Cannabis extracts are concentrates that are significantly more potent than standard cannabis buds.

Canna butter is a term used for butter that has been infused with THC cannabis and is a staple in cannabis cooking.

Charlotte's Web (CW) is a nonpsychoactive cannabis formula available in oil and capsules. CW received global attention when Charlotte Figi's story was featured in Dr. Sanjay Gupta's CNN documentary "Weed." Charlotte had suffered from over 300 seizures per week before taking CBD oil, and now she is a thriving student in her community.

CO_2 extraction oil is made from a supercritical extraction process utilizing high pressure to separate the cannabinoids from the plant matter. A similar CO_2 extraction process is also used in food, dry cleaning, and herbal supplement production.

Decarboxylation is a chemical reaction that removes the carboxyl group from the THC-A molecule and turns it into psychoactive THC.

Dronabinol is a synthetic cannabinoid for oral administration that is similar to tetrahydrocannabinol (THC). It is the active ingredient in Marinol®.

Dry sieve, also called dry sift, is a popular form of nonsolvent hash that has been run through a series of screens or sieves to eliminate all but the trichome heads. It is the easiest way to produce a quality dry sieve hash, which melts completely when exposed to heat.

Endocannabinoids are molecules that bind to and activate cannabinoid receptors. They are produced naturally by cells in the human body on an "as-needed basis."

Endocannabinoid system (ECS) is a biological system made up of endocannabinoids—arachidonoylethanolamine (commonly called anandamide) or AEA and 2-arachidonoylglycerol or 2-AE and others. They are lipid-based neurotransmitters that bind to cannabinoid receptors throughout the nervous system. The ECS is found in all vertebrate species.

Hash (Hashisch or Hasheesh) is made from the cannabis plant and has been around for centuries with many processes for production. The powdery kief that coats the cannabis flowers can be collected and pressed into hash. An ice water extraction is another common process used to create a nonsolvent hash by isolating the trichome heads which contain the essential oils. The finished product needs to be adequately dried to avoid mold and microbiological contamination. Alcohol is another means of effectively stripping the cannabis plant of its trichomes to be made into hash.

Hemp is the high-growing varieties of cannabis that are grown for fiber, oil, and seeds for refining into food, oil, paper, cloth, rope, or wax.

Intoxication occurs when a substance causes the loss of behavioral control due to direct effect on the brain (i.e., psychoactive effect of THC) or by indirectly causing damage to the body through toxicity.

Joint is slang for a cannabis cigarette.

Kief is the simplest of cannabis concentrates composed of dried resin trichomes (the crystalline structures coating the outside surface of the flowers). Trichomes are separated from the dried plant material using filtering screens. The THC content can vary from 20 to 60%. It can also be called crystal or pollen.

Marijuana is a Cannabis sativa plant product that is composed of the plant's dried leaves, stems, seeds, and buds. It was originally the Mexican term for "inebriation" and linked to the cannabis plant in the early 1930s by prohibitionists.

Nabilone is a synthetic cannabinoid for oral administration, similar to tetrahydrocannabinol (THC) that is the active component in Cesamet®.

National Cannabis Industry Association (NCIA) is a trade association in Washington, DC, working to develop and promote industry-wide standards and best practices.

Pistil (or stigma) is the female portion of the flower or pollen receptive part of the flower.

Pollen (trichomes) is the male fertilizing compound secreted by the cannabis glands which contains the highest levels of THC.

Psychoactive is a chemical substance that can enter the brain and directly affect the central nervous system.

Rick Simpson oil (RSO) is a whole plant cannabis oil for oral use but can also be topically applied and is convenient to use with rapid uptake through mucosal membranes in the mouth when taken in a sublingual form. Whole plant oil is derived from the cannabis plant (not the hemp plant), which is comprised of the buds/flower of the female plant and includes many different cannabinoids—THC, CBD, CBN, and others. It is named for the Canadian who was diagnosed with basal cell carcinoma after an asbestos exposure who thought he had nothing to lose trying cannabis. RSO is credited with curing his cancer.

Rosin is a solid form of resin that is obtained by adding pressure and vaporizing liquid terpenes.

Sativex® is a cannabis-based medicine that contains both THC and CBD.

Schedules of Controlled Substances

- **Schedule I:** These drugs are not safe, have no accepted medical use in the United States, and have a high potential for abuse. These drugs cannot be prescribed and are available only for research after special application to federal agencies. Examples: marijuana, heroin, LSD, peyote, and psilocybin.
- **Schedule II:** These drugs have a currently accepted medical use and have a high potential for abuse and dependence liability. A written prescription is required by a physician who is registered with the Drug Enforcement Administration (DEA). Telephones prescriptions are not allowed, and no refills are allowed. Examples: opium derivatives such as morphine, codeine, meperidine (Demerol), methadone, fentanyl, cocaine, and amphetamines (Dexedrine); short-acting barbiturates (e.g., Nembutal, Seconal); and dronabinol (Marinol-synthetic THC).
- **Schedule III:** Medicinal drugs with potential for abuse and dependence liability less than Schedule II but greater than Schedule IV. A telephoned prescription is permitted to be converted to written form by the dispensing pharmacist. Prescriptions must be renewed every six months, and refills are limited to five. Examples: paregoric, some appetite suppressants (e.g., Didrex, Tenuate), some hypnotics (e.g., glutethimide, methyprylon).
- **Schedule IV:** Medicinal drugs with less potential for abuse and dependence liability than Schedule III drugs. Prescription requirements are similar to Schedule III drugs. Examples: pentazocine (Talwin), propoxyphene (Darvon), benzodiazepines (e.g., Librium, Valium), meprobamate.
- **Schedule V:** Medicinal drugs with the lowest potential for abuse and dependence liability. Drugs requiring a prescription are handled the same way as any nonscheduled prescription drug. The buyer may be required to sign a log of purchase. Examples: codeine and hydrocodone in combination with other active, non-narcotic drugs usually in cough suppressants and antidiarrheal drugs.

Terpenes are compounds in cannabis that give the plant its unique smell.

Tetrahydrocannabinol (also known as delta-9-tetrahydrocannabinol or THC) is the most abundant phytocannabinoid in the cannabis plant and is a strong psychoactive compound.

- Tetrahydrocannabivarin (THCV) is found in some strains of cannabis with substitution of pentyl (5 carbon) for propyl (3 carbon) which may have effects in reducing panic attacks and suppressing appetite. It is CB1 antagonist.
- Tetrahydrocannabinolic acid (THCA) is the main constituent in raw cannabis that converts to THC when burned, vaporized or decarboxylated.

Tincture is an alcohol extract of cannabis plant material.

Trichomes are the resin containing growths on the surface of the plant, which are frequently called "hairs" or scales.

Appendix B: Recipes

CANNABIS MANGO PINEAPPLE SMOOTHIE

1 gram of dry cannabis buds or 8–10 fresh leaves
3/4 cup water
1 tablespoon coconut oil
1/4 fresh pineapple, cored and skinned, cut into cubes
1/2 mango, skinned and pit removed, cut into chunks
1/2 banana, peeled
2–3 ice cubes, optional

Grind cannabis buds in blender. Add rest of the ingredients, except ice cubes. Puree on high speed 1–2 minutes until smooth. Add ice cubes, if desired. Pour into tall glasses. Makes 2 servings.

RAW CANNABIS BLUEBERRY BANANA SMOOTHIE

15 cannabis leaves, rinsed well
2 fresh cannabis buds
1 banana, frozen
1 cup frozen blueberries
1/2 cup almond milk
1/2 cup coconut water
2 tablespoons hempseeds
1 tablespoon coconut oil

Juice cannabis leaves. Grind cannabis buds in blender or food processor. Add cannabis juice and rest of the ingredients to the blender. Puree until smooth. Pour into tall glasses. Makes 2 servings.

CANNABIS HEALTH JUICE

10–20 raw, green cannabis leaves (best from plant 60–70 days old)
2 raw cannabis buds
1/2 lime
2 green apples, cored and cut into chunks
4 carrots
1 pear, cored and cut into chunks

Juice 3 to 4 leaves at a time, followed by breaking up buds to juice with rest of ingredients. Pour into glass. Sip at 2- to 3-hour intervals throughout day.

CANNABIS HOT CHOCOLATE

I cup whole milk or milk substitute
2 teaspoons honey or sugar
1/8 ounce finely ground cannabis or 1/8 ounce of CBD oil
1-ounce unsweetened chocolate
Stick of cinnamon

Combine milk, honey, and cannabis in saucepan over low heat for fat in milk to release THC (when making THC canna milk) or dissolving CBD concentrate. Filter through coffee filter (when making CBD hot chocolate, skip this step). Combine canna milk and chocolate in saucepan, and heat until chocolate melts. Serve in mug with cinnamon stick. Makes 1 cup.

MOROCCAN MAJOUN JAM

1-1/2 teaspoons ground cannabis
1 cup chopped dates
1/2 cup raisins
1/2 cup finely chopped walnuts or almonds
1 teaspoon ground nutmeg
1 teaspoon ground anise
1 teaspoon ground ginger
1/2 cup honey
1/4 cup water
2 tablespoons canna THC butter or canna-CBD butter

Toast cannabis over low heat in dry skillet until aroma released. Add rest of the ingredients, and stir until well blended and canna butter is melted. Spoon into jar, and store in refrigerator until ready to serve with crackers or bread. Makes 2 cups.

Note: Morocco is a major producer of hashish, and over 10% of the country's land is devoted to growing it. Majoun is the traditional way Moroccans eat cannabis.

THC GUACAMOLE

1-1/2 teaspoons finely ground cannabis buds
1 lime, juiced
1 tablespoon extra-virgin olive oil
1 small red chili pepper, chopped (optional)
1/4 cup finely chopped onion
2 ripe avocados, peeled and chopped

Combine cannabis, lime juice, olive oil, and chili pepper in bowl. Let stand 40–60 minutes to enhance flavors and draw out THC. Add onion and avocados. Mash together until smooth by hand or in blender. Serve as dip or topping for tacos. Makes 1 cup.

Note: Guacamole—Medical Cannabis variation: Use above recipe except use CBD oil for olive oil and cannabis.

GREEN CBD CANNABIS DIP

1/3 cup chopped parsley
1/3 cup chopped fresh dill
1/3 chopped shallots or 1 green onion, chopped
1 tablespoon lemon juice
1 clove garlic, minced
1 cup Greek plain yogurt
4 ounces goat cheese
1 tablespoon CBD hemp oil
Salt and pepper to taste

Combine all ingredients in food processor and blend well. Serve dip with vegetables.

SPICY CANNA SALSA

1 small red onion, chopped
2 large tomatoes, seeds removed
1 small red chili pepper, minced
1 yellow bell pepper, chopped
1 green bell pepper, chopped
1 tablespoon fresh chopped cilantro
Juice of 1 lime
1/8 teaspoon dried ground cannabis bud

Combine all ingredients in bowl. Mix well and serve as side dish or snack. Makes 2 cups.

FRESH MARIJUANA SALAD

1/2 cucumber, chopped
1 ripe avocado, peeled, pitted, chopped
2 cups mixed salad greens
1/4 cup fresh cannabis leaves, finely chopped
1 scallion or green onion, sliced thin
1 tablespoon lemon juice or vinegar
1 tablespoon olive oil
4 cherry tomatoes
Salt and pepper to taste

Combine all ingredients in bowl and toss. Makes 2 servings.

CREAMY LEMON GARLIC CBD SALAD DRESSING

1-1/2 tablespoon CBD hemp oil
1/4 cup olive oil
1 tablespoon Dijon mustard
1/4 cup mayonnaise
1 clove garlic, peeled and minced
2 tablespoons lemon juice
2 tablespoons chopped parsley or cilantro

Combine all ingredients in bowl. Blend well and pour over salad greens. Store any leftover dressing in refrigerator to use within a week. Makes 1-1/2 cups.

CBD MUSTARD SALAD DRESSING

1–2 tablespoons Dijon mustard
4 tablespoons CBD olive oil
2 tablespoons balsamic vinegar
Salt and pepper to taste

Mix ingredients together in small bowl or glass bottle. Shake well or mix with wire whip to blend. Makes 1/2 cup.

CANNABIS MACARONI AND CHEESE

1 cup (4 ounces) dried elbow macaroni
1-1/2 cup grated Cheddar cheese
1/2 cup milk or dairy substitute
1/4 cup canna-THC butter
1 egg
Salt and pepper to taste

Cook macaroni in water until firm when you bite it. Meanwhile, combine rest of ingredients in bowl. When macaroni is cooked, drain off water and mix in canna-THC butter mixture. Place over low heat until butter and cheese are melted. Serve hot. Makes 4 servings.

SPAGHETTI SAUCE

2–4 garlic cloves (adjust to taste)
2 tablespoons olive oil
1/2 pound ripe tomatoes, chopped
1 teaspoon dried ground cannabis
1/4 cup fresh basil leaves
Salt and pepper to taste

Sauté garlic in olive oil. Add rest of ingredients, and simmer until mixture is thickened. Serve over spaghetti noodles or spaghetti squash. Makes 2 servings.

PIZZA

1/4 cup canna-THC butter or olive oil
1 medium onion, sliced
1 red bell pepper, chopped
1/4 cup sliced mushrooms
1 8-ounce can tomato sauce
2 teaspoons fresh or 1 teaspoon dried oregano
1 prepared pizza crust
2 cups (8 ounces) grated Mozzarella cheese

Sauté canna-THC butter, onion, bell pepper, and mushrooms in skillet. Add tomato sauce and oregano. Simmer until thickened. Spread tomato sauce over prepared crust. Sprinkle on cheese. Bake in 400°F. oven 10–15 minutes. Makes 4 servings.

MUSHROOM SAUTÉ

3 tablespoons canna-THC butter
2 cloves garlic, chopped
1 tablespoon fresh thyme or 1 teaspoon dried thyme leaves
1 tablespoon fresh oregano or 1 teaspoon dried oregano leaves
1 to 1-1/2 cups sliced mushrooms
1 tablespoon red wine vinegar
Salt and pepper to taste
Chopped fresh parsley

Sauté canna-THC butter, garlic, thyme, and oregano in skillet. Add mushrooms and cook over low heat until tender. Stir in vinegar, salt, pepper, and parsley. Makes 2–3 servings.

SWEET POTATO BISCUITS

1/2 cup cooked and mashed sweet potato
1/2 cup milk or dairy substitute
1 cup flour
1/2 teaspoon salt
1 tablespoon baking powder
1/3 cup cold canna-THC butter, cut into cubes

Combine sweet potatoes and milk in bowl. Beat until smooth. Mix together flour, salt, and baking powder in bowl. Add canna-THC butter and blend with fork or pastry blender until mixture is crumbly. Stir in sweet potato mixture. Form into smooth dough. Roll dough onto floured surface. Cut into desired shape. Lift onto oiled baking sheet. Bake in 400°F. oven 10–12 minutes or until golden brown. Makes 10 biscuits.

BROWNIE MARY SQUARES

Named for Mary Jane Rathbun, beloved volunteer at San Francisco General Hospital in late 1980s who provided AIDS patients with marijuana-laced brownies.

2 ounces unsweetened chocolate
1/4 cup canna-THC butter or THC oil
1/2 cup honey
2 eggs
1-1/2 cups flour
1 teaspoon baking powder
1 teaspoon vanilla extract

Melt chocolate and canna-THC butter over low heat. Stir in honey and eggs. Add flour, baking powder, and vanilla. Beat until batter is smooth. Pour into oiled 8-inch square baking pan. Bake in 350°F. oven 30–40 minutes or until toothpick inserted into center comes out clean. Cut into squares when cool. Makes 10–12 servings.

CANNABIS ENERGY BARS

1/4 cup canna-THC butter or canna-THC coconut oil
1/2 cup ground almonds
1-1/4 cup shredded unsweetened coconut
1/4 cup peanut butter
1 tablespoon honey
1/4 teaspoon salt
1/2 cup chocolate chips

Combine all ingredients into bowl. Press into oiled baking pan. Refrigerate until hardened. Cut into 4 bars.

CHOCOLATE CHIP HEMP COOKIES

1-1/2 cup hemp flour or all-purpose flour
1-1/2 teaspoon baking soda
1/2 teaspoon salt
1/2 cup canna-THC butter
1/2 cup coconut oil
1/4 cup honey
2 eggs
1 cup chocolate chips
1/2 cup chopped walnuts.

Combine flour, baking soda, and salt in bowl. Blend canna-THC butter, coconut oil, honey, and eggs in bowl and add to flour mixture. Beat well. Stir in chocolate chips and nuts. Drop by walnut-sized balls onto oiled cookie sheet. Bake in 375°F. oven 10–12 minutes until brown. Makes 36 cookies.

Note: Hemp Oatmeal Cookies: Use 1 cup oatmeal instead of chocolate chips and 1/2 cup raisins instead of walnuts.

CANNA-THC BUTTER BANANA BREAD

1/2 cup canna-THC butter
3/4 cup sugar
2 ripe bananas, peeled and mashed
1 egg
1 teaspoon ground cinnamon
2 teaspoons baking powder
1-1/2 cups flour
1/2 cup chopped nuts

Cream together canna-THC butter, sugar, bananas, and eggs. Combine rest of ingredients in bowl. Stir to mix. Add creamed mixture and beat until well combined. Pour into oiled baking pan. Bake in 350°F. oven 40–50 minutes or until toothpick inserted in center comes out clean. Cool on wire rack 10 minutes. Invert onto plate. Serve warm or cold. Makes 10 servings.

CANNABIS TRUFFLES

1-1/2 tablespoons canna coconut oil
2 tablespoons coconut flour or ground nuts
1/4 cup cocoa powder
4 large (1/2 cup chopped) dates
1 ripe avocado, peeled

Puree all ingredients in food processor or blender until silky smooth. Scoop one tablespoon of batter and roll into a ball. Roll into extra cocoa powder and place on plate. Repeat until all batter is rolled into balls. Refrigerate at least 2 hours until hardened. Keep chilled until ready to eat. Makes 12.

Index

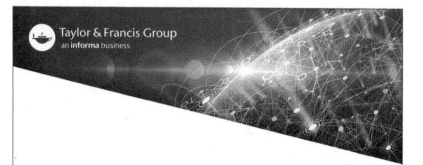